Pre-Screening Systems for Early Disease Prediction, Detection, and Prevention

Thierry Edoh
Technical University of Munich, Germany

Pravin Pawar
Philips Research, India

Sagar Mohammad
Philips Research, India

A volume in the Advances in Medical Diagnosis, Treatment, and Care (AMDTC) Book Series

IGI Global
DISSEMINATOR OF KNOWLEDGE

Published in the United States of America by
IGI Global
Medical Information Science Reference (an imprint of IGI Global)
701 E. Chocolate Avenue
Hershey PA, USA 17033
Tel: 717-533-8845
Fax: 717-533-8661
E-mail: cust@igi-global.com
Web site: http://www.igi-global.com

Library of Congress Cataloging-in-Publication Data

Names: Edoh, Thierry, 1968- editor. | Pawar, Pravin, 1978- editor. | Mohammad, Sagar, 1975- editor.
Title: Pre-screening systems for early disease prediction, detection, and prevention / Thierry Edoh, Pravin Pawar, and Sagar Mohammad, editors.
Description: Hershey, PA : Medical Information Science Reference, [2019] | Includes bibliographical references.
Identifiers: LCCN 2018016314| ISBN 9781522571315 (hardcover) | ISBN 9781522571322 (ebook)
Subjects: | MESH: Diagnosis, Computer-Assisted | Early Diagnosis | Remote Sensing Technology | Internet | Knowledge Bases
Classification: LCC RC78.7.D53 | NLM WB 141 | DDC 616.07/54--dc23 LC record available at https://lccn.loc.gov/2018016314

This book is published in the IGI Global book series Advances in Medical Diagnosis, Treatment, and Care (AMDTC) (ISSN: 2475-6628; eISSN: 2475-6636)

British Cataloguing in Publication Data
A Cataloguing in Publication record for this book is available from the British Library.

All work contributed to this book is new, previously-unpublished material.
The views expressed in this book are those of the authors, but not necessarily of the publisher.

For electronic access to this publication, please contact: eresources@igi-global.com.

Advances in Medical Diagnosis, Treatment, and Care (AMDTC) Book Series

ISSN:2475-6628
EISSN:2475-6636

MISSION

Advancements in medicine have prolonged the life expectancy of individuals all over the world. Once life-threatening conditions have become significantly easier to treat and even cure in many cases. Continued research in the medical field will further improve the quality of life, longevity, and wellbeing of individuals.

The **Advances in Medical Diagnosis, Treatment, and Care (AMDTC)** book series seeks to highlight publications on innovative treatment methodologies, diagnosis tools and techniques, and best practices for patient care. Comprised of comprehensive resources aimed to assist professionals in the medical field apply the latest innovations in the identification and management of medical conditions as well as patient care and interaction, the books within the AMDTC series are relevant to the research and practical needs of medical practitioners, researchers, students, and hospital administrators.

COVERAGE

- Critical Care
- Cancer Treatment
- Experimental Medicine
- Internal Medicine
- Emergency Medicine
- Chronic Conditions
- Disease Prevention
- Patient-Centered Care
- Medical Testing
- Patient Interaction

IGI Global is currently accepting manuscripts for publication within this series. To submit a proposal for a volume in this series, please contact our Acquisition Editors at Acquisitions@igi-global.com or visit: http://www.igi-global.com/publish/.

The Advances in Medical Diagnosis, Treatment, and Care (AMDTC) Book Series (ISSN 2475-6628) is published by IGI Global, 701 E. Chocolate Avenue, Hershey, PA 17033-1240, USA, www.igi-global.com. This series is composed of titles available for purchase individually; each title is edited to be contextually exclusive from any other title within the series. For pricing and ordering information please visit http://www.igi-global.com/book-series/advances-medical-diagnosis-treatment-care/129618. Postmaster: Send all address changes to above address.

Titles in this Series

For a list of additional titles in this series, please visit:
https://www.igi-global.com/book-series/advances-medical-diagnosis-treatment-care/129618

Effective Techniques for Managing Trigeminal Neuralgia
Steven Chang (Stanford University, USA) and Allen Ho (Stanford University, USA)
Medical Information Science Reference • ©2018 • 331pp • H/C (ISBN: 9781522553496) • US $225.00

Handbook of Research on Geriatric Health, Treatment, and Care
Barre Vijaya Prasad (Dharwad Institute of Mental Health and Neurosciences (DIMHANS), India) and Shamsi Akbar (King George's Medical University, India)
Medical Information Science Reference • ©2018 • 604pp • H/C (ISBN: 9781522534808) • US $375.00

Emerging Developments and Practices in Oncology
Issam El Naqa (University of Michigan, USA)
Medical Information Science Reference • ©2018 • 305pp • H/C (ISBN: 9781522530855) • US $245.00

Complementary and Alternative Medicine and Kidney Health
Mayuree Tangkiatkumjai (Srinakharinwirot University, Thailand) Annalisa Casarin (The NIHR Research Design Service East of England, UK) Li-Chia Chen (University of Manchester, UK) and Dawn-Marie Walker (University of Southampton, UK)
Medical Information Science Reference • ©2018 • 308pp • H/C (ISBN: 9781522528821) • US $265.00

Research-Based Perspectives on the Psychophysiology of Yoga
Shirley Telles (Patanjali Research Foundation, India) and Nilkamal Singh (Patanjali Research Foundation, India)
Medical Information Science Reference • ©2018 • 456pp • H/C (ISBN: 9781522527886) • US $225.00

For an entire list of titles in this series, please visit:
https://www.igi-global.com/book-series/advances-medical-diagnosis-treatment-care/129618

IGI Global
DISSEMINATOR OF KNOWLEDGE

701 East Chocolate Avenue, Hershey, PA 17033, USA
Tel: 717-533-8845 x100 • Fax: 717-533-8661
E-Mail: cust@igi-global.com • www.igi-global.com

Editorial Advisory Board

Table of Contents

Detailed Table of Contents

This chapter focuses on the screening for non-communicable diseases (NCDs), which in certain cases are likely caused by infectious diseases. The screening for NCDs in this specific case remains challenging since the convergence between both non-infectious and infectious diseases is less investigated. This chapter, therefore, aims at reviewing and addressing the challenges and limitation of the conventional methodologies for screening for diseases, in general. The chapter further proposes an innovative screening paradigm based on the internet of things technology. The chapter presents the state of the art on the conventional screening for diseases, discusses the fundamental difference between screening for diseases and diseases surveillance and monitoring, and the difference between screening for diseases and diseases diagnostics.

Change of disease patterns from communicable to chronic diseases has a tremendous impact on the healthcare ecosystem. For healthcare organizations to remain viable and economically sustainable during this transition, there is a desperate need of cost-effective solutions for chronic disease management. One important strategy for this is early diagnosis and management of diseases. With rapid technological advancements, IoT-based solutions are well-positioned to be an effective tool for disease screening and health monitoring provided that they are also able to bridge non-technical barriers in technology adoption. The three primary stakeholders for screening solutions are healthcare organizations, clinical fraternity, and end-users. The primary objective of this chapter is to review likely barriers in adoptions of the IoT solutions from the perspective of these three primary stakeholders.

Classification schemes have been applied in the medical arena to explore patients' data and extract a predictive model.This model helps doctors to improve their prognosis, diagnosis, or treatment planning processes.The aim of this work is to utilize and compare different decision tree classifiers for early diagnosis of Dengue. Six approaches, mainly J48 tree, random tree, REP tree, SOM, logistic regression, and naïve Bayes, have been utilized to study real-world Dengue data collected from different hospitals in the Delhi, India region during 2015-2016. Standard statistical metrics are used to assess the efficiency of the proposed Dengue disease diagnostic system, and the outcomes showed that REP tree is best among these classifiers with 82.7% efficient in supplying an exact diagnosis.

Prescreening and sensing of diseases offers a number of benefits that can help in prevention of major diseases. The aim of disease pre-screening is to detect possible disorders or diseases in people who do not have any symptoms. Earlier screening methods for the detection of diseases was invasive, complicated, and would require extensive tests. Some conventional methods used in clinical diagnoses include many invasive and potentially hazardous biopsy procedures, endoscopy, computed tomography; numerous innovative approaches have evolved to overcome the limitations of traditional techniques. Non-invasive biomedical sensor, genomics, electronic nose, nano-material, plasmonicsensor devices, microfabrication-based technologies, flat-panel detectors, digital breast object models, endomicroscopy, breath biopsy, and wavelet-based enhancement methods are some of the emerging frontiers in prescreening and sensing of diseases. This chapter will provide an in-depth discussion of the abovementioned innovative techniques related to prescreening and sensing of diseases.

Medical error is an adverse event of a failure in healthcare management, causing unintended injuries. Proper clinical care can be provided by employing a suitable clinical decision support system (CDSS) for healthcare management. CDSS assists the clinicians in identifying the severity of disease at the time of admission and predicting its progression. In this chapter, CDSS was developed with the help of statistical techniques. Modified cascade neural network (ModCNN) was built upon the architecture of cascade-correlation neural network (CCNN). ModCNN first identifies the independent factors associated with disease and using that factor; it predicts its progression. A case progressing towards severity can be given better care, avoiding later stage complications. Performance of ModCNN was evaluated and compared with artificial neural network (ANN) and CCNN. ModCNN showed better accuracy than other statistical techniques. Thus, CDSS developed in this chapter is aimed at providing better treatment planning by reducing medical error.

Screening for diseases is a medical process to predict, prevent, detect, and cure a disease in people at high risk. However, it is limited in the quality and accuracy of the outcomes. The reason for this is the lack of long-term data about the health condition of the patient. Launching modern information and communication technology in the screening process has shown promise of improving the screening outcomes. A previous study has shown that patient education can positively impact the patient behavior face to a disease and can empower the patient to adopt a healthy lifestyle and

in the diabetes investigation relating to genetic background and environment. With improving accuracy for early detection and prevention of diabetes, this chapter implemented a fuzzy linear and logistic regression model with fuzzy clustering for predicting early detection of diabetes.

This chapter presents a new methodology for detection and identification of cardiovascular diseases from a single-lead electrocardiogram (ECG) signal of short duration. More specifically, this method deals with the detection of the most common cardiac arrhythmia called atrial fibrillation (AF) in noisy and non-clinical environment. The method begins with appropriate pre-processing of ECG signals in order to get the RR-interval and heart rate (HR) signals from them. A set of indirect features are computed from the original and the transformed versions of RR-interval and HR signals along with a set of direct features that are obtained from ECG signals themselves. In all, 47 features are computed and subsequently they are fed to an ensemble system of bagged decision trees for classifying the ECG recordings into four different classes. The proposed method has been evaluated with 2017 PhysioNet/CinC challenge hidden test dataset (phase II subset) and the final F1 score of 0.81 is obtained.

Computers in disease prescreening are utilized to interpret medical information. This is known as computer-aided pre-screening tool (CAPST). CAPST helps in improving the accuracy of diagnosis in medicine. The medical experts usually take the outcome of the CAPST as a second opinion to make the final diagnostic decisions. Fast and accurate prediction of disease risk and diagnosis is crucial step for the successful treatment of an individual. The AI-based machine learning technology has undergone significant developments over the past few years and is successfully used in many intelligent applications covering problems of variety of domains. One of the most stimulating questions is whether these techniques can be successfully applied to medicine in disease pre-screening and diagnosis and what kind of data it requires to be trained and learned. There are so many real-time examples of the problems where machine learning methods are applied successfully, especially in medicine. Many of them showed significant improvement in classification accuracy.

Preface

INTRODUCTION

This book is an effort to look at the interdisciplinary field that combines two major domains – healthcare and ICT. The goal of disease pre-screening is to detect potential health disorders or diseases in people who do not have any symptoms of disease. The core goal of this book is, on one hand, to point out the limitations of existing methodologies and paradigms for diseases screening. On the other hand, this book aims at investigating the causes of these limitations and to propose new methodologies, paradigms, and policies to better take benefits from the screening for diseases. Advanced ICT techniques has the potential to solve many of the problems in health data collection (with focus on IOT/Crowd sensing), analysis (modern data analytics methods and Tools) and interpretation as well as improve existing health systems – in particular for pre-screening and sensing of diseases. Non-invasive biomedical sensor devices offer a variety of benefits such as early detection and thus prevention of the risk of infection, ease of use and suitability for long-term monitoring. This book is focused on bringing out the use of non-invasive biomedical sensor devices, IOT solutions, and knowledge database solutions for pre-screening of diseases so that the risk of disease is reduced, or it can be detected early enough to treat the disease most effectively. This book presents various case studies that deal with screening for as-yet-undiagnosed diseases in a better way, namely the pre-screening.

What are the differences between screening for diseases and pre-screening for diseases? This question is answered in the first chapter of the book. The author of the first chapter has discussed the different aspects of both paradigms.

The process of screening for diseases is voluntary-based and strictly follows a national program. Each country owns their specific screening program. The traditional screening programs make less use of modern information and communication technology. It is more focused on using traditional medical equipment to gather information which is used by medical doctors to perform analysis. In contrary to the screening for diseases, the pre-screening for diseases process autonomously and automatically collects gapless data and information on the health of individuals. During the screening phase, the medical doctor can additionally use the traditional medical equipment to perform some test and thus get the entire picture of the health status of the said individual. Table 1 summarizes the general differences between both the screening methodologies.

TECHNOLOGIES ENABLING THE PRE-SCREENING FOR DISEASES

The Internet of Things (IoT)

Istepanian et al. (2011) have discussed the benefits of using the Internet of m-health Things (m-IoT) for noninvasive glucose level sensing. m-IoT puts together the functionalities of m-Health and IoT. m-Health (mobile Health) is healthcare delivery supported by (smart) devices (i.e. Smartphones, etc.).

m-IoT is defined as an integration of objects, like thermometer in medical fields, with network connectivity from the digital and physical world (Edoh, 2017).

Table 1. Traditional screening vs. pre-screening for diseases

Characteristics	Conventional Screening for Diseases	Pre-Screening for Diseases
Data Gathering	Collected only during the screening process and often the data collected is patient-centered	Pervasively and ubiquitously collected
Data Completeness	Incomplete data	Complete and gapless data available
Patient-education	Does not include patient health education	Includes patient health education
Test-Outcomes Level	Depends on the sensitivity and specificity as well as test population	Highly independent of the test. Enough data and information are collected in earlier stage.
Error Rate Level	High rate of • False-Positive and • False-Negative test-outcomes	Minimal error rate
Technology and Equipments Used	Use only conventional equipment like • ECG • Radiography • Computer Tomography • MRT • Angiography • Etc.	Use modern technology like • Artificial Intelligence • Machine Learning • Internet of Things • Ubiquitous and Pervasive computing • Data Analytics and Prevention in addition to conventional equipment

In this book, the contributors have presented IoT-enabled screening systems, which have shown promise to improve the data gathering as well as the quality of the collected data. Furthermore, the barriers to implement IoT in pre-screening systems are also discussed.

The Artificial Intelligence (AI)

In Rigla, García-Sáez, Pons, and Hernando (2018), the authors define, according to Boden definition, the AI as "the ability to make computers do things that would require intelligence if done by humans." AI can be defined as the ability of a computer to simulate human cognitive capacity like read, writing, thinking (reasoning), and learning. It is debatable if the AI comprises the feeling capacity. There exist many sensors nowadays able to measure various parameters like temperature, air quality, etc. Though, the question is can a computer feels like a human being?

AI is used in several health or medical systems. In Rigla et al. (2018), the authors have presented a list of some health systems using the AI technology (see Table 1 in Rigla et al., 2018)). In Thrall et al., (2018) have discussed and analyzed the role of AI in medical Imaging and their impacts on radiology. They pointed out that the AI role in medical imaging and their impacts on radiologists are not clear yet. However, the AI has shown clear promise to improve the medical imaging.

Contributors of the book have discussed the use of the AI in the pre-screening for diseases paradigm. They show the benefits of using the AI technology and have presented cases studies.

The Machine Learning (ML)

ML is a subset of AI. It comprises the deep learning and categorize in supervised and unsupervised learning. All ML application are AI application, though, not all AI applications are ML applications. Figure below shows the relationship between AI, ML and DL.

The ML provides algorithms which allow a computer to learn from data and to predict events or to recognize patterns or objects. This book has discussed the usage of ML in the screening for diseases and pointed out diverse benefits by using ML in automated diseases detection.

The book is primarily targeted for researchers in health informatics, industry practitioners in health informatics, and academicians working in health informatics. This volume is also suitable as a reference book for graduate-level courses in Health Informatics.

Figure 1. Relationship between artificial intelligence, machine learning, and deep learning

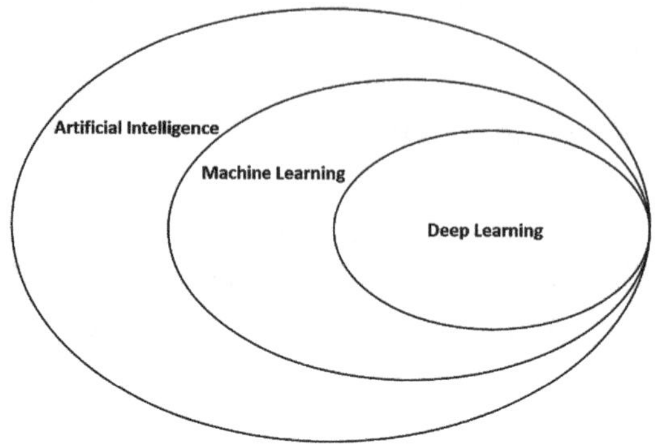

ORGANIZATION OF THE BOOK

The book is organized into 11 chapters that describe different cases studies and topics on the paradigm of pre-screening for diseases. In general, the chapters have discussed policies and recommendations for achieving high test-outcomes accuracy and technologies that could support the pre-screening paradigm. A brief description of each of the chapters follows:

Chapter 1, "Internet-of-Things-Enabled Pre-Screening for Diseases," is focusing on the screening for non-communicable diseases (NCDs), which in certain cases are likely caused by infectious diseases. The screening for NCDs in this specific case remains challenging since the convergence between both non-infectious and infectious diseases is less investigated. The chapter further presents new paradigm including the use of the Internet of Things to improve the conventional screening for diseases. This chapter, therefore, aims at reviewing and addressing the challenges and limitation of the conventional methodologies for screening for diseases, in general. The chapter presents the state-of-the-art on the conventional screening for diseases, discusses the fundamental difference between screening for diseases and diseases surveillance and monitoring and the difference between screening for diseases and diseases diagnostics.

Chapter 2, "Barriers to Adoptions of IoT-Based Solutions for Disease Screening," reviews the likely barriers in adoptions of the IoT solutions from perspective of the three primary stakeholders; healthcare organizations, clinical fraternity and end-users. Change of disease patterns from communicable to chronic diseases is going to have a tremendous impact on healthcare ecosystem. For healthcare organizations, to remain viable and economically sustainable during this transition there is a desperate need of cost-effective solutions for chronic disease management. One important strategy for this is early diagnosis and management of diseases. With rapid technological advancements, IoT-based solutions are well-positioned to be an effective tool for disease screening and health monitoring provided that they are also able to bridge non-technical barriers in technology adoption.

Chapter 3, "Early Diagnostics Model for Dengue Disease Using Decision Tree-Based Approaches," discusses and compare 6 different Decision Tree classifiers for early diagnosis of dengue. Classification schemes have been applied in the medical arena to explore patient's data and extract a predictive model. This model helps doctors to improve their prognosis, diagnosis or treatment planning processes. Six approaches mainly J48 tree, Random Tree, REP Tree, SOM, Logistic Regression and Naïve Bayes have been utilized to study real world Dengue data collected from different hospitals in the Delhi, India region during 2015-2016.Standard statistical metrics are used to assess the efficiency of the proposed dengue disease diagnostic system and the outcomes showed that REP tree is best among these classifiers with 82.7% efficient in supplying an exact diagnosis.

Chapter 4, "Innovative Approaches for Pre-Screening and Sensing of Diseases," covers various innovative techniques related to prescreening and sensing of diseases. Prescreening and sensing of diseases offers a number of benefits that can help in prevention and check of major diseases before its onset. The aim of disease pre-screening is to detect possible disorders or diseases in people who do not have any symptoms of disease. Earlier screening methods for the detection of diseases was invasive, complicated and would require extensive tests. Some conventional methods used in clinical diagnoses include many invasive and potentially hazardous biopsy procedures, endoscopy, computed tomography; numerous innovative approaches have evolved to overcome the limitations of traditional techniques. Non-invasive biomedical sensor, Genomics, electronic nose, Nano-material, plasmonic sensor devices, microfabrication-based technologies, flat-panel detectors, digital breast object models, endomicroscopy, breath biopsy and wavelet-based etc. are some of the emerging frontiers in prescreening and sensing of diseases.

Chapter 5, "Clinical Decision Support System for Early Disease Detection and Management," covers about clinical decision support systems (CDSS) and how CDSS assist the clinicians in identifying the severity of disease at the time of admission and predicting its progression. A CDSS developed with the help of statistical techniques is explained. Modified Cascade Neural Network (ModCNN) was built upon the architecture of Cascade-Correlation Neural Network (CCNN). ModCNN first identifies the independent factors associated with disease and using that factor; it predicts its progression. A Case, progressing towards severity can be given better care, avoiding later stage complications. Performance of ModCNN was evaluated and compared with Artificial Neural Network (ANN) and CCNN. ModCNN showed better accuracy than other statistical techniques. Thus, CDSS developed in this work is aimed at providing better treatment planning by reducing medical error.

Chapter 6, "Impact of Using Educational Materials From Online Health Communities for Patient Medical Education on Screening for Disease Outcomes," analyzes how medical education can contribute improving screening outcomes. Screening for Diseases is a medical process to predict, prevent, early detect, and cure a disease in people at high risk. However, it is limited in the quality and accuracy of the outcomes. The reason for this issue is the lack of long-term data about the health condition of the patient. Launching modern information and communication technology in the screening process has shown promise of improving the screening outcomes. A previous study has shown that patient education can positively impact the patient behavior face to a disease and can empower the patient to adopt a healthy lifestyle and thus avoid certain diseases. Offering medical education to the patient can positively impact screening outcomes since educated and empowered patient is more aware of certain diseases and can collect significant information. This can minimize the rate of false positive as well as false negative screening results.

Chapter 7, "Ubiquitous Wearable Healthcare Monitoring System Architectural Design for Prevention, Detection, and Monitoring of Chronic Diseases," provides a detailed description of subsystems, components, functionalities, requirements, and realization mechanisms along with their merits and demerits for Wearable Healthcare Monitoring Systems. Chronic diseases have become the leading cause of death and disability worldwide. Major chronic diseases currently account for almost 60% of all deaths and this contribution is expected to rise up to 73% by 2020. An integrated approach is needed for detection, prevention, and monitoring of these diseases. For better and specialized healthcare services, there is a need to develop a technology that should be fast, reliable, secure, accurate and economical. In this chapter, the authors have presented an architectural design for Wearable Healthcare Monitoring Systems. The main motivation behind this architectural design is to improve the efficiency, accuracy and generosity of WHMS. The architecture design divides the system into three layers or subsystems. The resolution of design issues like data fusion, data delivery, data processing, security, accuracy, and efficiency are the main points of this architecture design.

Chapter 8, "Fuzzy-Based Predictive Analytics for Early Detection of Diabetes," covers an assessment of the applications of machine learning algorithms and tools in the diabetes investigation relating to Genetic Background and Environment. Today, Diabetes is the most costly and burdensome chronic disease. The severity of diabetes is reducing with anticipation, premature recognition and the early supervision impediments in people. These symptoms are the optimization of the diagnosis phase of the disease through the process of evaluating symptomatic characteristics and daily habits of patients. Big data analytical tools play a useful task in executing significant real-time investigation on the huge volumes of data and are also used to foresee the crisis situations earlier than it occurs. With a target for improving accuracy for early detection and prevention of diabetes in this work, implemented a Fuzzy linear and logistic regression model with Fuzzy clustering for predicting early detection of diabetic.

Chapter 9, "A Fourier-Bessel Expansion-Based Method for Automated Detection of Atrial Fibrillation From Electrocardiogram Signals," presents a new methodology for detection and identification of cardiovascular diseases from a single-lead electrocardiogram (ECG) signal of short duration. More specifically, this method deals with the detection of the most common cardiac arrhythmia called atrial fibrillation (AF) in noisy and non-clinical environment. The method begins with appropriate pre-processing of ECG signals in order to get the RR-interval and heart rate (HR) signals from them. A set of indirect features are computed from the original and the transformed versions of RR-interval and HR signals along with a set of direct features that are obtained from ECG signals themselves. In all, 47 features are computed and subsequently they are fed to an ensemble system of bagged decision trees for classifying the ECG recordings into four different classes. The proposed method has been evaluated with 2017 PhysioNet/CinC Challenge hidden test dataset (Phase II subset) and the final F1 score of 0.81 is obtained.

Chapter 10, "Applications of Machine Learning in Disease Pre-Screening," covers the Application of computers in disease pre-screening with the example of a computer-aided pre-screening tool (CAPST). CAPST helps in improving the accuracy of diagnosis in medicine. Fast and accurate prediction of disease risk and diagnosis is crucial step for the successful treatment of an individual. The AI based machine learning technology has undergone through significant developments over the past few years and successfully used in many intelligent applications covering problems of variety of domains. One of the most stimulating questions is whether these techniques can be successfully applied to the medicine in disease pre-screening and diagnosis and what kind of data it requires to be trained and learned. There are so many real time examples of the problems where machine learning methods are applied successfully, especially in medicine. Many of them showed the significant improvement in classification accuracy.

Chapter 11, "Safety and Regulatory Aspects of Systems for Disease Pre-Screening," gives an over view of the medical device regulations and medical device safety. The definition of a medical device to the guideline of how a medical device is classified is then discussed. Pre-screening solutions for disease screening fall under medical device regulations because of the intended purpose of diagnosis. Hence the later part of the chapter covers the design control process with stages of user needs translating to requirements, the design process with the design outputs, design verification conforming that the design is right followed by design validation that proves that a right medical device is made. The risk management, usability engineering, and security & privacy risk management are part of the product realization process.

Having a clear regulatory strategy and plan beginning with country list and intended use followed by identification of all the applicable product standards is vital. The process thus culminates in the design and development file which is a formal document that describes the design history of the medical device.

CONCLUSION

As this is a book on the pre-screening for diseases, the readers will likely be familiar with the topic of screening for diseases, diseases diagnostics, diseases prediction, and prevention. This book aims to present modern technologies that may contribute to going one step earlier in the screening process to recognize the diseases at a very earlier stage. The concept of pre-screening is introduced by this book. This concept pursues the objectives to assist medical doctors and the population to gather significant and gapless data on their health and, thus, earlier detect and cure some medical conditions. It further assists the healthcare professionals in the screening process and contribute to providing sufficient, highly significant, and detailed medical, environmental, context-aware data that can positively impact the screening test-outcomes regarding the test accuracy and sensitivity as well as specificity.

The contributors in this book have presented a series of mechanism, technologies, and case studies of pre-screening for diseases and have shown the importance of pervasively collecting bio-parameters, monitoring the individual health conditions. This book would contribute to changing and improving the existing screening for diseases policies and paradigms with the objectives to reduce the rate of false-positive and false-negative test-outcomes.

REFERENCES

Edoh, T. (2017). Smart medicine transportation and medication monitoring system in EPharmacyNet. In *2017 International Rural and Elderly Health Informatics Conference (IREHI)* (pp. 1–9). Lomé: IEEE. 10.1109/IREEHI.2017.8350381

Istepanian, R. S. H., Hu, S., Philip, N. Y., & Sungoor, A. (2011). The potential of Internet of m-health things for non-invasive glucose level sensing. In *2011 Annual International Conference of the IEEE Engineering in Medicine and Biology Society* (pp. 5264–5266). IEEE. 10.1109/IEMBS.2011.6091302

Rigla, M., García-Sáez, G., Pons, B., & Hernando, M. E. (2018). Artificial Intelligence Methodologies and Their Application to Diabetes. *Journal of Diabetes Science and Technology*, *12*(2), 303–310. doi:10.1177/1932296817710475 PMID:28539087

Thrall, J. H., Li, X., Li, Q., Cruz, C., Do, S., Dreyer, K., & Brink, J. (2018). Artificial Intelligence and Machine Learning in Radiology: Opportunities, Challenges, Pitfalls, and Criteria for Success. *Journal of the American College of Radiology*, *15*(3), 504–508. doi:10.1016/j.jacr.2017.12.026 PMID:29402533

Acknowledgment

We would like to express our gratitude to all the people who have contributed to the realization of this book by way of providing encouragement and support, authoring book chapters, reviewing, and offering comments and assisting in the editing, proofreading and design.

We would like to thank Geetha M. from Philips Research, Chitra Iyer from Philips IP&S for providing their consent and motivating us to take on this journey.

We would like to thank the health informatics research community across the globe for welcoming this project, authoring manuscripts, accommodating reviewers' feedback and being our extended team for the peer review process. This book project wouldn't have been possible without your invaluable contributions.

Ms. Marianne Caesar from IGI Global has been instrumental in ensuring the success of this project. She has been with us from the inception to completion of this project and meticulously scrutinized every phase to improve the quality of the book content. We would also like to thank IGI Global for accepting our book proposal and providing us a platform to publish our aspiration.

Thierry Edoh
Technical University of Munich, Germany

Pravin Pawar
Philips Research, India

Sagar Mohammad
Philips Research, India

July 2018

Chapter 1
Internet-of-Things-Enabled Pre-Screening for Diseases:
A Novel Approach for Improving the Conventional Methodology and Paradigm for Screening for Non-Communicable Diseases

Thierry Edoh
Technical University of Munich, Germany

ABSTRACT

This chapter focuses on the screening for non-communicable diseases (NCDs), which in certain cases are likely caused by infectious diseases. The screening for NCDs in this specific case remains challenging since the convergence between both non-infectious and infectious diseases is less investigated. This chapter, therefore, aims at reviewing and addressing the challenges and limitation of the conventional methodologies for screening for diseases, in general. The chapter further proposes an innovative screening paradigm based on the internet of things technology. The chapter presents the state of the art on the conventional screening for diseases, discusses the fundamental difference between screening for diseases and diseases surveillance and monitoring, and the difference between screening for diseases and diseases diagnostics.

DOI: 10.4018/978-1-5225-7131-5.ch001

1. INTRODUCTION

Screening for diseases is a tool for predicting and/or early detecting diseases with the main objective of timely treating the detected diseases. It is, therefore, a key component of the care delivery system (Saquib, Saquib, & Ioannidis, 2015). The screening pursues the objective of reducing morbidity and mortality by early detecting, preventing, and predicting diseases is the main role assigned to the screening for diseases.

The screening for diseases rises various controversies and questions regarding its benefits or efficiency. Screening for diseases can be costly and people can be false-positive or false-negative screened (Lee, Huang, & Zelen, 2004), Hence, the follow-up treatment can be hazardous, or the disease would not at all be prevented. It is then worth investigating the underlying methodology for screening.

Nazmus Saquib et al. have reported cases where medical experts recommend against the screening for diseases. They discussed the role and benefit of screening and presented the case of screening for breast cancer in women aged from 40 to 49 years and screening for prostate in healthy men whose outcomes do not show any benefit (Saquib et al., 2015). In Maxim, Niebo, and Utell (2014b), Maxim et al. had pointed out the recommendation formulated by the Medicare Evidence Development and Coverage Advisory Committee (MEDCAC) against the screening procedure for certain patient group. They argued recommendation by the fact of lacking evidence supporting the benefits of screening of diseases in the target groups.

Despite the recommendation against the procedure of screening for diseases for a certain group of individuals and certain diseases, this study revealed a positive impact of the screening on the mortality. The question that arises here is to why this recommendation is made? Why there exist controversies regarding the screening for diseases? It is worth investigating the causes why screening procedure does not provide benefit to all patient groups. The inaccuracy of screening test outcomes undoubtedly plays an important role here. Though, what (negatively) impacts the quality of the test-outcomes?

1.1 Problem Statement and Analysis

Information Paucity and Lacking Long-Term Information

According to the literature review, the procedure of the Conventional Screening and Assessment (CSA) are strongly limited in the quality of the test-outcomes. The procedure of CSA foresees that health care units initiate the screening process. The procedure is holding among asymptomatic people who do not seek any medical attention because they do not present any symptoms of any diseases for which they are screened for (Strong, Wald, Miller, & Alwan, 2005b). Especially, the developing countries are being severely facing this limitation due to information paucity on one hand and due to medical fees (because of the lack of health insurance systems, which can cover the medical expenses). The high medical fees lead to poor access to healthcare and screening and assessment programs. Most people at risk of contracting or developing certain diseases, in general, do not take part to the offered screening programs because of the lack of symptoms since they really misunderstand the meaning on screening for diseases.

Traditionally, the procedure of screening for noncommunicable diseases is mostly based on investigating the individual's living style, age, body mass, and other physiological data. However, the data used in the scope of such medical examination are limited since they are short-term data that cannot really provide enough information to predict the occurrence of certain diseases. Some disease can remain undetected during a screening session, (Bergman, Neuhauser, & Provost, 2011). Bergman et al. (2011) have, therefore, proposed a longitudinal data collection to so easily detect such diseases. They concluded following;

Cancer screening is an illustrative example. If a fast-growing malign melanoma is growing without detection, the effectiveness of the diagnostic and treatment processes might be of little help. The citizens could be more actively engaged in monitoring their own health status. Longitudinal data are more useful if collected regularly. Daily measurement of hypertension or blood sugar can provide more information that can be collected once every few months in a doctor's office. (Bergman et al., 2011)

Inaccurate Screening Test-Outcomes, High Rate of False-Positive and False-Negative Test-Outcomes

Maxim et al. (2014a) conducted an exhaustive and comprehensive review of screening tests and concluded that screening tests outcomes can be false-positive or false-negative. They, therefore, recommended to carefully consider these aspects of the screening-outcomes by evaluating the advantages and disadvantages of the screening tests.

The conventional paradigm and methodology for screening for diseases are failing in delivering accurate test-outcomes (Maxim et al., 2014a; Di & Li, 2018; Yang, Zhang, Yao, & Fan, 2018). In Di and Li, (2018), the authors have figured out that test-outcomes of the Tuberculosis (TB) screening are impacted by the size of the participant cohort as well as by the factors like the patient age and the TB meningitis. The factor age has significantly impacted a specific group of individuals. The discussion conducted by the authors has shown the limitation of the conventional methodology for screening and the need for new policy and methodology improvement.

Another study (Yang et al., 2018), had also pointed to the patient age as one of the various factors impacting the test-outcomes. An earlier study work conducted by Nelson et al. (2016) have also pointed to the age as a factor associated with false-positive and false-negative screening-outcomes. That study has investigated the association between the rate of false-positive and false-negative screening-outcomes and the different age groups and found out similar factor association like in Di and Li, (2018). The rate of false-positive screening-outcomes is higher in the <49 years than >49 years group.

Beyond the factor age, the literature review has revealed other associating factors like multimorbidity. Multimorbidities associating non-infectious (also called non-communicable) diseases with infectious (also called communicable) diseases are frequent but less investigated. Often, Malaria tropica and/or other (tropical) infectious diseases are associated with cardiovascular or heart diseases (CVD) and/or diabetics HIV/Aids infection is associated with tuberculosis, etc. in several patients. Certain parasitic infections can be associated with significant morbidity and lead to mortality in regions of high endemicity (Hidron et al., 2010; Pusiol, Lavezzi, Radice, Alfonsi, & Matturri, 2014).

- **Morbidity and Multimorbidity:** The morbidity is defined as health condition or state. The multimorbidity is the extended concept of the comorbidity where comorbidity is the interaction between diseases or risk factors making the main disease worse. The World Health Organization (WHO) defines the multimorbidity as suffering from at least two chronic health conditions (Le Reste et al., 2015; Read, Sharpe, Modini, & Dear, 2017; WHO, 2016). The multimorbidity is also called the coexistence of at least two chronic conditions in the same person (WHO, 2016). The multimorbidity can, according to WHO (2016), impact on safety issues in the primary care. The question that arises here is how to reduce the impact of the different associating factors and, thus, reduce the rate of the false-positive/false-negative screening-outcomes? It is important to first understand the leading causes of false-positive and false-negative screening-outcomes and their prevalence in each screening category and age group, that means how the factors associated with the quality of the outcomes impact the results. A study (Renshaw & Gould, 2013), conducted in 2013 has shed light on most of the questions. The authors have investigated the leading causes by analyzing 8082 consults and found 0.3% false-positive and 0.7% false-negative cases and pointed out that the cases identified as false-negative concern a certain group of pathologies like breast, cytology, etc. with significant differences between the pathology-group. In contrary, no significant differences were found in false-positive cases. The authors claimed in the conclusion of the 9-years longitudinal research work that many false-positive cases could be avoided if the so-called immunohistochemistry method was used instead of requesting the review of a second pathologist. This study has shown the need for new paradigm and policy in general, but it is important to consider each pathology and disease group accordingly.

- **False-negative:** Screening outcomes are identified as false-negative when an individual is misclassified not having or not presenting any sign to develop or not at risk to contract the diseases for which she/he is screened. The misclassification leads to the false statement pretending that the screened individual is free of the given diseases. Mistakenly in this case, further recommended suitable medical examinations would not be provided to the individual. Hence, the given could be late detected with serious consequences for the individual. The individual is, therefore, facing an eventual risk of morbidity and mortality (Maxim et al., 2014a).
- **False-positive:** In contrary to a false-negative test-outcome, an individual is however misclassified having a given disease based on the screening test. The individual would, therefore, undergo unnecessary and costly recommended follow-up medical examinations and treatments and thus can suffer psychological consequences (Maxim et al., 2014a).

The terms of sensitivity and specificity are also used to qualify the screening test outcomes. The sensitivity of screening tests as the ratio of true-negative to {true-negative + false positive} and the specificity as the ratio of true-positive to {true-positive + false-positive}. The terms are interdependent.

Limitation of Screening for Diseases Policies

Ruth Etzioni et al. (2013) presented three limitations of a screening as follows:

- *First, screening policy development demands information about long-term benefits and harms because these policies generally pertain to interventions conducted over an individual's healthy lifetime. Unfortunately, most screening trials provide short-term results rather than the long-term outcomes generated by a typical population-based screening program.*
- *Second, screening trial results can be highly influenced by the trial population and by patterns of compliance with the trial protocol.*
- *Third, any inferences about screening benefit are limited to the screening strategy or strategies tested in the trial. This does not permit policymakers to identify and compare alternative policies that might be more acceptable."*

This study shows that the conventional screening for diseases has limitations to provide long-term results as requested by the policies. The fundamental reason why the current screening for disease is being outcoming short-prognostics is linked to the data inputs used for evaluating the risk. Mostly the inputs are composites of short-term and patient-centered information. No genetical and no long-term data about the health and activities of an individual are considered during the process. Today, it is well known that the genetics impacts the development of certain diseases. A recent study reveals the genetic susceptibility to lung cancer (Schwartz, Bailey-Wilson, & Amos, 2018). Several studies (Barer, 2017; Bluestone, Herold, & Eisenbarth, 2010; Chapman & Hill, 2012; Hunter, 2005) conducted prior by different authors have shown the link of the genetics to a predisposition to certain diseases and associated-effects.

Based on different works on the link between genes and diseases predispositions revealed in different studies, the present study has demonstrated the limitation of the screening policy that does not include the use of the genetical data in evaluating an individual's risk of developing a given disease.

Convergence Between Infectious and Non-Communicable Disease

Preventing a disease must not always include screening people at the high-risk factor but can also propose or use the available resources for population education about risk factors (e.g. reduce tobacco consumption to reduce the heart disease risks).

Furthermore, the screening for diseases does not consider another risk factor that may lead to developing a noncommunicable disease. Very few researchers were focused on finding out the causality and/or convergence between infectious and non-infectious (or noncommunicable) diseases. Cases of tropical infections, causing cardiovascular diseases, have been recently reported The authors in Chandra and Chandra (2011) have reported an interesting suspicious case of causality where a fatal complication of myocardial infarction in individuals appears by a delayed diagnosis of Plasmodium falciparum infection. Authors (Nieman et al., 2009) reported a similar case of causality regarding a complication of acute coronary after an experimental testing in individual a Plasmodium falciparum infection. The coronary syndrome was diagnosed after the successful treatment of the malaria infection. The convergence of tropical infectious diseases, such as malaria, and non-communicable diseases is neither trivial nor transient; but represents a phase in the epidemiological transition (Remais, Zeng, Li, Tian, & Engelgau, 2013), therefore, an improved early detection in asymptomatic or infected individuals is therefore highly motivated. The convergence of tropical infectious diseases, such as malaria, and non-communicable diseases is neither trivial nor transient; but represents a phase in the epidemiological transition

(Remais et al., 2013), therefore, an improved early detection in asymptomatic or infected individuals is therefore highly motivated.

Regarding the earlier reported cases of suspicious causality, it seems to exist a convergence of tropical infectious diseases and/or other non-communicable diseases. Remais et al. (2013) see in the convergence new challenges and opportunities to enact responsive changes in policy and research.

We are living nowadays in a globalized world. Traveling people are severely limited to timely get screened at their residence place. However, most people do not get screened on their trip due to language limitation, medical cost, or do not have time for that. Even, if they get screened during their journey since the global healthcare lacks ubiquitous patient medical and/or health records, the case-finding will not automatically be reported to the physician at home for further medical action. The care units of the global care system are not connected at all and the patient health and/or medical records are not shared among the different healthcare systems worldwide. The patient only can report the case-finding if he does not forget about it, then he does not fill sick yet.

People traveling to regions where certain infectious diseases are endemic can get infected back home with infection. During a screening for NCDs at home, the infection carried from aboard would not be considered. Only the infection control program will consider this infection.

1.2 Research Aims and Objectives

The main aims of this work are to tackle the controversies facing the screening for diseases. The controversies arise from the fact that the current paradigm of screening for diseases fails to show the benefits of screening for diseases. This is due to high rates of poor screening-outcomes.

Regarding the various controversies about the benefits of the screening for diseases the quality of the screening test outcomes (see subsection: Inaccurate Screening Test-Outcomes, High Rate of False-Positive and False-Negative Test-Outcomes), this research work aims at improving the procedure of the conventional screening for diseases on one hand in providing the healthcare professionals with high-quality data (patient-centric data and information, long-term data, medical health records) to overcome the data and information paucity. On the other hand, modern information and communication technology-based systems are used to support the procedure of the screening for diseases.

The main objectives being pursued in this ongoing study is to provide the public healthcare system with an improved tool for screening for diseases. The study will design and implement an IoT-Enabled screening tool called Pre-Screening that will be able to collect and sense day by day pervasive/ubiquitous physiological data and perform data analytics for early detection and prevention of multimorbidity, disability, the convergence of NCDs and CDs, and the death. The data collected using the proposed system will be exhaustive and comprehensive and include patient-centric and long-term data. Pre-Screening for diseases is a new paradigm and term launched in the scope of this study with the objectives to use the power of predictive and preventive analytics based on collected medical big data.

An Internet of Things-enabled Pre-Screening for diseases solution is, therefore, proposed and tested in a phase I. The results of the tests are compared with results of the tests conducted using the conventional. The experiment is still going on and the present results will be used for the phase II of the of the pilot study. This chapter presents the available results of the ongoing experiment. This approach further aims at overcoming the limitation of existing methodologies and tools for screening for diseases and diseases prevention. The proposed paradigm will focus especially on the convergence between (tropical) infectious diseases and non-communicable diseases in individuals at high risk of infectious diseases.

1.3 Chapter Layout

After the introduction section that presents and analyzes the problematic and the reasons why this study was conducted, the remainder of the chapter is structured the study methodology and material in section 2. In section 3 the backgrounds of the screening for diseases and definition of certain relating terms provided to help for a better understanding of the terminologies used in the chapter. Section 4 presents the implementation of the proposed solution. The resulting concept and the architectural view including a brief presentation of the key technologies underlying the proposed IoT-enabled Pre-Screening for diseases are discussed. The results of the conducted experiment are presented and discussed in section 6. Section 7 presents the further work and phases II and III tests which would be get done.

2. METHODOLOGY AND MATERIALS

2.1 Snowball Approach as Sampling Methodic

The snowball research methodology was the research approach used to build the different research cohort and the literature pool. This way of building study cohorts or population and literature pool eases to appropriately select or recruit, in a complex situation, people by interposed person and thus build the study cohort needed. The literature pool is also built in selecting suitable articles cited in an article that is already selected and put into the pool. This operation is repeated till the literature pool contains enough and recently published articles that can support an exhaustive and a comprehensive review of the literature.

A Snowball research approach is a low-cost research method and meaningful in specific cases (Acharya, Prakash, Saxena, & Nigam, 2013) like the current study where articles on challenges facing western healthcare systems relating to the poor access to the care services in certain regions are scarcely published. The snowball sampling is a method to select a research population or material through contact (social, virtual, or reference/recommendation). According to MacNealy, cited in Latham (2007), snowball sampling is defined as the use in rare cases when is hard for the researchers to identify selves the population of interest. Recruiting suited people for the research project is assigned to a person selected in the local population (MacNealy).

Mendeley was used to search and classify the recent literature on the topic. 150 materials (published papers) from different publication libraries: PubMed, Scopus, Google-scholar using the snowball process were reviewed.

Following words were sought in diverse databases: Predictive analysis, Screening for diseases, Pre-Screening, Non-Communicable diseases, infectious diseases, diseases convergence. diseases surveillance, patient-centricity, patient-centered care.

Beyond the references at the end of the chapter, following articles were also exploited (see Annex).

2.2 Testing-Cohort Sampling

Table 1 indicates the structure of built cohort, involving healthcare professionals only, to first determine the limitation of the conventional screening methodology and finally to prove the innovative proposed concept of Pre-Screening for diseases.

The main objective of the test is to find out to what extent the proposed concept can help to early detect diseases accurately than the conventional screening method and improve the sensitivity and specificity of screening.

A Pre-Screening for diseases, according to our concept, could be defined as pervasively sensing one's medical data using pervasive/ubiquitous computing paradigm and enabling technologies and tools like wearable, Internet of things, etc. The main objective is to accurately detect a medical condition and minimize as well as bring down to zero (0) the rate of false-positive and false-negative screening test's results.

The cohort size was 44 participants without any health condition issues. Due to the short-term experiment, only adults, aged between 40 and 55 and 2 infants, were selected.

Table 1. Participants structure

Participant's Category	Participants			Total
	University Hospital	Private Clinics	Medical Practice	
General Physician	13	3	5	14
In-Patient	10	2	4	21
Infant (pediatric)	2	0	0	02
Emergency-patient	5	0	0	07
Total				44

2.3 Data Collection

People who do not suffer from any infection for a long time before the test began were selected. The objective is to conduct short-term screening test on patients that that susceptible to contract malaria in order to figure out the impact of infectious on developing non-infectious diseases.

The selected cohort population were examined prior to the beginning of the test to make sure that they do not suffer from any non-infectious disease.

The test was conducted in the rainy season because people can easily be infected by malaria in this period of the year.

Vital parameters of the cohort population were daily remotely and/or onsite measured. The system collected automatically and autonomously all data from the bio-medical sensors placed on each participant. Unfortunately, it was not possible to measure the blood glucose level using the sensor. Therefore, once a day we measure this parameter on site.

- **Qualitative Research Approach:** Data is collected using the qualitative research approach. The results of Screening for diseases tests were collected and analyzed. The participants were selected based on criteria previously defined. The criteria are the participant should already be screened for non-communicable diseases and was suffering from an infectious disease during the screening phase. A further criterion is that the results of the test are clearly reported in the medical record. The record must clearly mention that the patient was suffering from an infection during the screening.
- **Quantitative Research Approach:** This approach was used in this study, to know how many people are false-positive and/or false-negative screened. This approach will show the importance of improving the screening for diseases methodology.

- **Collected Data:** A set of data is collected. This includes the following data
    - Daily blood sugar/glucose level
    - Body Temperature (twice a day – morning and afternoon -)
    - Breath Rhythm
    - Cardiac mechanical activities
    - Environmental contextual data (air humidity, pollution, attitude)
    - Individual's Activities
    - Health state (for example, did the participant develop an infectious disease during the study phase?)
    - Medicine used during the study phase

Questionnaire

A questionnaire (Table 2) has helped the participant to daily collect data and information that the system, in this implemented version, is limited to sense.

2.4 Study Limitation

The amount of collected data, the analyzed medical record, and the test period (about 1 ½ month) were qualitative, not satisfactory enough to conclude to a convergence between infectious and non-infectious diseases and to which extent an infectious disease can lead or link to an NCD.

Table 2. Questionnaire for gathering additional Information

Questions	Answers	Date: Hour
Do you use any medical and pharmaceutical product today?	○ yes ◉ no	**Why do you use it?**
Are you at risk to contract any infectious or parasites diseases?	○ yes ○ no	**Which risk?**
Any physical activities?	○ Nothing/ Seat ○ Sport/ Montain ○ Going to bed ○ Others **Others**	
Medical-related information you can report		

In contrary, the study confirms the limitation of the conventional screening methodology and show the promise of the proposed method to overcome these limitations-

2.5 Context and Ethical Approval

This subsection presents the study context. An ethical approval was applied and approved to conduct an experiment to prove the concept of the proposed approach.

Research Context

At the present stage, the study focuses on the convergence of infectious diseases and noncommunicable diseases. People living in the developing countries or people regularly traveling to regions with high infection endemicity are a target for the present study for two reasons (i) find out to what extent having infectious diseases can link to noncommunicable diseases and (ii) how to avoid noncommunicable diseases despite having been infected. The overall question is, is it possible to detect diseases or predict with high accuracy the risk of developing certain diseases using the proposed system?

Research Ethical Approval

Authorization and written informed participant consent are received from all major participants and parent of the young participants. We translate in a local tongue the participant consent for the illiterates.

An ad-hoc ethics committee at the involved clinics examined the request to conduct such a test involving patients and approved it.

3. BACKGROUND AND DEFINITIONS

This section provides a couple of definitions of themes related to the topic of the study with the objectives to help the reader to better perceive the difference between the different themes used in this chapter.

3.1 Methods of Screening for Diseases

A screening test is not intended to be diagnostic. A person with positive or suspicious findings must be referred to their physician for diagnosis and necessary treatment. (Wilson & Jungner, 1968)

The authors of the book (Wilson & Jungner, 1968) further state that "*screening also includes rapid physical examination*". What is rapid physical examination? What is a medical diagnosis? And finally, what is screening for diseases?

The term of "suspicious findings" shows already the limitation of the methodology. From my own experiences, those findings are mostly based on a patient-centered information. Based on an ongoing longitudinal study being conducted since 2015 in investigating the patient subjectivity and its impact on the patient-centered information, 1660 anonymized patient's cases files from the developing world and 535 anonymized patient's case files revealed that more than 80% are not confirmed by medical analyses. 89.11% of investigated cases revealed that patient-centered information is subjective and often leads to mitigated findings. 71% of investigated medical examinations that rely on such "suspicious findings" are not successful and the patient does get treated. In about 29% of the cases, the physician goes beyond the "suspicious findings" and proceed with another medical examination to detect the disease.

According to Wilson and Jungner (1968), screening can be classified in (i) mass screening, (ii) selective screening, and (iii) multiple or multiphasic screening.

Each disease shows different symptoms. A screening for diseases, therefore, looks for particular signs or early symptoms to early detect the given disease. Strong et al. (2005a) describe the screening as

Screening tests, while generally easier to perform and less expensive than diagnostic tests, yield indefinite results, indicating a probability of having or developing the disorder in question if positive and usually requiring the subsequent application of a diagnostic test. (Strong, Wald, Miller, & Alwan, 2005a)

The global healthcare system has defined a set of screening methodologies, which, however, is only valid for a given country. There exists no standardized screening. This is an issue that needs to be overcome (Strong et al., 2005a).

The existing screening categories independently of diseases and the trend in screening for diseases are discussed in various research works.

Opportunistic and Proactive Screening

The authors in Kariuki, Stuart-Shor, Leveille, and Hayman, (2015) discussed the so-called opportunistic and proactive screening programs. Opportunistic and proactive screening is a non-laboratory-based algorithm that can determine in few minutes the risk of developing a disease. This algorithm uses to estimate absolute risk basing on data like age, Body Mass Index, and diseases characteristic data like systolic blood pressure, antihypertensive medication use, current smoking, and diabetes status in the case of cardiovascular diseases. This methodology is cost-efficient and well adopted by the developing countries.

Strong et al. (2005a) figured out that the term of "opportunistic and proactive screening" is misused to define the term of screening. However, the methodology described in Kariuki et al., (2015) fits the definition K Strong et al. (2005a) have provided. Screening is to detect the risk of developing, and opportunistic as well as proactive screening do the same.

Clinical or Technical Screening (Laboratory Based Screening)

Wilson et al. (1968) have discussed a set of methodologies for screening. One of these methodologies is clinical screening, which consists of automated methods such as chemical tests. (Cf. to the article for more details)

Physical Examination Performed by a Physician

This test is based on patient-physician communication and medical examination conducted by a physician using various Technik. A physical examination is consisting of palpating, inspecting, and auscultating as well as measure blood-pressure, the glucose level in the blood, etc. The physician uses suggested or a questionnaire defined by and for a screening program to calculate or estimate the risk to develop a disease. The questionnaire aims to help the physician to track the medical history of the individual. This is called "self-screening". This methodology combines both the medical examination and the questionnaires to estimate the risk. However, this evaluation relies on short-term data that cannot really express the real health status of an individual.

Schmalfuss et al. (2013) conducted a review of methods of screening, which mostly is based on blood test using biomarker. They propose to use tissue samples to improve the early detection of oncological diseases.

3.2 Methods of Collecting Epidemiological Data

Collecting epidemiological data about emerging infectious diseases through the social media, or using wearable sensors systems, or mobile applications and data analysis is a trend in the diseases surveillance today.

In the age of Information and Communication Technology (ICT), many social web-platforms are used to collect epidemiological data to predict and prevent (emerging infectious) diseases. For example, Foodborne Chicago[1] and Flu Near You[2] are social media application used to collect diseases and health conditions related data (Christaki, 2015). Collecting data through social media applications, however, is limited in its "participatory" and/or voluntary aspect. Furthermore, they present a geographical surveillance gap due to limitations in communication infrastructures in low- and middle-income countries. To overcome this limitation, mobile phone application is using web-based surveillance tools and epidemic intelligence methods to collect epidemiological data on infectious diseases, since the mobile phone is widely distributed in these areas (Christaki, 2015). In Brownstein, Freifeld, Reis, and Mandl, (2008), the authors have discussed the limitations of the Internet-based diseases surveillance using the example of the Health Map System. The authors summarized the limitations of the HealthMap as follow:

...While Internet-based online media sources are becoming a critical tool for global infectious disease surveillance, important challenges still need to be addressed. Since regions with the least advanced communication infrastructure also tend to carry the greatest infectious disease burden and risk, system development must be aimed at closing the gaps in these critical areas. ...(Brownstein, Freifeld, Reis & Mandl, 2008)

3.3 Mass vs. Crowd Screening

Mass screening can be considered as crowd screening depending on the method and the technology used to perform the mass screening. Mass Screening is when a questionnaire is used to detect diseases in a group of individuals. It does matter which technology is used to. While crowd sensing or screening is when a group of individuals is participatory and/or opportunistically involved in collecting their health-related data.

Limitation of the Mass Screening

Collecting health-related data through questionnaires is limited since the responses are on voluntary base and further can be biased or incomplete. Beyond the questionnaires, mass-screening can be conducted following two different paradigms or approaches: (i) opportunistic approach and (ii) systematic approach. The authors of the study (Zink, Marx, Crijns, & Schotten, 2018) that has dealt with the opportunities and challenges of large scale screening had reported an example of an opportunistic screening conducted in Hong Kong where, within 12 months, 13,122 individuals were screened. The results (0,8% detected diseases among the cohort) had shown that this approach has limitation. The authors concluded that the impacts of this approach on diagnostics and treatment are unclear. The authors further presented a systematic large-scale screening study which took place in Sweden and last 28 months. In contrary to the opportunistic approach, the systematic shows more promise because this approach implies to preselect the cohort and repeatedly screen the participants. The term "Repeatedly screen" shows that the systematic approach also has limitation.

3.4 Selective Screening

Selective screening concerns high-risk groups in the population (Wilson & Jungner, 1968). In the early 1980s, at the beginning of the HIV-outbreak, certain groups of persons among the global population are targeted to be a high-risk group. These groups are regularly screened with the objectives to prevent the disease from spreading.

3.5 Multiple or Multiphasic Screening

Combines many screening examinations (at least two) to a mass. This art of screening is considered as cost-efficient.

3.6 Epidemiological Survey vs. Screening for Diseases

The trend today in diseases surveillance is consisting of epidemiological data collection about emerging infectious diseases using social media, wearable sensors systems, or mobile applications and data analysis. The survey does not pursue the objective to deliver the patients to a hospital for medical treatment, whereas the screening for diseases does. epidemiological survey cost-effective and enables rapid access to health care service. as discussed in Kasaie et al. (2017), a study on the impact of universal access to rapid tuberculosis diagnosis, appropriate epidemiological survey method has the potential to increase access to health care. A study (Yu et al., 2017) conducted in China had revealed patients preferences regarding which medical unit to visit when they caught infectious diseases. this behavior is due to the fact of the familiarity with the care units they visite. The familiarity means that the patients have developed some trust in such care units.

3.7 Case-Finding

The term "Case-Finding" is often used but its meaning is quite confused. Many authors have addressed the term and define it.

Examples of "case-finding" include

- *Communicable disease control*
- *Health systems data*
- *Opportunistic screening*

In Wald & Morris, (1996) the authors discussed the term and pointed out that the term is confusing and should be abandoned. The conducted basically the definition made by Wilson and Jungner:

Wilson and Jungner, in their original monograph, defined case-finding as "that form of Screening of which the main object is to detect disease and bring patients to treatment". (Wald & Morris, 1996)

Dr. Murad Ruf and Dr. Oliver Morgan in 2008, Dr. Kelly Mackenzie in 2017 define on

Case finding is a strategy for targeting resources at individuals or groups who are suspected to be at risk for a particular disease. It involves actively searching systematically for at-risk people, rather than waiting for them to present with symptoms or signs of active disease. Note the similarities to screening - both seek to risk stratify the population for further investigation.(Murad, Oliver, & Kelly, 2017)

On the weblog (Weblogs -WordPress-, 2016) the author of the blog stated has been failed to seek a difference between screening for diseases and case-finding. He also thinks that there is a confusion and wrote:

The line between the two concepts of screening and case finding is very gray. It is an important question

Confusion Between Screening and Case Finding

The main source of confusion in the everyday use of the term 'screening' is that it can mean any of the following terms that are often conflated, used interchangeably and differentially by different stakeholders:

- *A test offered opportunistically to one person*
- *A test offered systematically to a group of people or a whole population*
- *A set of loosely linked activities encompassing tests and interventions that roughly comprise a screening program*
- *A rigorously quality-assured and evidence-based screening programs encompassing all necessary steps for achievement of risk reduction.*

We believe that the lack of distinction between the terms "case finding" and "screening" matters (Weblogs -WordPress-, 2016).

3.8 Diseases Diagnostic

The "Businessdictionary," (2018) has defined the diagnostics for diseases as the process of identifying a health issue by medically analyzing an individual. This analysis relies on previous medical examination and mostly focuses on signs or symptom related to certain pathologies. The Diseases Diagnostics is, therefore, the process of determining the medical follow-up in term of medical treatment. The process of diagnosing a disease relies on well-defined workflow regarding the disease of concern. In Boulton et al. (2005) the authors have described the diagnostic criteria in the case of a diabetic neuropathy as examining the *Acute sensory neuropathy* and the *Chronic sensorimotor DPN(chronic sensorimotor* ***d****istal symmetric* ***p****oly****n****europathy (DPN)).* In the case of diabetes, World Health Organization (WHO) defines how the diagnosis of diabetes should be made in an asymptomatic individual. Abnormal blood glucose value is not sufficient to declare the person suffering from diabetes. An additional test is essential (WHO, 1999).

3.9 Diseases Surveillance

The goal of diseases surveillance is to collect and provide data and information about the prevalence of a disease or risks factors in the population (Strong et al., 2005a).

The healthcare systems in the developed countries have, unlike the developing world health systems, implemented policies and tools to control and monitor infectious diseases and antibiotics adverse among their populations (Paolotti et al., 2014; Kinoshita, Tokumasu, Tanaka, Kramer, & Kawakami, 2017). The implemented policies and tools are, however, limited to collecting data from patients who do not visit a doctor and thus deliver their infections related data. In Paolotti et al., (2014) the authors have shown this limitation and proposed a web-based data collection system, that overcomes the limitation of existing surveillance methods and systems. A study (Heil et al., 2017) carried out in the Netherlands that can be generalized to all European countries reveals also that the method, policies, and the surveillance tool in the case of pertussis surveillance are less accurate.

3.10 Patient Monitoring

Patient monitoring can be classified into two categories (i) inpatient monitoring and (ii) outpatient monitoring (Telemonitoring). In a previous work (Edoh, Pawar, & Brügge, 2016), a telemonitoring system was designed and implemented and showed through the conducted experiment the benefit of monitoring in-patient and outpatient. (Tele)monitoring consists of regularly check the vital parameters (physiological data) and health course regarding certain diseases with the objectives to quickly provide medical assistance in the case this is needed. The work presented in Ong et al., (2016) has demonstrated the benefit of monitoring patient. The authors present the case of patients with heart failure. These patients get benefits from telehealth that englobe telemonitoring of their heart parameter.

Kyriacos U. et al. evaluated in Kyriacos, Jelsma, and Jordan, (2011) various monitoring systems using warning scoring and found out safety issues for the patient, and concluded that recording vital parameters only is not enough. The patient's safety depends on the ability of the nurses. In a previous work (Edoh, Atchome, Alahassa, & Pawar, 2016), we discussed a Sensors Network enabled patient monitoring. We especially pointed the energy issues these systems can face and the impact on the patient outcomes. During the study, we have also noticed the safety issues a patient can face. Patient monitoring needs, therefore, to be improved. A new paradigm is long overdue since, *despite the increasing technical sophistication in vital signs monitoring in the developed world, monitoring problems persist* (Kyriacos et al., 2011).

Mirza Mansoor Baig et al. (2015) presented a tablet-based monitoring. They develop 5 tablet-based user interfaces (UI) for remote patient monitoring with the main objective to improve the patient care in integrating decision support algorithms into the patient monitoring system. Such a system integrating decision support algorithm in the patient monitoring can help to meet the safety issues described earlier since the healthcare professional in charge of the patient monitoring will be supported in decision making and thus, can rapidly react in providing the right care at the right time to the patient.

Roma Maguire et al. (Maguire et al., 2015) evaluated the impact of using mobile technology-enabled monitoring and found out that it is feasible and positively impact patient's outcomes. The evaluation especially concerned patients suffering from lung cancer.

3.11 Differences Between Diseases Diagnostics, Diseases Surveillance, and Screening for Diseases

Screening for diseases is often confused with diseases diagnosis. Examples include various cases of women who do not take part in the screening for breast cancer programs as the global care system recommends to women at a certain age, the same for certain men regarding the screening for prostate cancer.

Table 3 presents the fundamental differences between diagnostics, surveillance, and screening.

Table 3. Fundamental Differences between diseases diagnostics, surveillance, and screening for diseases

	Diseases Diagnostics	Diseases Surveillance	Screening for Diseases
Purpose	Confirm the presence or absence of a given disease based on visible symptoms	Prevention of emerging infectious diseases, disease outbreak	Detect a potential development of a given disease
Target population	1. Symptomatic individuals (people are already presenting some symptoms) 2. Individuals tested positive in the scope of a screening test	Large-scale or target population	Asymptomatic individuals at risk of developing a given disease. The national screening program defines the groups of individuals
Test method(s)	The medical doctor decides which medical examination he needs to confirm his suspicion. Several medical examinations could be conducted till the presence or absence of the disease is definitively confirmed. This kind is expensive and invasive.	Systematic data gathering and analysis for detecting undetected diseases among a population or to monitor any disease outbreak or spread. Following steps are required: 1. Case detection 2. Case registration 3. Case confirmation 4. Reporting 5. Data analysis and interpretation 6. Epidemic preparedness 7. Response and control 8. Feedback	The test follows a well-defined workflow and is most relied on structured question followed by a non-structured discussion between the healthcare professional and the individual.
Characteristics of the test outcomes	Test methods must present high sensitivity in order to detect any potential diseases	The test method must provide statistically significant data,	Test methods are chosen on basis of their specificity, accuracy, and precision
Means of the positive test outcomes	Indicate a potential presence of the given disease. The results may be confirmed through a supplementary test.	Measurement of risk caused by a disease on the basis of new cases in given period	Provide definitive diagnosis
Costs	Intensive; The costs can partially or fully be covered by the health insurance	Cost-intensive. The costs are covered by the national health care system.	Cheap Can be covered by the health insurance

4. IMPLEMENTATION

Since the pilot is ongoing, the coding, testing, and other development life cycle related activities are out of the scope of this section. A future paper will discuss the implementation, the components, and the performance test results.

Le paper will present the IoT based screening and how this implemented as well as how the system is non-invasive.

This section aims at presenting the concept of the system and the resulting architectural approach.

4.1 Enhancement Recommendations

This section enumerates a set of recommendation to improve the conventional screening for diseases process. Additionally, universal guidelines for screening for disease need to be implemented to enable a unicity in screening process independently of the country of residence of the patient.

The proposed approach covers all these recommended points.

Genetic Data

The method of screening for diseases should include the genetic data and related aspects like pharmacogenomics in clinical examination since the analysis of genetic predispositions can contribute to early diseases detection or prediction.

WHO had defined in 1968 the criteria and framework for screening for diseases. These criteria are well spread and widely used till today (Wilson & Jungner, 1968). However, the framework and criteria defined by WHO do not consider the genetic diversities among a population. It is now well known, for example, that intermittent ART therapy increases the cardiovascular disease risk in certain people living with HIV (PLWH), but not all. Is it due to the individual genomic? Therefore, it is recommended to include genetic data analysis in the screening process.

Pervasive Sensing Physical Bio-Signals

Patient-centricity, as well as patient-centered care delivery, have promised to enhance medical treatment. As defined earlier, patient-centric information emanates from the patient. Thus, screening for diseases will benefit from pervasive physical/physiological data sensing, which is known well advanced. This technology is to be used to improve the conventional screening, increasing the adherence to screening among the population and finally reducing and/or bringing down to zero the number of wrongly positive or negative screened individual. Certain disease modalities could be sensed at an early stage of the disease

Pervasive Sensing Mental Modalities

Mental diseases can lead to noncommunicable diseases. Various research works have discussed the topic. Screening for diseases can, therefore, take benefits from analyzing, in-depth, brain activities as well as other physiological modalities in individuals suffering from any mental disease. Most common solution approaches for sensing mental health are using video and web conferencing in mental health delivery (Kinley, Zibrik, Cordeiro, Lauscher, & Ho, 2012), also for facial gestures recognition. However, facial gestures cannot 100% reveal the mental health of an individual. Harris Georgiou has recently evaluated the number of active CPU cores in the human brain during the human brain is performing a simple task using a functional Magnetic Resonance Imaging (fMRI) (Haddadi, P. Healey, R. McCabe, 2014). This result is a fundament on which we can build further research for an innovative method of sensing mental health. Our hypothesis is that the number of parallel active processes in the human brain may determine the mental health of an individual.

Integrating the Medical Records in a Federated National Screening Database

Data collected from the population should be stored somewhere and call for analytics and decision tasks. This database can be a cloud (public or private). Though, the main question that arises here is about the place the collected have to be stored (persistently) and call for analysis and decision making.

The global healthcare system is facing an important challenge regarding the use of digital and ICT solution in their data management process. Few public healthcare systems are using medical and Health record systems (health records include medical records) (Edoh, 2018), This issue is more severe in the developing world.

This study proposes a federated database at the national level (centralized database) for storing and processing the screening data and concerns. It is also very important that each country adopts the usage of electronic medical records systems that can include replicates of screening data from the federated database.

4.2 Concept and Resulting Architectural View

Resulting Concept

The proposed innovative Pre-screening process is an interdisciplinary system combining two major domains (i) healthcare and (ii) information and communication technology (ICT) with the objective to implement a pervasive/ubiquitous IoT-enabled sensing for vital parameters system. The system, a non-invasive system, should efficiently sense health data, perform data analysis and interpretation as well as improve existing health systems – especially in developing countries. Especially body sensor (WBAN) would be used to automatically and autonomously screen individual (patient or asymptomatic) and to help to increase patient's adherence to screening programs.

The Internet of Things technology will be used to collect needed. The collected data should be transmitted to a national federated database for screening.

1. Proposed Screening Approach vs. Conventional Screening Approach

Based on the earlier recommendations and problem analysis, a system concept is made. The concept foresees to provide enough data and information from various sources to support an exhaustive and comprehensive analysis of an accurate test outcome. The objective is to bring down the high rate of false-positive and false-negative test outcomes the conventional approach is being produced. The data includes patient-centered and patient-centric data. Table 4 compares the conventional screening approach with the proposed IoT-enabled screening approach. The table shows that the proposed approach generates more data that can positively impact the analysis and the test outcomes. In contrary, the proposed approach is more supported by modern information and communication technology. The novel approach features functionalities like autonomous data analytics and ICT supported decision-making units. The medical doctor can then be assisted by the system in decision making and analyzing.

An important point regarding the difference is that the proposed approach enables a remote screening procedure, what the conventional approach does not. The methodology proposed includes the pervasive and ubiquitous data (vital parameters) sensing, 1:1 interview, and remote interview.

a. Patient-Centric and Patient-Centered Information Enabled Care

The terms of patient-centric and patient-centered are often used interchangeably and that leads to confusion. Many articles dealing with the topic have confused patient-centric with patient-centered. Regarding the definition the authors made in Barua, Liang, Lu, and Shen (2011), the interchangeable use or confusion about the term can be noted. This can explain why only a few articles handling with the topic are available.

Sven Stegemann et al. (2016) have defined the patient-centricity as "*The recognition of the needs of an individual patient or distinct patient populations and their specific needs as the focal point in the overall design of a medicine including the targeted patients' physiological, physical, psychological, and social characteristics*." The above definition seems to englobe patient-centered means and patient-centricity. Since, according to a post (Sheer, 2012) posted on March 2012 by David Lee Scher3, patient-centered care is based on information provided by the patient and his relatives as well as the respect of his needs; while patient-centricity is concern care based on information collected on the patient using technology like Wireless Sensors Networks (WSN)/ Wireless Body Area Network (WBAN). He wrote the following:

health care that establishes a partnership among practitioners, patients, and their families (when appropriate) to ensure that decisions respect patients' wants, needs, and preferences and solicit patients' input on the education and support they need to make decisions and participate in their own care.

Patient-centric healthcare differs in that the information and interactions emanate from the patient. Wireless technologies are built around the premise that personalized data and interactions prompted by the patient and managed by both the patient and provider. (Scher, 2012)

Neha Shankar Sharma (2015) described the role of the technology in driving patient-centricity and presented some existing systems, like Patient-Like Me, that are contributing in driving patient-centricity. This paper shows that patient-centricity more includes the usage of Information and Communication Technology (ICT) in collecting information on the patient. Athanasios et al.(2011) worked out a patient-centric diabetes management application and showed the importance of the User Interface (UI) for such application, This paper also clearly pointed out the involvement of ICT in a patient-centricity.

Patient-centricity offers a solid basis for personalized or individualized care in collecting patient's physiological data as well as social characteristics that enable to personalize the medical treatment. Hong et al. (2016) have investigated the impact of using web technology for driving patient-centricity and obtained significant and conclusive results.

Brand described (2012) a patient-centric approach to positive patient outcomes. The approach foresees to base health care on more evidence, more data, and experiences.

1. Patient-Centric Information Enabled Care

Patient-Centric Information is that information that emanates from the patient himself added to the data that are mined from the (electronic) medical and/or health records, which in turn must include genomic information, which enables to detect any disease predisposition.

The modern wireless technologies are used to collect the patient vital parameters as well as to filter clinical documents to gain patient-centric data. The use of Patient-Centric Information including genomic data in the healthcare is not established.

Medical records do not include genomic information yet (Bates & Bitton, 2010) and only few healthcare professionals are using electronic medical and/or health records (Edoh, 2018).

The conventional screening for diseases paradigm mostly relies on information the patient provides; thus, it is not a solid basis for a personalized healthcare. Unlike patient-centered information, patient-centric information enabled screening for disease presents various advantages like accurate data-driven analysis to detect disease in an embryonic state and furthermore perform a precisely predict the occurrence of a disease.

2. Patient-Centered Information Enabled Care

On the Weblog" Oneviewhealthcare.com" of May 15th, 2017, PCC is defined as:

.... Patient-centered care is the practice of caring for patients (and their families) in ways that are meaningful and valuable to the individual patient. It includes listening to, informing and involving patients in their care. The IOM (Institute of Medicine) defines patient-centered care as: "Providing care that is respectful of, and responsive to, individual patient preferences, needs and values, and ensuring that patient values guide all clinical decisions. (Oneview, 2018)

Barbara Starfield, MD, MPH defined in Starfield, (2011) the term of patient-centered care as visit-based. This means that patient-centered information is information the patient provides the physician with.

Patient-Centered Care is mostly initiated by the patient and thus called as care on-demand and with respect to the patient expectations. There exists no global or universal definition of the term. Though, most existing definitions emphasize certain core elements of what Patient-Centered Care is. Respecting the patient's choice and effective communication are the core elements in most definitions (Kitson, Marshall, Bassett, & Zeitz, 2013). Alison Kitson et al. (2013) conduct a narrative review on Patient-Centered Care and point out significant themes and sub-themes. They summarize these findings in three groups of themes: (i) Patient participation and involvement, (ii) Relationship between the patient and the health professional, and (iii) The context where the care is delivered.

The first theme requires to respect patient choice and to involve him in the care delivery process and procedure. The literature review revealed three (03) sub-themes in the first theme, *(1) Patient participating as a respected and autonomous individual, (2) Care plan based on patient's individual needs, and (3) Addressing a patient's physical and emotional needs.*

The second theme is subdivided into four sub-themes and is mostly concerning the communication between the patient and treating healthcare professionals, *(1) Genuine clinician-patient relationship, (2) Open communication of knowledge, personal expertise, and clinical expertise between the patient and the professional, (3) Health professionals have appropriate skills and knowledge, (4) A cohesive and co-operative team of professionals.*

The third and last theme is concerning the system issues that can be a barrier to Patient-Centered Care.

In (Tsuyuki & Krass, 2013), Tsuyuki et al. state the vision of PCC as:

It is a professional obligation to take responsibility for and provide care targeted to the individual patient's needs.

The responsibility includes six points like respect for the patient, communication by good listening to the patient, empower the patient, informing the patient, and assisting the patient in reaching his goals. The authors in Williams (2017) point out the same/similar findings.

Resulting Architecture

The system ecosystem is consisting, therefore, of a private cloud (belongs to the public health care system because of the sensible patient's data) and a web server, a client (intended for physicians and control/data centers – Application level -), a smartphone as a gateway (patient own device), raspberry pi.

MQTT (Message Queue Telemetry Transport), CoAP (Constrained Application Protocol), are the candidate data protocols. MQTT and CoAP are data protocols, which are suitable to the constrained environment. They support asynchronous communication via IP. MQTT enables to subscribe to the raspberry pi for data so that it publishes the received data from the sensors or perception sources.

For the communication layers, Bluetooth (short range, and low energy – communication between sensors and edge-gateway -), ZigBee (low Energy, higher range than BLE), WIFI (access to the Internet) are selected to enable communication between the end-point devices (for ex. sensors), the IoT-Gateway, and the Internet.

Noninvasive sensors are the best candidates as end-point devices that would be used to collect vital parameters during a medication and infection period since people would be hindered in the daily life by the non-invasive sensors system. The collected data are pre-processed and filtered at the edge (edge computing), at the fog (fog computing), and only relevant data is sent to cloud for long-term data processing and depth data analysis.

Table 4. Difference between the conventional and the proposed Approach

Category	Data Sources/Methodologies/Technical supports	Screening Approach	
		Conventional	Proposed
Data and Information	Data from structured and semi-structured interview	Yes	Yes
	Data/Information from available medical records file	Yes	Yes
	Data/Information from health medical records file	No	Yes
	Patient-centered information (provided by the patient self)	Yes	Yes
	Patient-centric information (Vital parameter measured and collected with the IoT end-point devices like sensors.)	No	Yes
	Genetical data	No	Yes
	Pervasive Sensing Mental Modalities	No	Yes
	Pervasive Sensing Physical Bio-signals	No	Yes
	Data from a Federated National Screening Database	No	Yes
	Short-term data	Yes	Yes
	Long-term data	No	Yes
	Contextual data	No	Yes
Methodology	1:1 Interview	Yes	Yes
	Remote Interview	No	Yes
	Pervasive/ubiquitous data sensing	No	Yes
	Automatic data analytics/operational data analysis	No	Yes
Technical Support	Business Intelligence /Operational Research	No	Yes
	Wearable/Pervasive/Ubiquitous computing	No	Yes
	Federated database system/databases system	No	Yes
	Autonomous data perception system (i.e sensors)	No	Yes
	Wireless Body Area Network	No	Yes
	Internet of Things Technology	No	Yes
Costs	Devices	Cheap	Not evaluated
	Services		
	Personel		

At the cloud, the analytics application will consider the results of the genome sequencing as well the patient dossier entries.

The system features a patient dossier (EMR – electronic medical record), where all patient medical data are recorded.

1. Infrastructure

The devices needed and used for the test are summarized in Table 5.

2. Key Enabling Technologies in IoT Enabled (Pre-) Screening for Diseases System (SDS)

a. Wireless Sensors Network(WSN)/Wireless Body Area Network (WBAN)

WSNs are now commonplace in the healthcare industry. Medical sensors are attached to a patient's body to measure bio-signal parameters such as body temperature, blood pressure, pulse oximetry, ECG, and breathing activity (Abed, Alkhatib, & Baicher, 2012). Remote medical centers can perform advanced monitoring of their patients via video and audio sensors (Abed et al., 2012).

A multi-tier WSN allows distributing tasks over nodes. Some nodes are used for simple tasks which reduces energy consumption. These nodes can last long and

Table 5. Test infrastructure

Infrastructure	Description
Data Acquisition (Sensors)	Following sensors were selected to be used to collect vital parameters, which will be sent to the cloud through and by diverse gateways (edge, IoT-gateways). • Respiratory, • Heart/ECG, • Blood pressure/pulse and oxygen, • Temperature, (v) air humidity, and • 5. Accelerometer/position sensor.
Web server	Web-Apache 2.4
Application server	Glassfish 4
Cloud	Cloud (Amazon AWS)
Edge Gateway	Edge/fog computing • Raspberry Pi
IoT Gateway	• Smartphone
Data protocols And Communication/ Transport Layer	• MQTT (Message Queuing Telemetry Transport) • CoAP • NB-IoT (NarrowBand-IoT) • Bluetooth Low Energy (BLE)

are suitable for data acquisition in healthcare applications. Multi-tier architectures have been used in similar applications like SenseEye (Kulkarni, Ganesan, Shenoy, & Lu, 2005) and IrisNet (Campbell et al., 2005)and have proved to be efficient. Kulkarni et al. (2005) and Campbell et al., (2005) argue that a camera sensor network containing heterogeneous elements provides numerous benefits over conventional homogeneous sensor networks. An experimental evaluation of prototype (Campbell et al., 2005) shows that as compared to a single-tier prototype, the multi-tier SensEye can achieve an order of magnitude reduction in energy usage while providing comparable surveillance accuracy while Kulkarni et al., (2005) highlights the fact that the richness of the data generated by multimedia sensors makes them useful for a wide variety of applications.

There are two methods of sensing bio-signals according to the position of the sensor: ex-situ and in-situ. The ex-situ sensors (such as video sensors) are those that do not touch the body of the patient. The video can be used to know the general conditions and appearance of the patient. The in-situ sensors (such as ECG sensors) are in direct contact with the patient. The acquisition of the bio-signals using in-situ sensors is an ongoing research field where a significant amount of research is reported (Bandodkar et al., 2015; Liakat et al., 2014; On & In, 2010; Yang et al., 2014). Yang et al., (2014) recognizes that acquiring information from the human body and spreading over multiple spatial and temporal scales is the first critical challenge in advanced health informatics. Bandodkar et al. (2015) and Liakat et al. (2014) developed non-invasive in vivo glucose sensors. A proof-of-concept demonstration of an all-printed temporary tattoo-based glucose sensor for non-invasive glycemia monitoring is developed in Bandodkar et al., (2015). Liakat et al., (2014) leveraged use mid-infrared quantum cascade laser spectroscopy. A platform which fuses IoT devices such as wearable sensors with in-home healthcare services for improved user experience and service efficiency is proposed in On and In, (2010).

M. Mazhar Rathore et al. (Wan et al., 2013) have discussed the presence of the Internet of things in the medical sector and the amount of data these systems produce. The wireless body area network (WBAN), a subset of the wireless sensor networks (WSNs), is using in the healthcare's applications to monitor the patient bio-signal (Wan et al., 2013). In a previous article, the author presents a wireless sensors network system used at a cardiologic intensive care unit (CICU) to monitor the cardiologic in-patient and the ambient air in the hospital rooms. The patients are attached to a WSN that collect in real-time the patients' vital parameters (Edoh et al., 2016). The experiment described in Edoh et al., (2016) has demonstrated the opportunities that the WSNs systems offer potentialities in collecting and retrieving medical data. The evaluated existing monitoring and/or surveillance system used at the CICU helps healthcare professionals to manually measure and process patient's physiological data every 15, 30, 45 or 60 minutes. Since the system in use does not enable automatic and continuous data collection, storage and processing, the medical data produced between two manual data collection phases is lost.

b. Internet of Things (IoT)/Internet of Health Things (IoHT)

Internet of Health Things (IoHT) integrates health objects with network connectivity from the digital and physical world. Furthermore. it combines personal health technologies and IoT and takes full advantages of IoT in expanding abilities to exchange useful data, improvements in context awareness. It also has the ability to initiate actions based on data that are collected and analyzed(Terry, 2016)

Istepanian et al. (2011) shown the benefits of using the Internet of m-health Things (m-IoT) for non-invasive glucose level sensing. m-IoT puts together the functionalities of m-Health and IoT. mHealth (mobile Health) is healthcare delivery supported by (smart) devices (i.e. smartphones, etc.). In Williams and McCauley, (2016), authors defined the Healthcare Internet of Things (IoHT – Internet of Health Things) as

...the new embedded sensing capabilities of devices together with the availability of always being connected, to improve patient care whilst reducing costs.

The Internet of Things (IoT) especially the Internet of Health Things (IoHT) affords significant enhancement in the medical care especially in disease prediction, prevention, and detection.

Information technology such IoT can help today to collect accurate data about an individual's health. In Riazul Islam, Daehan Kwak, Humaun Kabir, Hossain, & Kyung-Sup Kwak, (2015), the authors present a comprehensive survey on the usage of IoT in the medical field. The authors presented various healthcare sectors that take benefit of using IoT, for example handling efficiently the medical emergency, accurate data collection. The authors further present a medical record system that enables remote medical advice.

The IoT is facing various challenges such interoperability, security (authenticity, etc.) because of the diversity of objects that can be involved in an IoT system as well as the size of the network that can become security challenges. In Riazul Islam et al., (2015), a solution to overcome the interoperability challenges in IoT systems was approached. Interoperability can represent a barrier and especially an important issue in the emergency care. An IoT-enabled remote monitoring and management platform of healthcare information, similar to that presented and discussed in Edoh et al., (2016), is presented in Zhao, Wang, and Nakahira, (2012). This system describes the promise for enhancement by using in the healthcare the wireless sensors networks (WSNs), an IoT subset. Various advantages of using IoT in the healthcare have been described in Hu, Xie, and Shen, (2013). The authors present an interesting aspect „The Anti-counterfeit of Medical Equipment and Medication". Consuming counterfeit drugs can lead to certain non-communicable diseases; therefore, it is right if the modern technology can help to prevent counterfeit drug consumption.

The IoT ecosystem includes three layers: (i) data acquisition, (ii) network, and (iii) application layer. Figure 1 describes the different layers in an IoT ecosystem. The perception layer, composed of things, in context of IoT, and IoT-Gateways that are in charge to pre-process, filterless or not useful data, is the central point of the IoT. The IoT-Gateways perform the so-called edge/fog computing.

Edge computing pushes the data processing and filtering intelligence and capabilities to the edge gateway or appliance directly in devices like programmable automation controllers, while the fog computing pushes down the processing intelligence and capabilities to the IoT-Gateways or fog nodes.

The network layer consists of the cloud, data storage (persistent), and data analytics. This layer binds the IoT ecosystem to the Internet.

The third and last layer is the application and process layer. At this layer, the system user can interact with the system.

Figure 1. The seven and three layers of the system architecture
Source: (Edoh, 2018)

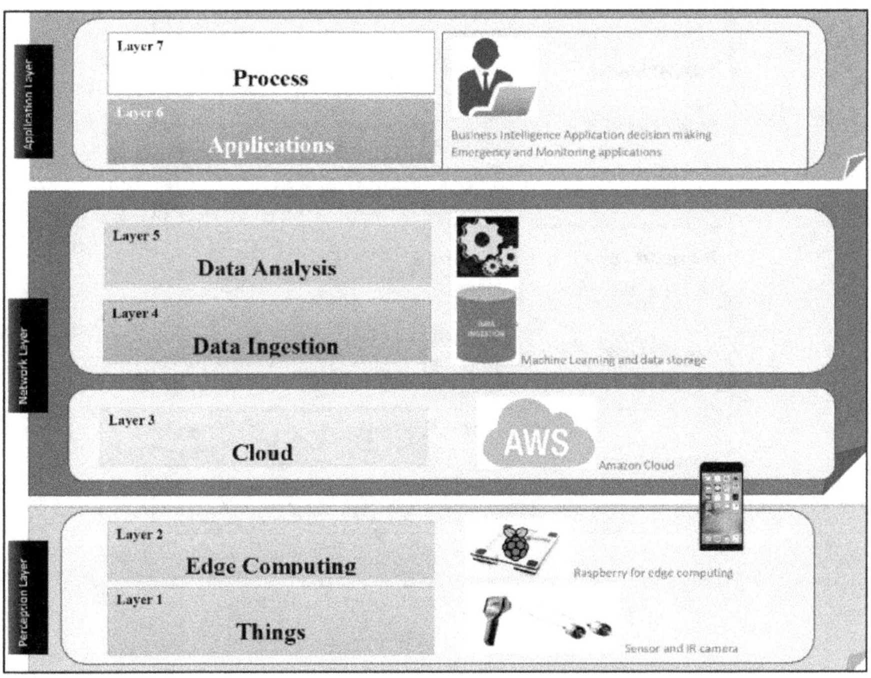

1. **Data Acquisition Layer:** Many non-invasive sensors are available at the market, which could be used such sensors and miniaturized devices so that the individual is not restricted in his daily activities. People carry pervasively on their smartphone. The smartphone can play the role of the gateway and will be connected to the cloud to forward all relevant data. We recommend using IoT infrastructure such as raspberry pi, which will be assigned to pre-processing tasks at the edge.
2. **Network Layer:** Figure 2 presents the different IoT stack at the network layer. Different protocols used at different layers are indicated here. A deep description of each protocol and how they are used, their restriction is out of the scope of this study.
3. **Application Layer:** The applications are located at this layer. The federated database (FD) is placed in the cloud whereas the FD-client application is at the application layer. Further implemented applications and services are located here. The WBAN system and associated applications are also located at this layer

Figure 2. IoT Standards
Source: https://www.linkedin.com/pulse/emerging-open-standard-protocol-stack-iot-aniruddha-chakrabarti/

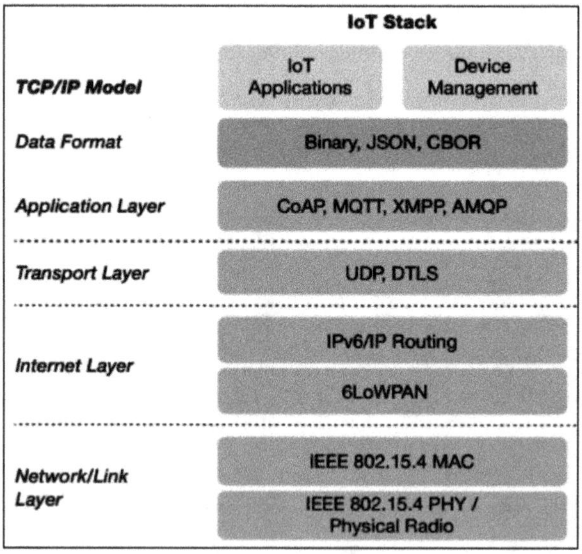

3. Electronic Medical Records (EMR)

Medical records are collected as well as sensing data on The use of Electronic Health Records (EHR) in the medical care delivery impacts positively the treatment outcomes (Kershaw et al., 2018; Bates & Bitton, 2010; Epstein, Fiscella, Lesser, & Stange, 2010). In Viswanathan, Baozhi, and Pompili, (2012) the authors have shown that context-aware data and patient-centric decision making are vital for personalized healthcare delivery. They discuss the challenges facing these new paradigms in wirelessly collecting physiological data, and consequently proposed patient-centric care delivery for ubiquitous healthcare. The study found out that the proposed patient-centric "will significantly improve the response time, quality, and relevance of data- and compute-intensive medical applications."

The comprehensive literature review has shown that only few research works have been done regarding the topic. However, the terms are often mixed up or confused. Earlier articles written on the topic have confused patient-centric with patient-centered. In Barua et al., (2011) one can note this regarding the definition the authors made. This can be the reason why only a few articles handle the topic.

4. Electronic Health Records (EHR)

The clinical documentation (CD) is a digital or analog record tracking all medical treatment and related activities. The health records are a superset information system containing patient medical records. The health records are federated databases (FDB), that means they include diverse record concerning a patient and are stored in a different part of a health care system.

An FDB is

a federated database system is a collection of independent, autonomous database systems, each with their own set of global users, which cooperate together to form an alliance or federation that enables global users to access data across the participating systems in a transparent manner. (Grimson et al., 1998)

The availability of medical and health records is ensured by the hospital information system (HIS). This information must stet be available, but also reliable, and the data privacy must be assured. Data accuracy and authenticity are beyond the data availability very important for accurate data-driven screening for diseases. Since the conventional screening for diseases is mostly based on short-term information that obviously is inefficient for conducting reliable screening, long-term data would afford enhancement in the screening performing any further medical activities. The medical records must be up-to-date and well written (in the case the practitioner likes to write a medical assessment into the record).

4.3 System Implementation

A rapid prototype of the system, like the system described in (T. O. C. Edoh et al., 2016), according to the concept was implemented to pervasively collect bio-signal. As an IDE eclipse running with Java 1.8 (Java ME 8) was used to implement a Java IoT using Bluetooth (BLE) as a communication protocol between the raspberry pi and the smartphone which sends the data to the cloud. The raspberry pi is connected to the different sensors and publishes the data collected by the sensors to the smartphone.

5. EXPERIMENTS AND RESULTS

5.1 Experiment

At this phase (phase I) of the ongoing study (pilot), 44 participants (30 patients and 14 medical doctors - see Table 1 -) were involved. Each participant is examined by 4 different medical doctors in the following scenarios: Two (02) medical doctors use the conventional methodology and the other two (02) medical doctors use the proposed approach to examine the patient. The results are compared with each other; conventional against conventional, proposed approach against the proposed approach, and finally, a cross-over comparison is performed. The comparison scenarios are in Table 5.

Table 6. Comparison Scenario

	RC1	RP1	RC12
RC2	1	0	0
RP2	0	1	0
RP12	0	0	1

Legend

1 means compared with each other

0 means no comparison

RC1 and RC2 are the results of the test using the conventional methodology. RCx is thrown if it presents biases.

RC12 is the outcome of comparing RC1 with RC2. RC12 is thrown if the difference between RC1 and RC2 is too significant.

RP1 and RP2 are the results of the test using the proposed approach. RPx is thrown if it presents biases.

RP12 is the outcome of comparing RP1 with RC2. RP12 is thrown if the difference between RP1 and RP2 is too significant.

5.2 Results and Discussion

- **Conventional Screening Methods:** The screening has followed the national paradigm. The participants were invited to pass a screening test. Only 13.05% (6 participants) of the cohort population went to the hospital and got screened. 1 participant got false positive screened. Precise medical exams have revealed that the test's results were false. The other 40 people (86,95%) could not visit the doctor because they were ill, suffering from malaria. The test was delayed.

They have then visited the medical doctors after recovering from malaria. The screening tests revealed no non-infectious diseases. Of course, the doctor was not aware of the collected data and the patients were not informed about any recorded data.

- **Pre-Screening Methods:** The data collection lasted six (06) weeks. The data analysis using Microsoft excel reveals that 86,95% of the participants have suffered from malaria during the test phase. The collected data have revealed that all participants who had suffered from malaria also suffered from acute hypoglycemia during the test. This medical condition was accompanied by temporary shortness of breath and high blood pressure.

Healthcare professionals state that an individual who is regularly facing such kind of disease can in the long develop such kind of NDCs.

- **Results:** The test shows promise for earlier detection and prevention of diseases using the proposed pre-screening paradigm. The system provides more information to the doctor so that he can better evaluate the health of an individual during a screening process.

On the basis of 30 screened people, 3.33% (N = 1) were false screened using the proposed approach against 16.6% (N = 5) using the conventional methodology.

6. CONCLUSION

This study reveals that the limitations of the conventional screening can be overcome using the proposed approach. It further shows that a data-driven (long-term) screening can pull down the rate of false-negative and false-positive screening test's results.

The Internet of things has shown promise to enhance the conventional screening methodology. Though due to the short-term experiment, the convergence between infectious and non-infectious was not statistically investigated, therefore, future works are needed to be conducted.

Data analytics, including machine learning and predictive analytics and modeling, in a form of predictive search (automated deduction or augmented reality. IoT technology and paradigms can be used or extended with the intelligence and capabilities of a data analytics processor for early detecting, surveillance, and monitoring of non-communicable diseases risks factors in individuals/patients with tropical infectious diseases.

Linking of wearable devices with big data analytics to provide feedback and a suggestion system for behavioral change is today well widespread (Wilson, 2013). The wearable devices have the capabilities to collect or sense data that can be published to an edge-gateway. The present study has used wearable IoT systems in determining causes of behavioral changes, to determine impacts of the behavioral changes in diseases treatment and vice-versa and factors of non-communicable diseases risks.

Data Analytics, including machine learning and predictive analytics and modeling, leads to understand and mitigate the behavioral, genetic and environmental causes of disease and treatment's failure. Machine learning methods are being used for large datasets to set up different patient groups, healthy, asymptomatic or sick, as well as to perform early symptoms analyses for early detection of acute NCDs and infection. The data sets could consist of genetic material and information and/or biophysical and mental conditions information collected from the patient.

7. FUTURE WORKS

As noted in section 2.4 Study Limitation, the present (ongoing) study has limitations. First, the test period is too short, Second the cohort at this phase I is relative ok but cannot produce statistically significant results regarding the convergence between noncommunicable and infectious diseases. Before a final claim can be made the pilot must go through 3 phases (phases I, phase II, and phase III). At the end of phase III, a comprehensive and exhaustive data analysis will be performed, and the final result will be presented. Therefore, the forthcoming work would consist to investigate in phase II (involving a large cohort) and in phase III (involving large-scale cohort) following:

1. Impacts of infectious diseases on NCDs outbreak
2. Impact of pharmacogenomics on NCDs outbreak

3. Efficiently and cost-effectively, pervasively sense the evidence of NCDs outbreak in an individual without genetic predisposition
4. Pervasively measure if ID affects the acceleration of NCDs outbreak
5. Monitor the adverse drug reactions that could provoke the NCDs outbreak.

In afterward, a novel policy for screening for disease will be implemented. Additionally, and based on the final result in form of requirements, a wearable solution combined with the Internet of Things technology will be designed, implemented, and deployed with respect to the resulting policy.

REFERENCES

Abed, A., Alkhatib, A., & Baicher, G. S. (2012). Wireless Sensor Network Architecture. *International Conference on Computer Networks and Communication Systems, 35*, 11–15.

Acharya, A. S., Prakash, A., Saxena, P., & Nigam, A. (2013). *Sampling: Why and How of it?* Academic Press.

Athanasios, T., Eleazar, G.-H., Ali, Y., & Benjamin, D. (2011). Designing patient-centric applications for chronic disease management. *Proceedings of the Annual International Conference of the IEEE Engineering in Medicine and Biology Society, EMBS*, 3146–3149. 10.1109/IEMBS.2011.6090858

Baig, M. M., GholamHosseini, H., & Linden, M. (2015). Tablet-based patient monitoring and decision support systems in hospital care. *Conference Proceedings: ... Annual International Conference of the IEEE Engineering in Medicine and Biology Society. IEEE Engineering in Medicine and Biology Society. Annual Conference, 2015*, 1215–8. 10.1109/EMBC.2015.7318585

Bandodkar, A. J., Jia, W., Yardımcı, C., Wang, X., Ramirez, J., & Wang, J. (2015). Tattoo-based noninvasive glucose monitoring: A proof-of-concept study. *Analytical Chemistry, 87*(1), 394–398. doi:10.1021/ac504300n PMID:25496376

Barer, M. (2017). *Why are Some People Healthy and Others Not?* (M. Barer, Ed.). New York: Routledge.

Barua, M., Liang, X., Lu, R., & Shen, X. (2011). ESPAC: Enabling Security and Patient-centric Access Control for eHealth in cloud computing. *International Journal of Security and Networks, 6*(2/3), 67. doi:10.1504/IJSN.2011.043666

Bates, D. W., & Bitton, A. (2010). The future of health information technology in the patient-centered medical home. *Health Affairs*, *29*(4), 614–621. doi:10.1377/hlthaff.2010.0007 PMID:20368590

Bergman, B., Neuhauser, D., & Provost, L. (2011). Five main processes in healthcare: a citizen perspective. *BMJ Quality & Safety*, *20*(Suppl_1), i41-2. doi:10.1136/bmjqs.2010.046409

Bluestone, J. A., Herold, K., & Eisenbarth, G. (2010). Genetics, pathogenesis and clinical interventions in type 1 diabetes. *Nature*, *464*(7293), 1293–1300. doi:10.1038/nature08933 PMID:20432533

Boulton, A. J. M., & Vinik, A. J. (2005). AI and Brief Clinical. *Diabetes Care*, *28*(4), 956–962.

Brand, C. S. (2012). Management of retinal vascular diseases: A patient-centric approach. *Eye (Basingstoke)*, *26*(S2), S1–S16. doi:10.1038/eye.2012.32 PMID:22495396

Brownstein, J. S., Freifeld, C. C., Reis, B. Y., & Mandl, K. D. (2008). Surveillance sans frontières: Internet-based emerging infectious disease intelligence and the HealthMap project. *PLoS Medicine*, *5*(7), 1019–1024. doi:10.1371/journal.pmed.0050151 PMID:18613747

Businessdictionary. (2018). Retrieved from http://www.businessdictionary.com/definition/diagnosis.html

Campbell, J., Gibbons, P., Nath, S., Pillai, P., Seshan, S., & Sukthankar, R. (2005). IrisNet: an internet-scale architecture for multimedia sensors. In *Proceedings of the 13th annual ACM international conference on Multimedia* (pp. 81–88). ACM Digital Library. 10.1145/1101149.1101162

Chandra, S., & Chandra, H. (2011). *Myocardial Infarction Associated with Plasmodium Falciparum Malarial Infection*. Academic Press.

Chapman, S. J., & Hill, A. V. S. (2012). Human genetic susceptibility to infectious disease. *Nature Reviews. Genetics*, *13*(3), 175–188. doi:10.1038/nrg3114 PMID:22310894

Christaki, E. (2015). New technologies in predicting, preventing and controlling emerging infectious diseases. *Virulence*, *6*(6), 558–565. doi:10.1080/21505594.2015.1040975 PMID:26068569

Di, L., & Li, Y. (2018). The risk factor of false-negative and false-positive for T-SPOT.TB in active tuberculosis. *Journal of Clinical Laboratory Analysis*, *32*(2), e22273. doi:10.1002/jcla.22273 PMID:28594104

Edoh, T. (2018). Risk Prevention of Spreading Emerging Infectious Diseases Using a HybridCrowdsensing Paradigm, Optical Sensors, and Smartphone. *Journal of Medical Systems*, *42*(5), 91. doi:10.100710916-018-0937-2 PMID:29633021

Edoh, T. O., Pawar, P. A., Brügge, B., & Teege, G. (2016). A Multidisciplinary Remote Healthcare Delivery System to Increase Health Care Access, Pathology Screening, and Treatment in Developing Countries. *International Journal of Healthcare Information Systems and Informatics*, *11*(4), 1–31. doi:10.4018/IJHISI.2016100101

Edoh, T. O. C. (2018). *Advanced Systems For Improved Public Healthcare And Disease Prevention Emerging Research And Opportunities* (A. Moumtzoglou, Ed.). IGI Global, Medical Information Science Reference (an imprint of IGI Global). doi:10.4018/978-1-5225-5528-5

Edoh, T. O. C., Atchome, A., Alahassa, B. R. U., & Pawar, P. (2016). Evaluation of a Multi-Tier Heterogeneous Sensor Network for Patient Monitoring – The Case of Benin. In *MMHealth '16 Proceedings of the 2016 ACM Workshop on Multimedia for Personal Health and Health Care* (pp. 23–29). Amsterdam, The Netherlands: ACM Digital Library. 10.1145/2985766.2985772

Epstein, R. M., Fiscella, K., Lesser, C. S., & Stange, K. C. (2010). Analysis & commentary: Why the nation needs a policy push on patient-centered health care. *Health Affairs*, *29*(8), 1489–1495. doi:10.1377/hlthaff.2009.0888 PMID:20679652

Etzioni, R., Cooperberg, M. R., Penson, D. M., Weiss, N. S., & Thompson, I. M. (2013). *Limitations of basing screening policies on screening trials: The US Preventive Services Task Force and prostate cancer*. Academic Press. doi:10.1109/TMI.2012.2196707.Separate

Grimson, J., Grimson, W., Berry, D., Stephens, G., Felton, E., Kalra, D., … Weier, O. W. (1998). A CORBA-based integration of distributed electronic healthcare records using the synapses approach. *IEEE Transactions on Information Technology in Biomedicine, 2*(3), 124–138. doi:10.1109/4233.735777

Haddadi, Healey, & McCabe. (2014). *Healthcare informatics for mental health: recent advances and the outlook for the future*. Ment. Health Found.

Heil, J., ter Waarbeek, H. L. G., Hoebe, C. J. P. A., Jacobs, P. H. A., van Dam, D. W., Trienekens, T. A. M., ... Dukers-Muijrers, N. H. T. M. (2017). Pertussis surveillance and control: Exploring variations and delays in testing, laboratory diagnostics and public health service notifications, the Netherlands, 2010 to 2013. *Eurosurveillance*, *22*(28), 1–8. doi:10.2807/1560-7917.ES.2017.22.28.30571 PMID:28749331

Hidron, A., Vogenthaler, N., Santos-Preciado, J. I., Rodriguez-Morales, A. J., Franco-Paredes, C., & Rassi, A. (2010). Cardiac involvement with parasitic infections. *Clinical Microbiology Reviews*, *23*(2), 324–349. doi:10.1128/CMR.00054-09 PMID:20375355

Hong, S. H., Lee, W., & AlRuthia, Y. (2016). Health care applicability of a patient-centric web portal for patients' medication experience. *Journal of Medical Internet Research*, *18*(7), 1–22. doi:10.2196/jmir.5813 PMID:27450362

Hu, F., Xie, D., & Shen, S. (2013). On the application of the internet of things in the field of medical and health care. *Xplore IEEE - 2013 IEEE International Conference on Green Computing and Communications and IEEE Internet of Things and IEEE Cyber, Physical and Social Computing, GreenCom-IThings-CPSCom 2013*, 2053–2058. 10.1109/GreenCom-iThings-CPSCom.2013.384

Hunter, D. J. (2005). Gene-environment interactions in human diseases. *Nature Reviews. Genetics*, *6*(4), 287–298. doi:10.1038/nrg1578 PMID:15803198

Istepanian, R. S. H., Hu, S., Philip, N. Y., & Sungoor, A. (2011). The potential of Internet of m-health Things “m-IoT” for non-invasive glucose level sensing. In *2011 Annual International Conference of the IEEE Engineering in Medicine and Biology Society* (pp. 5264–5266). IEEE. 10.1109/IEMBS.2011.6091302

Kariuki, J. K., Stuart-Shor, E. M., Leveille, S. G., & Hayman, L. L. (2015). Methodological Challenges in Estimating Trends and Burden of Cardiovascular Disease in Sub-Saharan Africa. *Cardiology Research and Practice*, *2015*, 1–6. doi:10.1155/2015/921021 PMID:26697260

Kasaie, P., Sohn, H., Kendall, E., Gomez, G. B., Vassall, A., Pai, M., & Dowdy, D. W. (2017). Exploring the epidemiological impact of universal access to rapid tuberculosis diagnosis using agent-based simulation. In 2017 Winter Simulation Conference (WSC) (pp. 1097–1108). IEEE. doi:10.1109/WSC.2017.8247858

Kershaw, C., Taylor, J. L., Horowitz, G., Brockmeyer, D., Libman, H., Kriegel, G., & Ngo, L. (2018). Use of an electronic medical record reminder improves HIV screening. *BMC Health Services Research*, *18*(1), 1–8. doi:10.118612913-017-2824-9 PMID:29316919

Kinley, A., Zibrik, L., Cordeiro, J., Lauscher, H. N., & Ho, K. (2012). *TeleHealth for Mental Health and Substance Use*. Academic Press.

Kinoshita, T., Tokumasu, H., Tanaka, S., Kramer, A., & Kawakami, K. (2017). Policy implementation for methicillin-resistant *Staphylococcus aureus* in seven European countries: A comparative analysis from 1999 to 2015. *Journal of Market Access & Health Policy*, *5*(1), 1351293. doi:10.1080/20016689.2017.1351293 PMID:28804601

Kitson, A., Marshall, A., Bassett, K., & Zeitz, K. (2013). What are the core elements of patient-centred care? A narrative review and synthesis of the literature from health policy, medicine and nursing. *Journal of Advanced Nursing*, *69*(1), 4–15. doi:10.1111/j.1365-2648.2012.06064.x PMID:22709336

Kulkarni, P., Ganesan, D., Shenoy, P., & Lu, Q. (2005). SensEye : A Multi-tier Camera Sensor Network. In *MULTIMEDIA '05 Proceedings of the 13th annual ACM international conference on Multimedia, Hilton, Singapore* (pp. 229–238). Hilton, Singapore: ACM Digital Library. 10.1145/1101149.1101191

Kyriacos, U., Jelsma, J., & Jordan, S. (2011). Monitoring vital signs using early warning scoring systems: A review of the literature. *Journal of Nursing Management*, *19*(3), 311–330. doi:10.1111/j.1365-2834.2011.01246.x PMID:21507102

Latham, B. (2007). Sampling: What is it? *Quantitative Research Methods*, 1-13. Retrieved from http://webpages.acs.ttu.edu/rlatham/Coursework/5377(Quant))/Sampling_Methodology_Paper.pdf

Le Reste, J. Y., Nabbe, P., Rivet, C., Lygidakis, C., Doerr, C., Czachowski, S., ... Van Royen, P. (2015). The European general practice research network presents the translations of its comprehensive definition of multimorbidity in family medicine in ten European languages. *PLoS One*, *10*(1), 1–13. doi:10.1371/journal.pone.0115796 PMID:25607642

Lee, S., Huang, H., & Zelen, M. (2004). Early detection of disease and scheduling of screening examinations. *Statistical Methods in Medical Research*, *13*(6), 443–456. doi:10.1191/0962280204sm377ra PMID:15587433

Liakat, S., Bors, K. A., Xu, L., Woods, C. M., Doyle, J., & Gmachl, C. F. (2014). Noninvasive in vivo glucose sensing on human subjects using mid-infrared light. *Biomedical Optics Express*, *5*(7), 2397. doi:10.1364/BOE.5.002397 PMID:25071973

Maguire, R., Ream, E., Richardson, A., Connaghan, J., Johnston, B., Kotronoulas, G., ... Kearney, N. (2015). Development of a novel remote patient monitoring system: The advanced symptom management system for radiotherapy to improve the symptom experience of patients with lung cancer receiving radiotherapy. *Cancer Nursing*, *38*(2), E37–E47. doi:10.1097/NCC.0000000000000150 PMID:24836956

Maxim, L. D., Niebo, R., & Utell, M. J. (2014). Screening tests: A review with examples. *Inhalation Toxicology*, *26*(13), 811–828. doi:10.3109/08958378.2014.955932 PMID:25264934

Murad, R., Oliver, M., & Kelly, M. (2017). *Differences between screening and diagnostic tests and case finding*. Retrieved March 18, 2018, from https://www.healthknowledge.org.uk/public-health-textbook/disease-causation-diagnostic/2c-diagnosis-screening/screening-diagnostic-case-finding

Nelson, H. D., O'Meara, E. S., Kerlikowske, K., Balch, S., & Miglioretti, D. (2016). Factors associated with rates of false-positive and false-negative results from digital mammography screening: An analysis of registry data. *Annals of Internal Medicine*, *164*(4), 226–235. doi:10.7326/M15-0971 PMID:26756902

Nieman, A.-E., de Mast, Q., Roestenberg, M., Wiersma, J., Pop, G., Stalenhoef, A., ... van der Ven, A. (2015, November). … van der Ven, A. (2009). Cardiac complication after experimental human malaria infection: A case report. *Malaria Journal*, *8*(1), 277. doi:10.1186/1475-2875-8-277 PMID:19958549

On, R., & In, E. (2010). Editorial Note on the Processing. *Storage*, *14*(4), 895–896. PMID:20687242

Oneview. (2018). *The Eight Principles of Patient-Centered Care*. Retrieved from https://www.oneviewhealthcare.com/the-eight-principles-of-patient-centered-care/

Ong, M. K. (2016). Effectiveness of Remote Patient Monitoring After Discharge of AMA Intern Med Hospitalized Patients With Heart Failure: The Better Effectiveness After Transition–Heart Failure (BEAT-HF) Randomized Clinical Trial. *Jama Interm Med.*, *314*(19), 2034–2044. doi:10.1001/jama.2015.7712

Paolotti, D., Carnahan, A., Colizza, V., Eames, K., Edmunds, J., Gomes, G., ... Vespignani, A. (2014). Web-based participatory surveillance of infectious diseases: The Influenzanet participatory surveillance experience. *Clinical Microbiology and Infection*, *20*(1), 17–21. doi:10.1111/1469-0691.12477 PMID:24350723

Pusiol, T., Lavezzi, A. M., Radice, F., Alfonsi, G., & Matturri, L. (2014). Unsuspected imported malaria in a case of sudden infant death. *World Journal of Clinical Infectious Diseases*, *4*(2), 5–8. doi:10.5495/wjcid.v4.i2.5

Read, J. R., Sharpe, L., Modini, M., & Dear, B. F. (2017). Multimorbidity and depression: A systematic review and meta-analysis. *Journal of Affective Disorders*, *221*, 36–46. doi:10.1016/j.jad.2017.06.009 PMID:28628766

Remais, J. V., Zeng, G., Li, G., Tian, L., & Engelgau, M. M. (2013). Convergence of non-communicable and infectious diseases in low- and middle-income countries. *International Journal of Epidemiology*, *42*(1), 221–227. doi:10.1093/ije/dys135 PMID:23064501

Renshaw, A. A., & Gould, E. W. (2013). Reducing false-negative and false-positive diagnoses in anatomic pathology consultation material. *Archives of Pathology & Laboratory Medicine*, *137*(12), 1770–1773. doi:10.5858/arpa.2013-0012-OA PMID:24283857

Riazul Islam, S. M., Daehan Kwak, Humaun Kabir, M., Hossain, M., & Kyung-Sup Kwak. (2015). The Internet of Things for Health Care: A Comprehensive Survey. *IEEE Access: Practical Innovations, Open Solutions*, *3*, 678–708. doi:10.1109/ACCESS.2015.2437951

Saquib, N., Saquib, J., & Ioannidis, J. P. A. (2015). Does screening for disease save lives in asymptomatic adults? Systematic review of meta-analyses and randomized trials. *International Journal of Epidemiology*, *44*(1), 264–277. doi:10.1093/ije/dyu140 PMID:25596211

Scher, D. L. (2012). *How Patient-Centric Care Differs from Patient-Centered Care*. Retrieved from https://davidleescher.wordpress.com/2012/03/03/how-patient-centric-care-differs-from-patient-centered-care-2/

Schmalfuss, F., & Kolominsky-Rabas, P. L. (2013). Personalized medicine in screening for malignant disease: A review of methods and applications. *Biomarker Insights*, *8*, 9–14. doi:10.4137/BMI.S11153 PMID:23471146

Schwartz, A. G., Bailey-Wilson, J. E., & Amos, C. I. (2018). 6 – Genetic Susceptibility to Lung Cancer. *IASLC Thoracic Oncology*, 46–51. doi:10.1016/B978-0-323-52357-8.00006-8

Sharma, N. (2015). Patient centric approach for clinical trials: Current trend and new opportunities. *Perspectives in Clinical Research*, *6*(3), 134. doi:10.4103/2229-3485.159936 PMID:26229748

Sheer, D. L. (2012). *How Patient-Centric Care Differs from Patient-Centered Care*. Retrieved from https://davidleescher.wordpress.com/2012/03/03/how-patient-centric-care-differs-from-patient-centered-care-2/

Starfield, B. (2011). Is patient-centered care the same as person-focused care? *The Permanente Journal, 15*(2), 63–69. doi:10.7812/TPP/10-148 PMID:21841928

Stegemann, S., Ternik, R. L., Onder, G., Khan, M. A., & van Riet-Nales, D. A. (2016). Defining Patient Centric Pharmaceutical Drug Product Design. *The AAPS Journal, 18*(5), 1047–1055. doi:10.120812248-016-9938-6 PMID:27317470

Strong, K., Wald, N., Miller, A., & Alwan, A. (2005a). Current concepts in screening for noncommunicable disease: World Health Organization Consultation Group Report on methodology of noncommunicable disease screening. *Journal of Medical Screening, 12*(1), 12–19. doi:10.1258/0969141053279086 PMID:15825234

Strong, K., Wald, N., Miller, A., & Alwan, A. (2005b). Current concepts in screening for noncommunicable disease : World Health Organ .... *The Library, 12*(1), 12–19.

Terry, N. (2016). Will the Internet of Health Things Disrupt Healthcare? *Vanderbilt Journal of Entertainment & Technology Law, 19*(2), 28–31. doi:10.2139srn.2760447

Tsuyuki, R. T., & Krass, I. (2013). What is patient-centred care? [que sont les soins axes sur le patient?]. *Canadian Pharmacists Journal, 146*(4), 177–180. doi:10.1177/1715163513494591

Viswanathan, H., Baozhi, C., & Pompili, D. (2012). Research challenges in computation, communication, and context awareness for ubiquitous healthcare. *Communications Magazine, IEEE, 50*(5), 92–99. doi:10.1109/MCOM.2012.6194388

Wald, N. J., & Morris, J. K. (1996). Editorials What is case-finding? *Journal of Medical Screening, 3*(1), 1996. doi:10.1177/096914139600300101 PMID:8861041

Wan, J., Zou, C., Ullah, S., Lai, C.-F., Zhou, M., & Wang, X. (2013). Cloud-enabled wireless body area networks for pervasive healthcare. *IEEE Network, 27*(5), 56–61. doi:10.1109/MNET.2013.6616116

Weblogs-WordPress. (2016). *Is screening different to case finding in high risk groups*. Retrieved March 18, 2018, from https://gregfellpublichealth.wordpress.com/2016/02/20/is-screening-different-to-case-finding-in-high-risk-groups/

WHO. (2016). Multimorbidity. In *Technical Series on Safer Primary Care* (pp. 1–28). World Health Organization. Retrieved from http://apps.who.int/iris/bitstream/handle/10665/252275/9789241511650-eng.pdf;jsessionid=563FC8FC1EB37789B5F44978759EF4C4?sequence=1

Williams, P. A. H., & McCauley, V. (2016). Always connected: The security challenges of the healthcare Internet of Things. In *2016 IEEE 3rd World Forum on Internet of Things (WF-IoT)* (pp. 30–35). IEEE. 10.1109/WF-IoT.2016.7845455

Williams, S. J. (2017). *Improving Healthcare Operations*. Cham: Springer International Publishing; doi:10.1007/978-3-319-46913-3

Wilson, H. J. (2013). Wearables in the Workplace. *Harvard Business Review*, 1–6.

Wilson, J. M., & Jungner, Y. G. (1968). Principles and practice of screening for disease. *Boletin de La Oficina Sanitaria Panamericana. Pan American Sanitary Bureau*, *65*(4), 281–393. doi:10.1001/archinte.1969.00300130131020

Yang, C., Zhang, S., Yao, L., & Fan, L. (2018). *Evaluation of risk factors for false-negative results with an antigen-specific peripheral blood-based quantitative cell assay (T-SPOT. TB) in the diagnosis of active tuberculosi : A large-scale retrospective study in China*. Academic Press. doi:10.1177/0300060518757381

Yang, G., Xie, L., Mäntysalo, M., Zhou, X., Pang, Z., Xu, L., & Da. (2014). A Health-IoT platform based on the integration of intelligent packaging, unobtrusive bio-sensor, and intelligent medicine box. *IEEE Transactions on Industrial Informatics*, *10*(4), 2180–2191. doi:10.1109/TII.2014.2307795

Yu, C., Yang, J., Pang, C., Dai, M., Wang, Z.-S., & Wang, Y.-W., … Lu, Y. (2017). Behavior analysis of epidemiological patients for medical site treatment from a spatial perspective. In *2017 International Conference on Machine Learning and Cybernetics (ICMLC)* (pp. 311–316). IEEE. 10.1109/ICMLC.2017.8107782

Zhao, W., Wang, C., & Nakahira, Y. (2012). Medical application on internet of things. *IET Conference Publications IET International Conference on Communication Technology and Application, ICCTA 2011 Elsevier, 2011*(586 CP), 660–665. Retrieved from http://www.scopus.com/inward/record.url?eid=2-s2.0-84864915621&partnerID=tZOtx3y1

Zink, M. D., Marx, N., Crijns, H. J. G. M., & Schotten, U. (2018, December). Opportunities and challenges of large-scale screening for atrial fibrillation. *Herzschrittmachertherapie + Elektrophysiologie*, 57–61. doi:10.100700399-017-0550-y

ADDITIONAL READING

Aring, A. M., Jones, D. E., & Falko, J. M. (2005). Evaluation and prevention of diabetic neuropathy. *American Family Physician*, *71*(11), 2123–2130. PMID:15952441

Bandodkar, A. J., Jia, W., Yardımcı, C., Wang, X., Ramirez, J., & Wang, J. (2015). Tattoo-based noninvasive glucose monitoring: A proof-of-concept study. *Analytical Chemistry*, *87*(1), 394–398. doi:10.1021/ac504300n PMID:25496376

Barua, M., Liang, X., Lu, R., & Shen, X. (2011). ESPAC: Enabling Security and Patient-centric Access Control for eHealth in cloud computing. *Int. J. Secure. Networks*, *6*(2/3), 67. doi:10.1504/IJSN.2011.043666

Bates, D. W., & Bitton, A. (2010). The future of health information technology in the patient-centered medical home. *Health Affairs (Project Hope)*, *29*(4), 614–621. doi:10.1377/hlthaff.2010.0007 PMID:20368590

Bind, S., Tiwari, A. K., & Sahani, A. K. (2015). A Survey of Machine Learning Based Approaches for Parkinson Disease Prediction. *Int. J. Comput. Sci. Inf. Technol.*, *6*(2), 1648–1655.

Capriotti, E., & Altman, R. B. (2011, October). A new disease-specific machine learning approach for the prediction of cancer-causing missense variants. *Genomics*, *98*(4), 310–317. doi:10.1016/j.ygeno.2011.06.010 PMID:21763417

Epstein, R. M., Fiscella, K., Lesser, C. S., & Stange, K. C. (2010). Analysis & commentary: Why the nation needs a policy push on patient-centered health care. *Health Affairs (Project Hope)*, *29*(8), 1489–1495. doi:10.1377/hlthaff.2009.0888 PMID:20679652

Gilbert, B. J., Patel, V., Farmer, P. E., & Lu, C. (2015, June). Assessing Development Assistance for Mental Health in Developing Countries: 2007–2013. *PLoS Medicine*, *12*(6), e1001834. doi:10.1371/journal.pmed.1001834 PMID:26035429

Growth, P., Growth, E., Proliferative, W., & Retinopathy, D. (2002). Intravitreous Levels significantly correlated with intravitreous VEGF levels in both PDR patients (r ϭ 0.824. *Blood Pressure Monitoring*, *25*(12), 575–583.

Growth, P., Growth, E., Proliferative, W., & Retinopathy, D. (2002). Intravitreous Levels significantly correlated with intravitreous VEGF levels in both PDR patients (r ϭ 0.824. *Blood Pressure Monitoring*, *25*(12), 575–583.

Ichiho, H. M., & Aitaoto, N. (2013). Assessing the system of services for chronic diseases prevention and control in the US-affiliat-d Pacific Islands: Introduction and methods. *Hawai'i Journal of Medicine & Public Health: a Journal of Asia Pacific Medicine & Public Health*, *72*(5Suppl 1), 5–19. PMID:23901363

Ichiho, H. M., Demei, Y., Kuartei, S., & Aitaoto, N. (2013). An assessment of non-communicable diseases, diabetes, and related risk factors in the Republic of Palau: A systems perspective. *Hawai'i Journal of Medicine & Public Health: a Journal of Asia Pacific Medicine & Public Health, 72*(5Suppl 1), 98–105. PMID:23901368

Ketkar, A. R., Veluswamy, S. K., Prabhu, N., & Maiya, A. G. (2015). Screening for noncommunicable disease risk factors at a workplace in India: A physiotherapy initiative in a healthcare setting. *Hong Kong Physiotherapy Journal, 33*(1), 3–9. doi:10.1016/j.hkpj.2014.12.001

Kuhn, M. (2008). Building Predictive Models in R Using the caret Package. *Journal of Statistical Software, 28*(5), 1–26. doi:10.18637/jss.v028.i05 PMID:27774042

Kume, S., Thomas, M. C., & Koya, D. (2012). Nutrient Sensing, Autophagy, and Diabetic Nephropathy. *Diabetes, 61*(1), 23–29. doi:10.2337/db11-0555 PMID:22187371

Kume, S., Thomas, M. C., & Koya, D. (2012). Nutrient Sensing, Autophagy, and Diabetic Nephropathy. *Diabetes, 61*(1), 23–29. doi:10.2337/db11-0555 PMID:22187371

Liakat, S., Bors, K. A., Xu, L., Woods, C. M., Doyle, J., & Gmachl, C. F. (2014). Noninvasive in vivo glucose sensing on human subjects using mid-infrared light. *Biomedical Optics Express, 5*(7), 2397. doi:10.1364/BOE.5.002397 PMID:25071973

Mai, M., Wang, K., Huber, G., Kirby, M., Shattuck, M. D., & O'Hern, C. S. (2015, August). Outcome Prediction in Mathematical Models of Immune Response to Infection. *PLoS One, 10*(8), e0135861. doi:10.1371/journal.pone.0135861 PMID:26287609

Malik, R. A. (2014). Which Test for Diagnosing Early Human Diabetic Neuropathy? *Diabetes, 63*(7), 2206–2208. doi:10.2337/db14-0492 PMID:24962918

Malik, R. A. (2014). Which Test for Diagnosing Early Human Diabetic Neuropathy? *Diabetes, 63*(7), 2206–2208. doi:10.2337/db14-0492 PMID:24962918

Manca, D. P., Campbell-Scherer, D., Aubrey-Bassler, K., Kandola, K., Aguilar, C., Baxter, J., ... Grunfeld, E. (2015). Developing clinical decision tools to implement chronic disease prevention and screening in primary care: The BETTER 2 program (building on existing tools to improve chronic disease prevention and screening in primary care). *Implementation Science; IS, 10*(1), 107. doi:10.118613012-015-0299-9 PMID:26238338

Mittag, F., Römer, M., & Zell, A. (2015, August). Influence of Feature Encoding and Choice of Classifier on Disease Risk Prediction in Genome-Wide Association Studies. *PLoS One*, *10*(8), e0135832. doi:10.1371/journal.pone.0135832 PMID:26285210

Press, F. (2010). Research news 1. *Fraunhofer Press*, *37*(3), 153–167.

Raghu, A., Praveen, D., Peiris, D., Tarassenko, L., & Clifford, G. (2015, August). Implications of Cardiovascular Disease Risk Assessment Using the WHO/ISH Risk Prediction Charts in Rural India. *PLoS One*, *10*(8), 1–13. doi:10.1371/journal.pone.0133618 PMID:26287807

Remais, J. V., Zeng, G., Li, G., Tian, L., & Engelgau, M. M. (2013, February). Convergence of non-communicable and infectious diseases in low- and middle-income countries. *International Journal of Epidemiology*, *42*(1), 221–227. doi:10.1093/ije/dys135 PMID:23064501

Sun, F., Kuo, C., Cheng, H., Buthpitiya, S., Collins, P., & Griss, M. (2012). Activity-aware Mental Stress Detection Using Physiological Sensors. *Mob. Comput. Appl. Serv.*, *76*, 1–20.

U. S. F. Service and R. Mountain. (2002). Comparing Five Modelling Techniques. *Ecological Modelling*.

Viswanathan, H., Baozhi, C., & Pompili, D. (2012). Research challenges in computation, communication, and context awareness for ubiquitous healthcare. *Commun. Mag. IEEE*, *50*(5), 92–99. doi:10.1109/MCOM.2012.6194388

Wilson, J. M., & Jungner, Y. G. (1968). Principles and practice of screening for disease. *Boletin de la Oficina Sanitaria Panamericana*, *65*(4), 281–393. PMID:4234760

ENDNOTES

1 www.foodbornechicago.org

2 https://flunearyou.org

3 David Lee Scher, MD is Founder and Director at DLS HEALTHCARE CONSULTING, LLC, which specializes in advising digital health technology companies, their partners, investors, and clients. As a cardiac electrophysiologist and pioneer adopter of remote patient monitoring, he understood early on the challenges that the culture and landscape of healthcare present to the development and adoption of digital technologies. He is a well-respected

thought leader in mobile and other digital health technologies. Scher lectures worldwide on relevant industry topics including the role of tech in Pharma, patient advocacy, standards for development and adoption, and impact on patients and healthcare systems from clinical, risk management, operational and marketing standpoints. He is a Clinical Associate Professor of Medicine at Penn State College of Medicine. [https://davidleescher.wordpress.com/2012/03/03/how-patient-centric-care-differs-from-patient-centered-care-2/]

Chapter 2
Barriers to Adoptions of IoT-Based Solutions for Disease Screening

Sujitkumar Hiwale
Philips Research India, India

Shrutin Ulman
Philips Research India, India

Karthik Subbaraman
Philips Research India, India

Change of disease patterns from communicable to chronic diseases has a tremendous impact on the healthcare ecosystem. For healthcare organizations to remain viable and economically sustainable during this transition, there is a desperate need of cost-effective solutions for chronic disease management. One important strategy for this is early diagnosis and management of diseases. With rapid technological advancements, IoT-based solutions are well-positioned to be an effective tool for disease screening and health monitoring provided that they are also able to bridge non-technical barriers in technology adoption. The three primary stakeholders for screening solutions are healthcare organizations, clinical fraternity, and end-users. The primary objective of this chapter is to review likely barriers in adoptions of the IoT solutions from the perspective of these three primary stakeholders.

DOI: 10.4018/978-1-5225-7131-5.ch002

INTRODUCTION

Availability of precise and continuous medical data has been identified for a long time as one of the important prerequisites for effective clinical management. Such data is also required for optimal practice of evidence based medicine as well as for planning patient-specific treatment regimes. This has led to ever increasing deployment of Internet-of-Things (IoT)-based solutions in the healthcare sector due to their unique ability to automatically gather and share physiological data in real-time. By 2020, it is estimated that out of 30 billion IoT devices, 40% would be used in healthcare for disease-screening, diagnosis and management (Bauer, Patel, & Veira, 2014). When combined with rapidly evolving predictive and classification capabilities of machine learning algorithms, the IoT devices are likely to minimize subjective errors in assessment, reduce inefficiencies, and enable more robust remote–monitoring thereby reducing the overall cost of patient-management—and save lives (Dimitrov, 2016). This is especially important for healthcare systems that are over-burdened with ever-increasing number of patients with chronic diseases who consume a greater share of limited healthcare resources.

The Internet of Medical Things (IoMT) refers to the connected system of medical devices and applications that collect and share healthcare data through online networks. The concept of an electronic device that captures or monitors data and shares it using internet connection is not new as such, but has evolved tremendously over a period of time due to accelerated progress in hardware and embedded software development. The introduction of newer technologies such as wearable electro-chemosensors, nanomaterial-enabled wearable sensors (Yao, Swetha, & Zhu, 2018) has made the IoT devices even more powerful and reliable tool for the disease-screening and long-term monitoring of the chemical, biological, and physical systems in real-time (Haghi, Thurow, & Stoll, 2017). These technological advancements have also made it possible to have miniaturized, lightweight, transparent, ultrathin, high flexibility, and stretchable sensors, which can be conformally attached on the surface of organs or skin, thereby enabling health-monitoring in a non-obtrusive and more convenient way (Trung & Lee, 2016). The decline in the overall cost and energy requirement has also made it possible to deploy increasing number of IoT solution for practical applications. A report by Allied Market Research predicts that the IoMT healthcare market will reach US$136.8 billion worldwide by 2021. These developments in the IoT sensors along with computational and algorithmic advancements are well-positioned to create newer, unforeseen possibilities for disease screening and health monitoring in the 21st century.

Disease screening is very important aspect of healthcare continuum, as it provides an opportunity of early diagnosis, which could ultimately lead to better disease management for individual and for healthcare organizations. This is the reason that a number of digital solutions starting form web-based application to smartphone-based apps have been proposed and tested for disease prescreening. In the recent-past, smartphone-based applications have played a predominant role in coming up with connected solutions for healthcare. These solutions range from simple SMS-based reminders (Uy et al., 2017) to sophisticated machine learning algorithms for risk-prediction based on plethora of external and smartphone's inbuilt sensors (Lowres et al., 2014). However, despite being in existence for more than three decades, these solutions are still bogged with low adoption by the clinical fraternity and the end-users (Li, Land, & Ray, 2008). As Winston Churchill once famously said "The farther back you can look, the farther forward you are likely to see." In the same way, it is important to have a critical review of past and present digital methods of disease prescreening in order to understand barriers in adoption to ensure success of the future IoT-based solutions. Moreover, lack of sufficient literature on barriers for adoption and use of the IoT solution also makes such an analyses important. The three primary stakeholders for screening solutions are healthcare organizations, clinical fraternity and end-users. All of these stakeholders have different expectation from solutions and use different criteria to evaluate them. This makes it essential to understand the barrier for adoption of screening solutions from each stakeholder's perspective.

The primary objective of this chapter is to review factors which are likely to impact success or failure of the IoT-based solutions form perspective of healthcare organizations, clinical fraternity and end users. The first section of the chapter discusses the need and challenges of disease screening from perspective of public healthcare organizations; it also discusses cost-effectiveness evidence of digital solution for disease screening. Section two deals with the factors, which influence adoption of digital technology by healthcare providers. The end-use perspective in acceptance of technology is covered in section three. The overall conclusion and recommendation for the IoT-based solution for disease screening are provided in the section four.

DISEASE SCREENING AND PUBLIC HEALTHCARE ORGANIZATIONS

Life-expectancy has increased significantly across the globe, and with that came diseases of lifestyle like diabetes mellitus, hypertension, chronic obstructive pulmonary disease, and their complications. As an end result people have started living longer but with morbidities. This impacts the healthcare organizations significantly as it has been observed that the overall healthcare expenditure burden of a person increases exponentially as the person ages (US Centers for Medicare and Medicaid

Services, 2017). As the world ages and the population increases, the world is rapidly being engulfed in the dual spectre of an epidemic of chronic diseases and a rigid healthcare system, which is tuned to deal with emergency care and acute diseases and therefore grappling with cost-effective ways to manage chronic diseases.

Throughout the world, leaders of government health agencies, heads of private healthcare companies, and even patients/consumers—collectively, the shapers of the modern healthcare system—behold the growth of healthcare spending with alarm as it is expected that by 2025, global annual healthcare expenditure will almost double to US$13.9 trillion from US$7.8 trillion in 2013. For almost 50 years, healthcare spending has grown by two percentage points in excess of Gross Domestic Product (GDP) growth across all the member countries of the Organization for Economic Co-operation and Development (OECD). Going by the historic growth rate, healthcare will consume an ever-growing proportion of the developed nations' wealth, reaching 30% of GDP in the United States in 2040, and 30% of the median OECD GDP by 2070. If left unchecked, (by 2100) it could take up 97% of GDP in the United States and more than 50% of GDP in most other OECD countries—astonishing proportions (OECD, 2017). This clearly indicates that the current healthcare systems are not efficient and are unsustainable in long term.

To understand the current healthcare organizations, it is important to study history of disease profiles, inventions and their impact on healthcare systems. Antibiotics, vaccines, imaging modalities like ultrasonography, Computed Tomography (CT) scans and Magnetic Resonance Imaging (MRI), dialysis, stents, heart-lung machine, heart transplant and nuclear medicine can be rated as the greatest innovations in medicine in the last century (Le Fanu, 2011). Of these the greatest impact has been that of antibiotics and vaccinations; they have been able to significantly reduce the global burden of communicable diseases as they prevent or treat diseases in early stages of disease progression. High prevalence of communicable diseases and availability of these inventions had a great impact on shaping the modern healthcare as an acute condition focused entity. However, emergence of chronic disease has rattled healthcare systems and there is a desperate need of new age solutions to deal with this problem as conventional ways of working has found to be inadequate and unsustainable.

Chronic diseases need a different strategy to deal with them. The healthcare system needs to address this issue by considering various methodologies, which primarily should include: (1) risk stratification-identifying people at the highest risk; (2) identifying preventive strategies for persons based on their "risk profile" (3) working out a cost benefit analysis to select the best strategy to optimize health care delivery at the lowest cost; and (4) continuous monitoring and improvement in strategies.

Logically, stratifying the population into various risk categories for diseases is likely to be the best initial step in formulating a strategy to prevent the disease or detect it as soon as possible. However, risk stratification of a general population especially when many facts about very early stages of the disease are unknown is still a daunting task. Thus, leveraging the technologies on the horizon and evolving a system for patient screening, care and management is the need of the hour. Genetic tests, metabolic screening tests, wearables devices for tracking physical activities, etc. are all the newer tools that can be leveraged to stratify risk and also attempt at detecting early signs of disease. Genetic and metabolic tests are still evolving and will take some time to be available for general purpose screening in a cost-effective manner. On other hand, with availability of several nanotechnologies based IoT sensors for tracking and storing clinical data along with advanced risk stratification algorithms a lot of IoT solution have been already developed and deployed for disease screening.

It is important that risk stratification should go hand in hand with appropriate preventive or curative strategies. There is no point in risk stratification, unless we have a clear idea on how to prevent or manage the risk. e.g. if there is a program for screening children with celiac disease then there should be a provision to prevent or treat long term health complications associated with the disease. This has been an onerous task, e.g. a child born with Leigh's syndrome has a genetic defect in its mitochondria and this disease is progressive until the child dies. This disease has no proven treatment yet, so having a population screening initiative for such diseases will raise a lot of ethical questions. On the other hand, screening and primary prevention is likely to be beneficial for diseases where risk factors and ways to modify them are well-known and proven. Sedentary behavior, obesity, tobacco-smoking, alcohol-consumption are known risk factors for a number of diseases. These factors not only impact an individual but country as well. The World Health Organization (WHO) has estimated that globally, smoking alone causes over US$500 billion in economic damage each year (Ekpu & Brown, 2015). Therefore, a wide variety of digital solutions have been proposed to screen and monitor these risk factors. Moreover, there is an increasing evidence that such interventions can be effective in reducing and monitoring these risk factors such as sedentary behavior (Stephenson, McDonough, Murphy, Nugent, & Mair, 2017), smoking cessation (Chen et al., 2012) etc.

A number of governments around the world are also supporting digital technologies and have committed huge investments for it such as the "meaningful use" program in the United State of America for the adoption and implementation of Electronic Health Records (EHRs). Similarly, in 2015, companies have invested almost US$6 trillion for IoT solutions, expecting a US$13 trillion return over investment by 2025 (Business Insider, 2016). However, it is important to note that financial investments do not always lead to a favorable change in medical practices and outcomes if the new technology or intervention are not implemented with a clear objectives and thorough cost-effective analysis. One notable example for this is National Health Service's (NHS) National Programme for IT in the United Kingdom for deployment of EHR systems in trust hospitals, which was ultimately dismantled by the government after spending over US$24 Billion due to poor design and implementation ("Dismantling the NHS National Programme for IT - GOV.UK," 2011). This also emphasizes importance of continuous monitoring and improvement of the healthcare initiatives.

The healthcare organizations are very important stakeholders for IoT devices. For high adoption of IoT devices in healthcare, and especially for disease screening, it is important that IoT devices align themselves with the broader strategy of healthcare organizations. In this regard, it is important that the IoT solution should target a problem, which is relevant for the healthcare organizations and has well known early risk factors or markers. Secondly, the IoT solution should not be limited to data collection only but should provide practical inputs for clinical decision making. Finally, the solution should be cost-effective so that an individual and organization can afford it. For IoT solutions or for that matter for any digital solutions in healthcare cost-effectiveness is one of the most important barriers and therefore need thorough consideration.

Cost-Effectiveness of Digital Solutions for Disease Screening

In 1968, the WHO published guidelines on the principles and practice of screening for disease. One of the principles in this guideline states that the total cost of finding a case should be economically balanced in relation to medical expenditure as a whole (Wilson, Jungner, & Organization, 1968). This principle clearly highlights the importance of cost-effectiveness aspect of a screening solution. This makes it important to evaluate available literature on IoT devices from cost-effectiveness perspective. This analysis can also help in formulating recommendations for building cost effective IoT devices. Outcome of the cost-effectiveness analysis is measured in treatment-response and are usually summarized in cost-effectiveness ratios (CER), where the costs in the numerator are related to a single common measure of effectiveness in the denominator (e.g. abstinence from alcohol/smoking) (Kraemer, 2007). When comparisons between two interventions are made using this ratio, this is called the incremental cost-effectiveness ratio (ICER). Cost-effectiveness can also be presented in terms of cost for one year gained living with disability (YLD) averted. Cost-utility ICERs refers to the cost of one quality of life year (QALY) gained in the experimental treatment compared to the control condition (Hedman et al., 2011).

Along the care-continuum, screening for chronic disease states using IoT promises greatest cost-benefits since IoT solutions have the potential to, (1) decrease the overall cost of disease diagnosis, treatment and management; (2) enable more robust remote–monitoring by utilizing skill-sets that are not specialized, or those that are easily transferrable; and (3) reduce inefficiencies by extending services beyond traditional hospital care setups (Dimitrov, 2016). However, as of now, very limited literature is available for the IoT solutions' cost-effectiveness, which can be largely attributed to technology focused nature of the current studies (Westerlund, Leminen, & Rajahonka, 2014). Therefore, the evidence available for other digital eHealth solutions need to be considered to understand cost-effectiveness aspects of IoT solutions, which are logical extension of the existing digital solutions.

Although, a lot of work has already been done in this area, conflicting results from different studies due to varied application areas, and solutions make it complicated to understand the overall cost-effectiveness of digital solutions in healthcare in general. In a systematic review of more than 60 Randomized Control Trials (RCT) to assess effectiveness and cost-effectiveness of computer and other electronic aids for smoking cessation Chen et al., have found small but significant impact of computer and other electronic aids on smoking cessation (Chen et al., 2012). They have indicated that some form of digital intervention is likely to be cost-effective when added to non-electronic behavioral support. The upper limit for such benefit has been estimated to be around £ 2000-3000 per person. On other hand, in a review of RCT to evaluate the cost effectiveness of guided Internet-based interventions for depression compared to controls, Kolovos et al. found that guided Internet-based interventions are not cost effective (Kolovos et al., 2018).

Similarly, for disease screening a number of new approaches have been introduced; in one such attempt Lowres et al., have proposed use of iPhone-based electrocardiography (iECG) for community–based screening for atrial fibrillation (Lowres et al., 2014). In their study with 1,000 subjects they have reported the incremental cost-effectiveness ratio of extending screening into the community, would be US$ 4,066 per QALY gained and US$ 20,695 for preventing one stroke. They have further noted that cost-effectiveness improved with increased treatment adherence and have concluded that screening with iECG is both feasible and cost-effective measure. In the same way, for the population-wide Chlamydia trachomatis screening of sexually active women under 26 years of age, when two different screening strategies, self-sampling via the a dedicated Website and traditional, clinic-based screening were comparted it was found that internet-based screening strategy prevented 35.5 more cases of pelvic inflammatory disease and saved an additional US$41,000 in direct medical costs as compared with the clinic-based screening strategy (Huang, Gaydos, Barnes, Jett-Goheen, & Blake, 2011).

Although, there is a substantial uncertainty regarding the most effective approach for screening, available studies points toward increasing evidence of feasibility and cost-effectiveness of eHealth solutions from screening perspective. However, still more research is required in this field to fully assess potential and short and long term impact of such solutions. All these factors need due consideration when a community-based screening method needs to be introduced. Generally, the cost-effectiveness of IoT solutions can be enabled by increasing the outreach of healthcare services beyond the traditional model.

CLINICAL FRATERNITY AND DIGITAL SOLUTIONS FOR DISEASE SCREENING

Being a crucial link between medical solutions and end-users, healthcare providers are a key driving force of healthcare initiatives. Introduction of any new eHealth/mHealth solution is likely to disturb the health care provider's workflow; therefore, the way in which a solution addresses this workflow disturbance and healthcare providers' response to it largely determines success or failure of such solution. This is the reason that a number of sociology, psychology, and consumer behavior theory based models such as the Technology Acceptance Model (TAM), Unified Theory of Acceptance and Use of Technology (UTAUT), have been used to understand technology adoption barriers and usage in healthcare providers (Tavares & Oliveira, 2017). In a systematic review of more than 93 studies on health care providers' adoption of eHealth, Li et al., have identified 40 factors, which influence the health care providers' acceptance of eHealth solutions (Junhua Li, Talaei-Khoei, Seale, & MacIntyre, 2013). These factors are subsequently grouped into seven clusters based on underlying themes. The review highlights that adoption of new technology is influenced by a number of factors and technical design and specification of a solution is just one aspect of it. Similar findings have been observed in other studies for adoption of different digital technologies such as electronic health record (Tavares & Oliveira, 2017), mHealth-based solution (Wu, Wang, & Lin, 2007) etc. Such studies provide valuable information on barriers and critical success factors for technology development and adoption.

Based on findings of these studies it is possible to further simplify the healthcare providers' acceptance of eHealth solutions into three broad categories; (1) individual characteristics of a healthcare provider including his social-network and medical practice; (2) usability and perceived usefulness of a solution; and (3) technical aspects of the solution. Individual characteristics of a healthcare provider such as demographic characteristics and prior experience with digital solutions are important aspects for adoption of any healthcare solution. Similarly, social factors such as a doctor's perception about end-users' perspectives, organizational and leadership support for digital initiatives, and influence from doctors own personal network also play important role in a doctor's acceptance of any new technology (Junhua Li et al., 2013). Regarding medical practice, factors such as hospital-type, location, size, access to data, ability to transfer information are important for technology adoption (Kruse, Kothman, Anerobi, & Abanaka, 2016). In-depth understanding of underlying problems, socio-cultural factors and workflows are crucial to appreciate healthcare provider related factors during design of a solution.

The second category includes factors related to usability and perceived usefulness of a solution. Usability of a solution is determined by its ease of use and associated operational complexities. The perceived usefulness of a solution is linked with appropriateness of the solution from a healthcare provider's job perspective and the clinical and financial advantages associated with it. The factors in this category basically deals with how a particular solution is designed and integrated in an existing clinical workflow and how it is likely to impact the outcome in short and long term. This require not only thorough understanding of underlying workflows but also requires frequent and systematic feedback from clinical fraternity on various aspects of solution throughout development phase of a solution. The third category is related to the technology related factors such as availability of digital infrastructure, interoperability, business process alignment, legal and regulatory requirements etc. These factors mostly fall in technology domain and should be thoroughly studied and implemented in context of an IoT solution especially from legal and ethical point of views. The practical learning from these findings are important for success of any IoT solution.

Lack of a proper scientific evidence on effectiveness is another important factor, which is responsible for low adoption of digital solutions among clinical fraternity. Although, the smartphone apps have increased exponentially in number and popularity in recent time, they still have not been thoroughly evaluated for their possible clinical impact in a scientific manner. To address this issue, Covolo et al., have recently published a systematic review of RCTs to evaluate role of mobile phone apps as a driver for promoting healthy lifestyles from a public health perspective (Covolo, Ceretti, Moneda, Castaldi, & Gelatti, 2017). In their review, they found that only 25% of total selected RCTs had statistical difference between intervention and control groups with most of the studies having a short follow-up and a very small sample size. Overall they found only modest efficacy of apps in health promotion. Similarly, Buechi et al., have recently published a systematic review to investigate the diagnostic value of available smartphone-based health applications (Buechi et al., 2017). They found that out of more than 165,000 medical apps available on iOS and Android platforms only nine percent are actually related to topics of screening, diagnosis and monitoring. They further noted that a large majority of these apps have not undergone any scientific evaluation before release. Moreover, for the apps where studies are available they are either very small or have low methodological quality. This points toward lack of scientific evidence of clinical usefulness of mobile apps and call for thorough evaluation of such apps.

Well-designed observation studies and focused-group discussions conducted during the initial stages of the solution's development could be very useful tools to understand healthcare providers concerns and barriers for adoption in detail. The IoT solution should be designed with due consideration of these factors. Furthermore, not much literature is available on scientific validity of IoT-based solution as of now. However, taking learning from mobile apps it is important that any IoT-based solutions should undergo thorough evaluation with well-established protocol and methodology for asserting its potential and possible clinical usefulness for acceptance from a larger clinical fraternity. All these evidences points toward need of a holistic approach in design and implement of any IoT solution.

END-USER PERSPECTIVES IN DISEASE SCREENING

In the last two decades, digital healthcare solutions have witnessed an interesting trend in regard to end-users' acceptance for technology. In the early years of these technologies, users were quite enthusiastic about digital technology and believed that it would improve healthcare quality. However, as issues such as privacy and security arose, end-users started becoming more restrictive in their approach towards digital health solutions (Ancker, Brenner, Richardson, Silver, & Kaushal, 2015; Richardson & Ancker, 2015). The perception has started to change again with better design of solutions and implementation of strict privacy and confidentiality features. This trend underscores that how quickly end-users' perception can change and how important it is in the success of any digital heath solution. Therefore, capturing consumer attitudes has been recognized as a key factor for identifying potential opportunities and barriers for technology adoption (Ohno-Machado, 2013). This has also led to the development of many consumer centered acceptance models for IoT (Attié & Meyer-Waarden, 2017).

In the context of the IoT-based solutions, end-users' perception towards technology is far more important as it is patients' own health data which is collected and shared by such devices. Therefore, patients' attitude and concerns are critical factors and have the potential to affect design and future of health information exchange (HIE) systems in digital solutions and consequently require a thorough analysis. A literature review conducted by Esmaeilzadeh and Sambasivan has identified seven key factors that influence patients' support for HIE systems; these include (1) perceived benefits, (2) perceived concerns, (3) patient characteristics, (4) patient participation level in HIE, (5) type of health information, (6) identity of recipients, and (7) patient preferences regarding consent and features (Esmaeilzadeh & Sambasivan, 2017).

Each one of these factors need detailed deliberation to understand their impact on acceptance of digital health solution.

Perceived benefits is one of the first factors considered by any user for adoption of new technology. Over a period of time end-users have witnessed several perceived benefits associated with digital technologies such as convenience, faster care due to information sharing, high quality care, and reduced healthcare bill (Unertl, Johnson, & Lorenzi, 2011). All these factors have contributed in wider adoption of digital solutions by end-users. Care providers' attitude and adoption of digital health solutions have also been shown to influence patients' perception toward benefit of new technology (Esmaeilzadeh & Sambasivan, 2017). It has also been observed that perceived benefits in turn also influence patients' attitude towards other factors like privacy and security with patient more willing to adopt new technology if they believe that perceived benefits outweigh the concerns. This makes it very important for IoT solutions to have elaborated explanation on end-user benefits with relevant evidences so as to instilled belief in end-user about the solution.

Privacy and security aspects of the collected data have been identified as one of the most important concerns regarding the digital solutions from end-users' viewpoint (Kim, Joseph, & Ohno-Machado, 2015). If not addressed properly they become an important barrier of adoption of digital solutions (Wen, Kreps, Zhu, & Miller, 2010). Concerns regarding what type of data get exchanged and with whom has been also identified as important factors from patients' perceptive. Overall lack of transparency in which clinical data is used, shared and stored is one of the important root causes for these issues. Having a solution with well-designed control access, proper architectural frameworks for scalability and interoperability, trustworthy security and privacy mechanisms are paramount important to build trust with the end-users (Papoutsi et al., 2015; Rezaeibagha, Win, & Susilo, 2015). Providing end-users all relevant information on solution, architecture, measures implemented for protection, and keeping end-users well informed about data are equally important for trust building.

A number of factors such as patient's age, gender, education, income etc. have been implied to impact patients attitude for technology (Esmaeilzadeh & Sambasivan, 2017). The studies have also reported that social framework and cultural factors also influence end-users' decision for technology adoption (Hoque & Bao, 2015). In a systematic review Montague & Perchonok have shown that how technology can be used to positively affect the health of historically underserved populations; however, they have cautioned that technology must be tailored toward the intended population, as personally relevant and contextually situated health technology is more likely than broader technology to create behavior changes. (Montague & Perchonok, 2012). As these factor show significant variation and there is no consensus in literature on exact role of such factors these factors need to be duly considered based on context of a solution.

The patients' participation in any digital solution is heavily influenced by a patient's prior experience with such technologies. Similarly, factors linked to ease of use, ergonometric factors also influence the patient's perception. Overall, it has been observed that acceptance of eHealth solution can be increased by letting end-users practice with the application; especially those with less education and who have not used such solutions before (de Veer et al., 2015). Patient engagement requires pro-active participation from the individual in his welfare and need appropriate support from the solution as well. The person needs to be compliant with preventive measures and also motivated enough on a long term basis; solution should also help to enable these virtues. The type of healthcare information being collected is also very important aspects, which determines patient's' attitude towards a digital solution. In many studies confidentiality and privacy of information such as disease status has been identified as a crucial factor in acceptance and feasibility of a digital solutions (Nachega et al., 2016). Other equally important factors are measures undertaken to safeguard identity of recipients, and their voluntary and informed participation in a study via a valid and informed consent. The IoT designers should carefully study these factors and should involve the end-users in development process from early on.

DISCUSSION

The world has witnessed a tectonic shift in disease profiles in the past five decades with emergence of chronic diseases as the leading cause of morbidity and mortality. The conventional healthcare systems, which are healthcare provider centric and are geared for treating acute conditions have not been fully able to cope with this change. The healthcare systems must re-design and re-create themselves to meet the challenges of the future. This is especially important as the traditional healthcare models have shown to be either redundant or unaffordable, and therefore unviable. Screening could be a very important tool in dealing with these new problems and it is one of the most economical ways to deal with it. The IoT devices are likely to play an important role in screening program by virtue of their ability to continuously monitor data in a systematic manner.

Even though the healthcare industry has been slower to adopt new age technologies such as IoT than other industries, the IoMT is poised to transform how we keep people safe and healthy, especially as the demand for solutions to lower healthcare costs increase in the coming years. This require a new approach for disease screening.

Network medicine is a new branch of medicine, which looks at the networks of the cellular ecosystem, biochemical processes, genetic linkages and social networks, for prediction of disease onset. Leveraging data from IoT devices potentially could help us to weave together a network of genetic make-up, dietary choices, physical activities, social/economic/geographic networks of the people, for risk stratification, prediction of disease onset and ultimately for personalization of therapy. This needs a multi-disciplinary approach and continuous monitoring to piece together a solution that individualizes therapy and addresses the challenges in the individual's ecosystem to make behavior change and stick to it.

To fulfill its potential for screening the IoT device will need to overcome many challenges both on technical and implementation front. On technical front, there are still several challenges such as standardization, interoperability, networking issues, addressing and sensing issues, power and storage restrictions, privacy and security (Haroon et al., 2016). Even for wearable sensors, challenges such as long-term stability, biocompatibility, comfort level, system integration, and costs need to be addressed to improve their performance (Qian & Long, 2017). Similarly, even after tremendous progress in machine learning and dig data analysis domain there are still significant challenges in processing the large-scale sensing data gathered from different IoT sensors into meaningful inputs for real-world applications.

Recommendation for IoT Solutions

From implementation perspective it is important that IoT solutions should pay due attention to all three primary stakeholders, "healthcare organizations", "clinical fraternity" and "end-users" and incorporate their feedback in the solution. From the healthcare organizations' perspective, cost-effectiveness is very crucial factor for any screening solution. The solution should be able to detect or predict disease in early phase of disease progression so that appropriate measures can be taken to control it. The IoT solution hold a lot of potential in this regard. However, they should be designed with due consideration to make them an ideal tool for cost-effective disease screening. From care providers' perspectives it is important that a solution is designed with consideration of individual and social characteristics of healthcare providers with emphasis on usability and perceived usefulness. The IoT solution should instill confidence in clinical fraternity by addressing their concerns and should have valid and thorough scientific evidence to support its potential benefits. For end-users the solution should be user centric with emphasis on privacy and security.

CONCLUSION

IoT-based solutions have a long way to go before they can become a preferred solution for disease screening and monitoring. Thorough understanding of barriers for adoption of IoT-based solutions is very important aspect in this journey. Although a lot of work has been already done on this but none of the existing source provides a comprehensive overview of these barriers from primary stakeholders' perspectives'. The major strength of this chapter lies in being a first literature source where all important barriers to adoption are summarized in one document. This is likely to help the IoT developer to have a holistic view of adoption barriers from each stakeholders' perspective. However, given vastness of the topic it was not possible to cover all the aspects of the topic in-depth. To cover the topic comprehensively and systematically we have used systematic reviews as a primary source for information for this chapter but critical appraisal of case studies is also important source to understand practical issues in implementation and success of IoT-based solutions. Therefore, we recommend a detailed assessment of appropriate case studies to cover the relevant adoption barriers from a practical view point. Similarly, cost-effectiveness of digital solution for disease screening and possible method to achieve it also need more detailed assessment. We further recommend that the IoT developer should assess the relevant barriers with due consideration of their solution and ecosystems.

To summarize, the IoT-based solutions should address a well-defined problem, which is relevant for the individual and community with a practical and cost-effective approach. The healthcare systems and care providers both have central roles in creating an effective ecosystem for such changes. Within this, the leveraging of healthcare information technology and mobility can be a conduit to bridging the divide between patients and providers. Especially with the shifts in the health system toward wellness and preventive care — but also with the shifts toward value-based reimbursement — patient engagement will continue to grow as a focal point issue.

REFERENCES

Ancker, J. S., Brenner, S., Richardson, J. E., Silver, M., & Kaushal, R. (2015). Trends in Public Perceptions of Electronic Health Records During Early Years of Meaningful Use. *The American Journal of Managed Care*, *21*(8), e487–e493. PMID:26625503

Attié, E., & Meyer-Waarden, L. (2017). *The Impacts of Social Value*. Cognitive Factors and Well-Being on the Use of the Internet of Things and Smart Connected Objects.

Bauer, H., Patel, M., & Veira, J. (2014, December). *The Internet of Things: Sizing up the opportunity*. McKinsey & Company. Retrieved February 21, 2018, from https://www.mckinsey.com/industries/semiconductors/our-insights/the-internet-of-things-sizing-up-the-opportunity

Buechi, R., Faes, L., Bachmann, L. M., Thiel, M. A., Bodmer, N. S., Schmid, M. K., ... Lienhard, K. R. (2017). Evidence assessing the diagnostic performance of medical smartphone apps: A systematic review and exploratory meta-analysis. *BMJ Open*, *7*(12), e018280. doi:10.1136/bmjopen-2017-018280 PMID:29247099

Chen, Y.-F., Madan, J., Welton, N., Yahaya, I., Aveyard, P., Bauld, L., … Munafò, M. R. (2012). Effectiveness and cost-effectiveness of computer and other electronic aids for smoking cessation: a systematic review and network meta-analysis. *Health Technology Assessment (Winchester, England), 16*(38), 1–205, iii–v. doi:10.3310/hta16380

Covolo, L., Ceretti, E., Moneda, M., Castaldi, S., & Gelatti, U. (2017). Does evidence support the use of mobile phone apps as a driver for promoting healthy lifestyles from a public health perspective? A systematic review of Randomized Control Trials. *Patient Education and Counseling*, *100*(12), 2231–2243. doi:10.1016/j.pec.2017.07.032 PMID:28855063

de Veer, A. J. E., Peeters, J. M., Brabers, A. E. M., Schellevis, F. G., Rademakers, J. J. D. J. M., & Francke, A. L. (2015). Determinants of the intention to use e-Health by community dwelling older people. *BMC Health Services Research, 15*(1), 103. doi:10.118612913-015-0765-8 PMID:25889884

Dimitrov, D. V. (2016). Medical Internet of Things and Big Data in Healthcare. *Healthcare Informatics Research*, *22*(3), 156–163. doi:10.4258/hir.2016.22.3.156 PMID:27525156

Dismantling the NHS National Programme for IT - GOV.UK. (2011, September). Retrieved March 2, 2018, from https://www.gov.uk/government/news/dismantling-the-nhs-national-programme-for-it

Ekpu, V. U., & Brown, A. K. (2015). The Economic Impact of Smoking and of Reducing Smoking Prevalence: Review of Evidence. *Tobacco Use Insights*, *8*, 1–35. doi:10.4137/TUI.S15628 PMID:26242225

Esmaeilzadeh, P., & Sambasivan, M. (2017). Patients' support for health information exchange: A literature review and classification of key factors. *BMC Medical Informatics and Decision Making*, *17*(1), 33. doi:10.118612911-017-0436-2 PMID:28376785

Haghi, M., Thurow, K., & Stoll, R. (2017). Wearable Devices in Medical Internet of Things: Scientific Research and Commercially Available Devices. *Healthcare Informatics Research*, *23*(1), 4–15. doi:10.4258/hir.2017.23.1.4 PMID:28261526

Haroon, A., Shah, M. A., Asim, Y., Naeem, W., Kamran, M., & Javaid, Q. (2016). Constraints in the IoT: The world in 2020 and beyond. *Constraints*, *7*(11).

Hedman, E., Andersson, E., Ljótsson, B., Andersson, G., Rück, C., & Lindefors, N. (2011). Cost-effectiveness of Internet-based cognitive behavior therapy vs. cognitive behavioral group therapy for social anxiety disorder: Results from a randomized controlled trial. *Behaviour Research and Therapy*, *49*(11), 729–736. doi:10.1016/j.brat.2011.07.009 PMID:21851929

Hoque, M. R., & Bao, Y. (2015). Cultural Influence on Adoption and Use of e-Health: Evidence in Bangladesh. *Telemedicine Journal and E-Health: The Official Journal of the American Telemedicine Association*, *21*(10), 845–851. doi:10.1089/tmj.2014.0128 PMID:26348844

Huang, W., Gaydos, C. A., Barnes, M. R., Jett-Goheen, M., & Blake, D. R. (2011). Cost-effectiveness analysis of Chlamydia trachomatis screening via Internet-based self-collected swabs compared to clinic-based sample collection. *Sexually Transmitted Diseases*, *38*(9), 815–820. doi:10.1097/OLQ.0b013e31821b0f50 PMID:21844736

Kim, K. K., Joseph, J. G., & Ohno-Machado, L. (2015). Comparison of consumers' views on electronic data sharing for healthcare and research. *Journal of the American Medical Informatics Association*, *22*(4), 821–830. doi:10.1093/jamia/ocv014 PMID:25829461

Kolovos, S., van Dongen, J. M., Riper, H., Buntrock, C., Cuijpers, P., Ebert, D. D., ... Bosmans, J. E. (2018). Cost effectiveness of guided Internet-based interventions for depression in comparison with control conditions: An individual-participant data meta-analysis. *Depression and Anxiety*, *35*(3), 209–219. doi:10.1002/da.22714 PMID:29329486

Kraemer, K. L. (2007). The cost-effectiveness and cost-benefit of screening and brief intervention for unhealthy alcohol use in medical settings. *Substance Abuse*, *28*(3), 67–77. doi:10.1300/J465v28n03_07 PMID:18077304

Kruse, C. S., Kothman, K., Anerobi, K., & Abanaka, L. (2016). Adoption Factors of the Electronic Health Record: A Systematic Review. *JMIR Medical Informatics*, *4*(2), e19. doi:10.2196/medinform.5525 PMID:27251559

Le Fanu, J. (2011). *The rise and fall of modern medicine*. Hachette, UK.

Li, J., Land, L., & Ray, P. (2008). *Humanitarian Technology Challenge (HTC)-electronic health records perspective.* A Report of Joint Project of IEEE and United Nations Foundation.

Li, J., Talaei-Khoei, A., Seale, H., Ray, P., & MacIntyre, C. R. (2013). Health Care Provider Adoption of eHealth: Systematic Literature Review. *Interactive Journal of Medical Research, 2*(1), e7. doi:10.2196/ijmr.2468 PMID:23608679

Lowres, N., Neubeck, L., Salkeld, G., Krass, I., McLachlan, A. J., Redfern, J., ... Freedman, S. B. (2014). Feasibility and cost-effectiveness of stroke prevention through community screening for atrial fibrillation using iPhone ECG in pharmacies. The SEARCH-AF study. *Thrombosis and Haemostasis, 111*(6), 1167–1176. doi:10.1160/TH14-03-0231 PMID:24687081

Montague, E., & Perchonok, J. (2012). Health and wellness technology use by historically underserved health consumers: Systematic review. *Journal of Medical Internet Research, 14*(3), e78. doi:10.2196/jmir.2095 PMID:22652979

Nachega, J. B., Skinner, D., Jennings, L., Magidson, J. F., Altice, F. L., Burke, J. G., ... Theron, G. B. (2016). Acceptability and feasibility of mHealth and community-based directly observed antiretroviral therapy to prevent mother-to-child HIV transmission in South African pregnant women under Option B+: An exploratory study. *Patient Preference and Adherence, 10*, 683–690. doi:10.2147/PPA.S100002 PMID:27175068

OECD. (2017). *Health at a Glance 2017*. OECD Publishing. doi:10.1787/health_glance-2017-

Ohno-Machado, L. (2013). Sharing data for the public good and protecting individual privacy: Informatics solutions to combine different goals. *Journal of the American Medical Informatics Association: JAMIA, 20*(1), 1. doi:10.1136/amiajnl-2012-001513 PMID:23243087

Papoutsi, C., Reed, J. E., Marston, C., Lewis, R., Majeed, A., & Bell, D. (2015). Patient and public views about the security and privacy of Electronic Health Records (EHRs) in the UK: Results from a mixed methods study. *BMC Medical Informatics and Decision Making, 15*(1), 86. doi:10.118612911-015-0202-2 PMID:26466787

Qian, R., & Long, Y. (2017). Wearable Chemosensors: A Review of Recent Progress. *ChemistryOpen, 7*(2), 118–130. doi:10.1002/open.201700159 PMID:29435397

Rezaeibagha, F., Win, K. T., & Susilo, W. (2015). A systematic literature review on security and privacy of electronic health record systems: Technical perspectives. *Health Information Management: Journal of the Health Information Management Association of Australia, 44*(3), 23–38. doi:10.1177/183335831504400304 PMID:26464299

Richardson, J. E., & Ancker, J. S. (2015). Public Perspectives of Mobile Phones' Effects on Healthcare Quality and Medical Data Security and Privacy: A 2-Year Nationwide Survey. *AMIA ... Annual Symposium Proceedings - AMIA Symposium. AMIA Symposium, 2015*, 1076–1082. PMID:26958246

Stephenson, A., McDonough, S. M., Murphy, M. H., Nugent, C. D., & Mair, J. L. (2017). Using computer, mobile and wearable technology enhanced interventions to reduce sedentary behaviour: A systematic review and meta-analysis. *The International Journal of Behavioral Nutrition and Physical Activity, 14*(1), 105. doi:10.118612966-017-0561-4 PMID:28800736

Tavares, J., & Oliveira, T. (2017). Electronic Health Record Portal Adoption: A cross country analysis. *BMC Medical Informatics and Decision Making, 17*(1), 97. doi:10.118612911-017-0482-9 PMID:28679423

Trung, T. Q., & Lee, N.-E. (2016). Flexible and Stretchable Physical Sensor Integrated Platforms for Wearable Human-Activity Monitoringand Personal Healthcare. *Advanced Materials (Deerfield Beach, Fla.), 28*(22), 4338–4372. doi:10.1002/adma.201504244 PMID:26840387

Unertl, K. M., Johnson, K. B., & Lorenzi, N. M. (2011). Health information exchange technology on the front lines of healthcare: Workflow factors and patterns of use. *Journal of the American Medical Informatics Association, 19*(3), 392–400. doi:10.1136/amiajnl-2011-000432 PMID:22003156

US Centers for Medicare and Medicaid Services. (2017). *National health expenditure data*. Author.

Uy, C., Lopez, J., Trinh-Shevrin, C., Kwon, S. C., Sherman, S. E., & Liang, P. S. (2017). Text Messaging Interventions on Cancer Screening Rates: A Systematic Review. *Journal of Medical Internet Research, 19*(8), e296. doi:10.2196/jmir.7893 PMID:28838885

Wen, K.-Y., Kreps, G., Zhu, F., & Miller, S. (2010). Consumers' perceptions about and use of the internet for personal health records and health information exchange: Analysis of the 2007 Health Information National Trends Survey. *Journal of Medical Internet Research, 12*(4), e73. doi:10.2196/jmir.1668 PMID:21169163

Westerlund, M., Leminen, S., & Rajahonka, M. (2014). Designing business models for the internet of things. *Technology Innovation Management Review, 4*(7).

Wilson, J. M. G., Jungner, G., & Organization, W. H. (1968). *Principles and practice of screening for disease*. Academic Press.

Wu, J.-H., Wang, S.-C., & Lin, L.-M. (2007). Mobile computing acceptance factors in the healthcare industry: A structural equation model. *International Journal of Medical Informatics*, *76*(1), 66–77. doi:10.1016/j.ijmedinf.2006.06.006 PMID:16901749

Yao, S., Swetha, P., & Zhu, Y. (2018). Nanomaterial-Enabled Wearable Sensors for Healthcare. *Advanced Healthcare Materials*, *7*(1), 1700889. doi:10.1002/adhm.201700889 PMID:29193793

Chapter 3
Early Diagnostics Model for Dengue Disease Using Decision Tree-Based Approaches

Shalini Gambhir
SRM University, India

Yugal Kumar
Jaypee University of Information Technology, India

Sanjay Malik
SRM University, India

Geeta Yadav
Manav Bharti University, India

Amita Malik
Deenbandhu Chhotu Ram University of Science and Technology, India

ABSTRACT

Classification schemes have been applied in the medical arena to explore patients' data and extract a predictive model.This model helps doctors to improve their prognosis, diagnosis, or treatment planning processes.The aim of this work is to utilize and compare different decision tree classifiers for early diagnosis of Dengue. Six approaches, mainly J48 tree, random tree, REP tree, SOM, logistic regression, and naïve Bayes, have been utilized to study real-world Dengue data collected from different hospitals in the Delhi, India region during 2015-2016. Standard statistical metrics are used to assess the efficiency of the proposed Dengue disease diagnostic system, and the outcomes showed that REP tree is best among these classifiers with 82.7% efficient in supplying an exact diagnosis.

DOI: 10.4018/978-1-5225-7131-5.ch003

INTRODUCTION

Dengue is a life threatening disease prevalent in several developed as well as developing nations. This is a virus born disease caused by the breeding of Aedes mosquitoes. Presently, in most regions of the tropics, epidemics are near peak transmission before they are acknowledged and supported as a viral infection.It is mostly too late to implement effective preventive steps that could represent an efficient impact on transmission.To master this situation the surveillance and diagnosis of Dengue should be proactive.The most important concern in developing the dengue diagnostic model is timely prediction of the disease, as its initial symptoms are similar to some other infections (Santosh Kumar et al., 2017; Chopra et al., 2014; Muniaraj, 2014; World Health Organization, 2009,2007). The aim of the survey is to diagnose patients as "Dengue Positive" group or "Dengue Negative'' on the basis of preliminary symptoms. To address this concern different machine learning techniques for dengue fever classification are used such as Naïve Bayes (NB) classifier (Tu et al., 2009) Decision Tree (DT) (Palaniappan & Awang, 2009), K-Nearest Neighbor (KNN) Technique (Jonsson & Wohlin, 2004), Multilayered Technique, Support Vector Machines (SVM) (Andreeva, 2006) and so along. These techniques can then be assessed based on several performance measures like Accuracy, Precision, Sensitivity, Specificity and Negative rate. This chapter offers a Decision Tree (DT) based dengue diagnostic model. This model can help medical staff to forecast early and accurate diagnosis of dengue using health and medical related data of patients. Moreover, this information can analyze data in different situations and also draws out a pattern of behaviors of patients. The primary aim of Decision Tree (DT) based diagnostic system is to create a model for early detection and diagnosis of dengue disease. Further, three different tree classifiers namely J48, Random tree and REP tree were evaluated and compared with SOM, Logistic regression and Naïve Bayes for precise diagnosis of dengue positive patients. The aims of the proposed chapter by using the real world dengue disease data from the different hospitals located in Delhi (India) are as follows:

1. Using the real world dengue disease data from the different hospitals located in Delhi (India).
2. To apply the DT technique for precise detection of dengue positive patients.
3. To develop a diagnostic model based on machine learning techniques for early detection and diagnosis of dengue disease and furthermore for the assistance of physicians.
4. To validate the results of the proposed diagnostic model.

RELATED WORKS

E-Diagnostic Model

Machine Learning approaches have been found to have a great applicability for diagnosis and prediction of diseases. For cardiovascular diseases,Das, Turkoglu, and Sengur, (2009), proposed the NN ensemble method enhanced with SAS enterprise miner 5.2 for heart disease diagnosis and evaluated their scheme with accuracy, sensitivity and specificity parameters. Hongmei et al. (2006) offer a medical DSS established on the Multilayer Perceptron to identify and diagnose heart diseases. Their model performance was cross-validated, checked out and bootstrapped to provide more than 90% accuracy in classifying heart disease. Austin et al. (2012) applied bagging, boosting, Random forests, and Support Vector Machine techniques on cardiovascular dataset. Results indicated the higher accuracy rate of Random forest method over all other methods. In case of Chest infections, Tuberculosis and Liver diseases, Yong et al., (2008) used F-test, KNN-ES and FSVM-ES methods to identify HBV-induced Liver failure. Amongst these, the performance of FSVM-ES were found to be superior on accuracy parameter. Kumar and Sahoo (2013) developed a Rule based classification model to anticipate different types of liver diseases and claimed the higher accuracy rate of DT-based classification model. In continuation of their work, Sahoo, Anoop, and Kumar(2014). Applied five Machine learning approaches to evaluate seminal quality and observed that PSO-SVM approach provides better resolution over the MLP, DT, NB and SVM approaches. Orhan and Temurtas, (2012) used the Artificial Immune (AI) technique to examine Chest infections, separating the Chest disease patient's dataset and compared it to Multilayer, Probabilistic, Learning Vector Quantization, and Generalized Regression NNs. The results predicted the better classification accuracy of the AI method. Orhan, Temurtas, and Tanrıkulu, (2010) developed the two MLNN models for the diagnosis of tuberculosis disease, in which one model uses a single hidden layer while another uses two hidden layers. In evaluating the accuracy parameter of both the models, the MLNN with two hidden layers were found to provide better accuracy. Karabatak and CevdetInce (2009) suggested a novel model, grounded along the association rule and NN, to diagnose the breast cancer. Threefold method parameter was used to evaluate the performance of the proposed model and the classification rate. Evaluation of the novel method was performed against the NN model. The results demonstrated the better classification rate of the proposed model. Recently, Chung-Ho et al., (2011) developed a novel model based on the random forest, support vector machine and ANN to diagnose acute appendicitis and evaluated the models in terms of AUC, Sensitivity, Specificity, True predictive and Negative predictive values. The performance of the random forest was found to be the best. Ozcift (2011) used random forest ensemble classifiers to create a diagnostic model for enhancing cardiac arrhythmia diagnosis and the accuracy rate. Yadav, Kumar, and Sahoo (2012) applied three popular machine learning approaches such as tree, statistical and SVM classifiers to detect Parkinson's disease affected patients. The results concluded the more respectable functioning of the logistic regression classifier.

Machine Learning Based Dengue Diagnostic System

In this section, we will focus on literature related to machine learning techniques for dengue prediction. Rahmawati and Huang, (2016) predicted the dengue disease outbreak by using the C-Support Vector Classification. Here, location, air temperature, and daily precipitation attributes were considered the primary factors responsible for the occurrence of dengue. The RBF kernel based C-Support Vector Classification provided better prediction accuracy for the dengue fever outbreak. Mulyani, Rahman and Riza (2016) produced a specialist framework incorporating the Dempster Shafer (DS) and NB procedures for the accurate prediction of dengue fever. In this work, the ES Dempster Shafer theory was adopted to design the rules, whereas the machine learning part was implemented using NB. The proposed ES obtained 70% accuracy in the training phase while the accuracy in the testing phase was calculated to be 56%. Shaukat, Masood, Mehreen and Azmeen, (2015) carried out work with various attributes such as fever, bleeding, flu, and a few others. The authors utilized NB, REP Tree, Random tree, J48 and SOM methods for accurate prediction of dengue and reported that both NB and J48 yield better outcomes than other methods. Similarly, Albinati, Meira, and Pappa, (2016) proposed a Gaussian-based early warning framework for dengue outbreak based on attributes such as humidity, rainfall, temperature, dengue incidence rate. Results witnessed the efficiency of the proposed model to predict the dengue infection rate. Siriyasatien et al. (2016) published a report on significant factors responsible for dengue considering the K-H model, SVM, and ANN in forecasting dengue. It was understood that temperature, rainfall, humidity, wind speed, aedesaegypti larvae infection rate, female mosquito infection rate, male mosquito infection rate, season, and population attributes are main in analyzing dengue infection. Cheong, Leitão, and Lakes (2014) applied boosted regression trees to asses the land use factors associated with dengue. In this work, fifteen attributes such as coconut and cocoa plantation, animal farming, mixed horticulture, plantation and farm, tea plantation, mining, oil palm plantation, neglected grassland, rubber plantation, paddy field, swamp forest, woodland, open state, human settlements and water bodies, used for dengue prediction. It was reported that boosted regression trees can be used as an effective tool to connect the land use factors and dengue. Indeed, a risk map could also be projected for the same use. Althouse et al. (2011) applied step-down linear regression, generalized boosted regression, negative binomial regression, logistic regression and SVM models to predict dengue spread. It was proposed that the SVM-based model yields a higher accuracy rate over other models. Faisal, Ibrahim and Taib (2010) presented an intelligent approach for the detection of dengue by combining MLNNs and SOM with their proposed approach. They establish that the proposed approach provides 70% accuracy rate. Altogether, various soft computing approaches used in the healthcare arena in the last decade for predicting dengue and its diagnosis are discussed in Gambhir, Malik and Kumar (2016) while in Gambhir, Malik and Kumar (2017), a similar study of dengue diagnosis using machine learning algorithms is discussed.

DATASET DESCRIPTION

The details of dengue disease data set are described in this section. The actual data is accumulated from the different hospitals located in Delhi during 2015-2016.A detailed questionnaire is developed to get the relevant data about the patients which is given in Annexure-1. The discretion of dengue dataset is summarized in Table 1. This data set consists of 110 data instances with sixteen attributes and having two classes such dengue positive and negative. The attributes of dengue dataset are Age (years), Sex (M/F), Temperature, Pulse, Platelet count, Fever, Vomit, Abdominal pain, Chills, Body ache, Headache, Weakness, Dengue Antigen (NS1), IgM, IgG, Dengue NS1 Antigen (Elisa). The aim of this data set is the early diagnosis of Dengue disease. It is a two-class problem with class label dengue positive and negative. The dengue positive class describes a dengue affected person, whereas, dengue negative class specifies not affected person. There are 85 samples of dengue positive and 25 samples of dengue negative. The aim of the work is to look into the relationship between the dengue diagnostic result, environmental, and physiological parameters. The normalized values of all attributes of dengue data set are represented in Table 2. Moreover, Figure 1 presents the visual representation of the attributes of dengue data set.

TREE BASED CLASSIFIERS AND OTHER MACHINE LEARNING METHODOLOGIES

This section describes the tree based classifier as one of the prominent machine learning methodologies for resolving the classification problems. These are powerful and popular tools for classification and prediction. These are usually applied for data mining tasks such as ID3, ID4, ID5, C4.5, C5.0, and CART (Quinlan, 1986,1993;

Table 1. Characteristics of dataset

Data Set	Number of Samples	Input Attribute	Output Attribute	Output Classes	Number of Attributes	Missing Attributes	Noisy Attribute
Dengue Disease	110	16	1	2	17	No	No

Table 2. Description of various attributes of dengue dataset

S. No.	Attributes		Data Type	S. No.	Attributes		Data Type
1	Non Clinical	Age	Numeric	10	Clinical	Platelet count	Numeric
2		Gender	Binary	11		Temperature (F)	Numeric
3		Vomit	Binary	12		Heart rate (bpm)	Numeric
4		Abdomen Pain	Binary	13		Dengue Antigen (NS1)	Numeric
5		Chills	Binary	14		IgM	Numeric
6		Bodyache	Binary	15		IgG	Numeric
7		Headache	Binary	16		Dengue NS1 Antigen (Elisa)	Numeric
8		Weakness	Binary				
9		Fever	Numeric				

Utgoff, 1988,1989; Breiman, 1984). The tree classifiers goal is to create a model that predicts the value of a target class for an unseen test instance based on several input features (Loh & Shih, 1997; Safavian & Landgrebe, 1991; Turney, 1995). Hence, it takes off with a source node generating a lot of nodes typically having only one incoming and one outgoing edge (internal clients) with the ease of the guests having no outgoing edges (end nodes or leaf nodes). DT is thus a classifier that forms a tree structure, in which each node is either a leaf node that indicates the value of the target attribute (class) or a decision node that specifies several tests to be carried away on a single attribute value, with one branch and sub-tree for each possible outcome of the test. Among other data mining methods, DTs have various advantages such as (1) it is simple to interpret; (2) it is easy to implement, requiring little prior knowledge; (3) it is able to handle both numerical and categorical data; (4) it is robust; and (5) it can portion out with large and noisy data sets. Compared to other AI methods, DTs represent rules. In fact, these rules can be easily expressed so that everyone can understand them. Likewise, these principles can be used straight off in a database. In some domain instances, the main concern is the accuracy of a

Figure 1. Visual representation of dengue dataset attributes

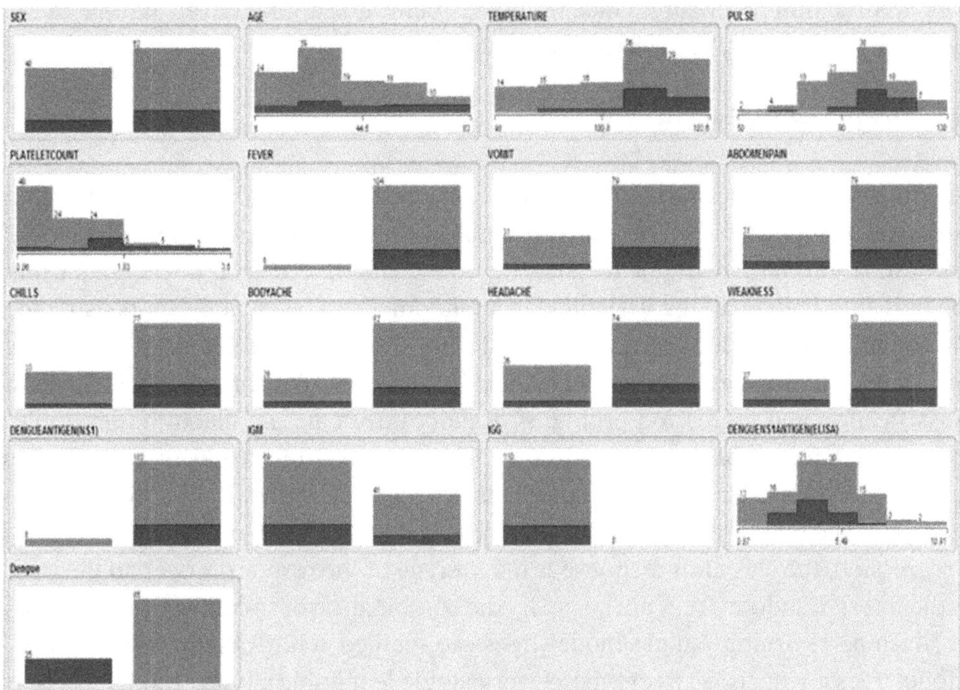

classification or prediction technique whereas, in other cases, the ability to explain the reason for a decision is important. For instance, to predict the male fertility potential, one has to follow, the ingredients involved so that others can employ this knowledge for a successful prediction. Therefore, the domain experts must identify or modeled the crucial parameters fueling this discovered knowledge. Many decision tree algorithms such as the classification and regression tree (CART) (Breiman, Friedman, Stone & Olshen, 1984), the chi-square automatic interaction detector decision tree (CHAID) (Kobayashi, Takahashi, Arioka, Koga, Fukui, 2013), ID3 (Quinlan, 1986), and C4.5 (Quinlan, 1993) have been presented in recent years. Out of these, we would be concentrating on mainly three Tree classifiers, i.e. J48 Tree, Random Tree and REP Tree.

J48 Tree

J48 classifier is a simple C4.5 decision tree for classification and is experienced as an evolution and elaboration of the ID3 algorithm (Interactive Dichotomize 3) with good classification accuracy (Quinlan, 1993; Breiman, Friedman, Stone & Olshen, 1984). It creates a binary tree. The decision tree approach is the most useful in classification problem. With this technique, a tree is constructed to model the classification procedure. Once the tree is built, it is applied to each tuple in the database and results in classification for that tuple.

Random Tree Classifiers

Random Tree is a supervised Classifier; it is an ensemble learning algorithm that generates many individual scholars. It employs a bagging idea to create a random set of data for constructing a decision tree. In standard tree each node splits using the best split among all the variables. In a random forest, each node splits using the best among the subset of predicators randomly chosen at that node. Random trees were introduced by Leo Breiman and Adele Cutler. The algorithm can deal with both classification and regression problems. Random trees are a collection (ensemble) of tree predictors that is called as forest. The classification works as follows: the random tree classifier takes the input feature vector, classifies it with every tree in the forest, and outputs the class label that received the majority of "votes". In case of a regression, the classifier response is the average of the responses over all the trees in the forest. Random Trees are basically the combination of two existing algorithms in Machine Learning: single model trees are merged with Random Forest ideas. Model trees are decision trees where every single leaf holds a linear model which is optimized for the local subspace described by this leaf. Random Forests have shown to ameliorate the functioning of single decision trees considerably: tree diversity is brought forth by two ways of randomization.Start the training data sample with replacement for each single tree like in Bagging.Secondly, when growing a tree, instead of always working out the best possible rent for each node only a random subset of all properties is taken at every node, and the best split for that subset is computed.Such trees are applied to classify Random model trees for the first time by combining model trees and random forests.Random trees employ this for split selection and thus induce reasonably balanced trees where one global context for the ridge value works across all leaves, therefore simplifying the optimization process.

REP Tree

REP Tree uses the regression tree logic and creates multiple trees in different iterations. After that it selects the best one from all the generated trees. That will be considered as the representative. In pruning the tree, the measure used is the mean square error on the predictions made by the tree. Basically Reduced Error Pruning Tree ("REPT") is fast decision tree learning and it builds a decision tree based on the information gaining or reducing the variance. REP Tree is a fast decision tree learner, which constructs a decision/regression tree using information gain as the splitting criterion, and prunes it uses reduced error pruning. It only sort values for numeric attributes once. Missing values are dealt with using C4.5 method of using fractional instances.

Self-Organizing Map

A self-organizing map (SOM) or self-organizing feature map (SOFM) is a type of artificial neural network (ANN) that is trained using unsupervised learning to produce a low-dimensional (typically two-dimensional), discretized representation of the input space of the training samples, called a map, and is therefore a method to do dimensionality reduction. Self-organizing maps differ from other artificial neural networks as they apply competitive learning as opposed to error-correction learning (such as backpropagation with gradient descent), and in the sense that they use a neighborhood function to preserve the topological properties of the input space.

Logistic Regression

In statistics, the logistic model (or logit model) is a statistical model that is usually taken to apply to a binary dependent variable. In regression analysis, logistic regression or logit regression is estimating the parameters of a logistic model. More formally, a logistic model is one where the log-odds of the probability of an event is a linear combination of independent or predictor variables. The two possible dependent variable values are often labelled as "0" and "1", which represent outcomes such as pass/fail, win/lose, alive/dead or healthy/sick. The binary logistic regression model can be generalized to more than two levels of the dependent variable: categorical outputs with more than two values are modelled by multinomial logistic regression, and if the multiple categories are ordered, by ordinal logistic regression, for example the proportional odds ordinal logistic model.

Naive Bayes

In machine learning, naive Bayes classifiers are a family of simple "probabilistic classifiers" based on applying Bayes' theorem with strong (naive) independence assumptions between the features.It was introduced under a different name into the text retrieval community in the early 1960s, and remains a popular (baseline) method for text categorization, the problem of judging documents as belonging to one category or the other (such as spam or legitimate, sports or politics, etc.) with word frequencies as the features. With appropriate pre-processing, it is competitive in this domain with more advanced methods including support vector machines. It also finds application in automatic medical diagnosis.

Proposed Model

This subsection identifies the proposed diagnostic model to detect the dengue disease earlier using decision tree based approaches.The working of the diagnostic model is split into three stages. In the first phase, dengue disease dataset is constructed by collecting information through patients. In this stage, all clinical and non-clinical parameters are projected which are responsible for earlier detection of dengue disease.After gathering information, it is converted into target code using missing information, sampling and preprocessing methods.In the second stage, the different decision tree approaches such as J48, random tree classifier and REP tree is planted in a diagnostic model for more accurate and earlier detection of dengue disease.In this phase, k-cross validation method is likewise used to validate the public presentations of machine learning advances. In the third phase of diagnostic model, performances of tree classifiers and other machine learning approaches are tested using some performance measures. These measures are accuracy, sensitivity, specificity and error rate and resulted in the best performing approach. Figure 2 shows the proposed diagnostic model for earlier detection of dengue disease.

RESULTS AND ANALYSIS

Performance Measures

This subsection describes the various performance measures which are considered in evaluating the performance of the different decision tree based approaches. These performance standards are described as below.

- **Accuracy:** Accuracy of a model is defined as the total positive cases of the model are divided by the total number of cases. Accuracy parameter provides the percent of correctly classified cases. The accuracy of model is defined as

$$Accuracy\left(\%\right) = \frac{TP + TN}{TP + FP + TN + FN}.$$

- **Sensitivity:** This parameter is used to determine the degree of the attributes to correctly classify the person with the disease and is defined as

$$Sensitivity\left(\%\right) = \frac{TP}{TP + FN}$$

- **Specificity:** This parameter is used to determine the degree of the attributes to correctly classify the person without disease and is defined as

$$Specificity(\%) = \frac{TN}{TN + FP}$$

- **Error Rate:** Error rate (ERR) is calculated as the number of all incorrect predictions divided by the total number of the dataset and is defined as

$$Error\ Rate = \frac{FP + FN}{TP + TN + FN + FP}$$

RESULTS AND DISCUSSION

This subsection presents the results of our study. Table 3 illustrates the Confusion Matrix obtained for Dengue dataset using J48, Random Tree and REP Tree techniques. The Confusion Matrix is used to derive the result of performance measures used in this chapter. This matrix contains actual and predicted values of all data instances of Dengue disease. Table 4 depicts the comparative analysis of the results of J48, Random Tree, REP Tree, SOM, Logistic function and Naïve Bayes techniques using different performance criteria. It is seen that REP Tree approach provides better solutions in comparison to other approaches. The REP tree based diagnostic model achieves higher Accuracy, Sensitivity and Specificity rate. While, Random Tree approach exhibits worst performance among all. Moreover, the ranking of each approach is computed with each performance measure. It is observed that the REP tree approach gets the first rank for all parameters. Figure 3-5 represents various Decision trees generated using J48, Random Tree and REP Tree.

Figure 7 presents the performance of different techniques in the graphical manner. It depicts the comparing of the Accuracy, Sensitivity, Specificity and Error Rate parameters of all the six techniques.It is discovered that the REP tree achieves higher accuracy rate, 82.7% respectively.Hence, it is revealed that significant differences occur between the execution of the above mentioned attacks.In conclusion, it can be concluded that REP Tree based diagnostic model is more efficiently capable of observing and diagnosing dengue disease in earlier stage.

Figure 2. Proposed diagnostic model for earlier detection dengue disease

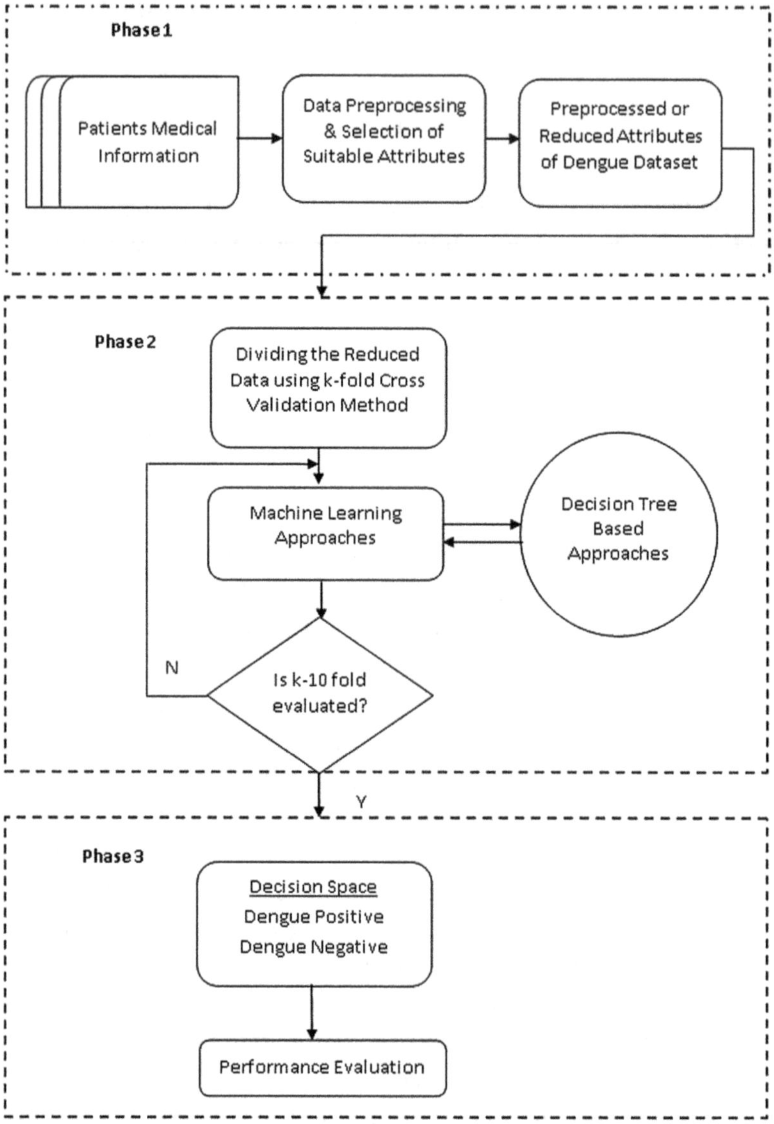

Table 3. Confusion Matrix for J48, Random Tree, REP Tree, SOM, Logistic Regression and Naïve Bayes

Confusion Matrix		J48		Random Tree		REP Tree		SOM		Logistic Regression		Naïve Bayes	
		Predicted											
Actual	Dengue (+)	12	13	8	17	12	13	5	20	15	10	17	8
	Dengue (-)	9	76	16	69	9	76	4	81	8	77	12	73

Table 4. Performance comparison of J48, Random Tree, REP Tree, SOM, Logistic Regression and Naïve Bayes

Parameters	Techniques					
	J48	Random Tree	REP Tree	SOM	Logistic Regression	Naïve Bayes
Accuracy	80	73.66	82.7	78.1	80.6	81.8
Rank	4	6	1	5	3	2
Sensitivity	89.4	81.1	92.9	83.4	90.5	91.3
Rank	4	6	1	5	3	2
Specificity	84.4	82.55	89.9	83.7	85.0	85.8
Rank	4	6	1	5	3	2
Error Rate	20	26.34	17.3	23.8	19.1	18.5
Rank	4	6	1	5	3	2
Overall Rank	4	6	1	5	3	2

Figure 3. Decision tree generated using J48

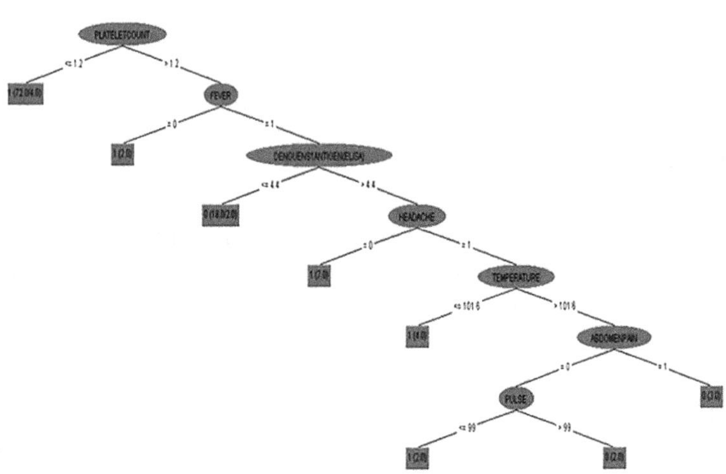

Figure 4. Decision tree generated using Random Tree

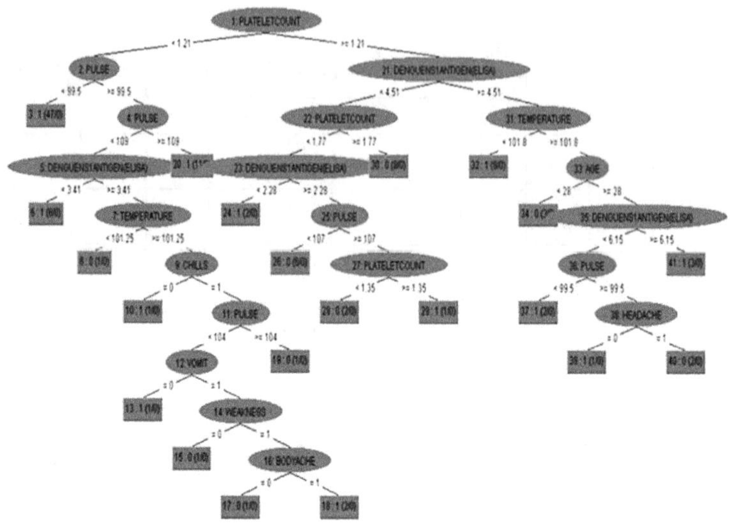

Figure 5. Decision tree generated using REP Tree

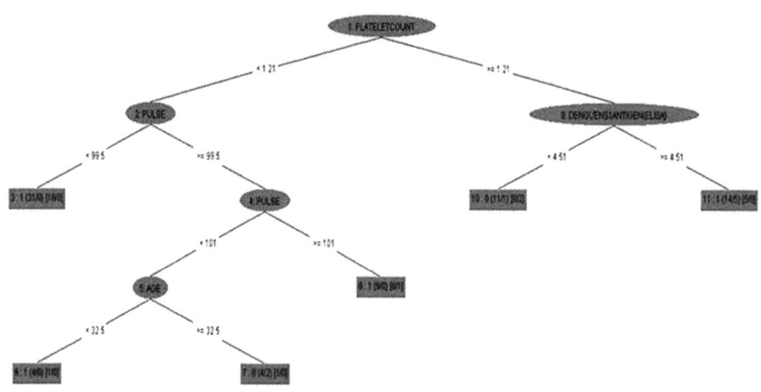

CONCLUSION

The aim of this work is to produce a diagnostic model for earlier detection and precise prediction of dengue disease using different Decision Tree approaches and compare their performance with other machine learning approaches.To achieve the same, three popular Decision Tree approaches such as J48, Random Tree and REP tree are selected to get the desired effect and they are also compared with other machine learning approaches like SOM, NB, and Logistic Regression.In this study, real world Dengue disease data are compiled from different hospitals located in Delhi

Figure 6. ROC generated using Logistic Function, SOM, Naïve Bayes, J48 Random Tree and REP Tree

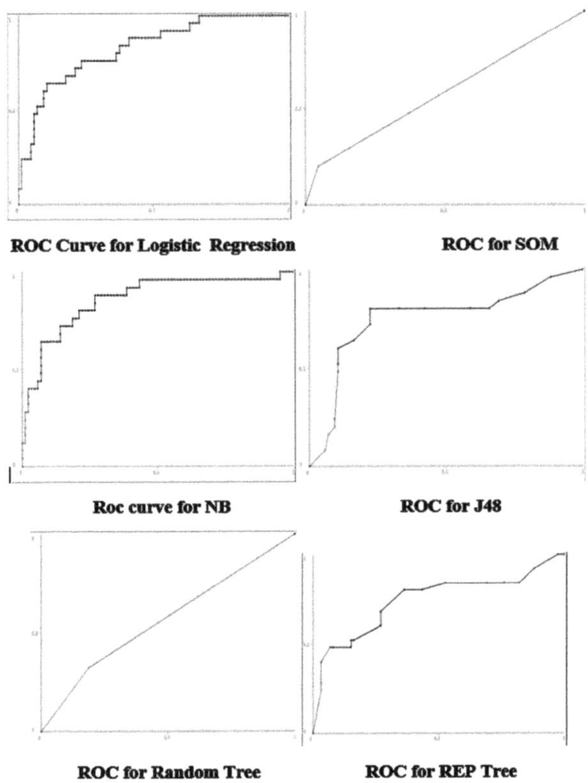

Figure 7. Performance comparison of Accuracy, Sensitivity, Specificity and Error rate parameters for J48, Random Tree, REP Tree, SOM, Logistic Function and NB

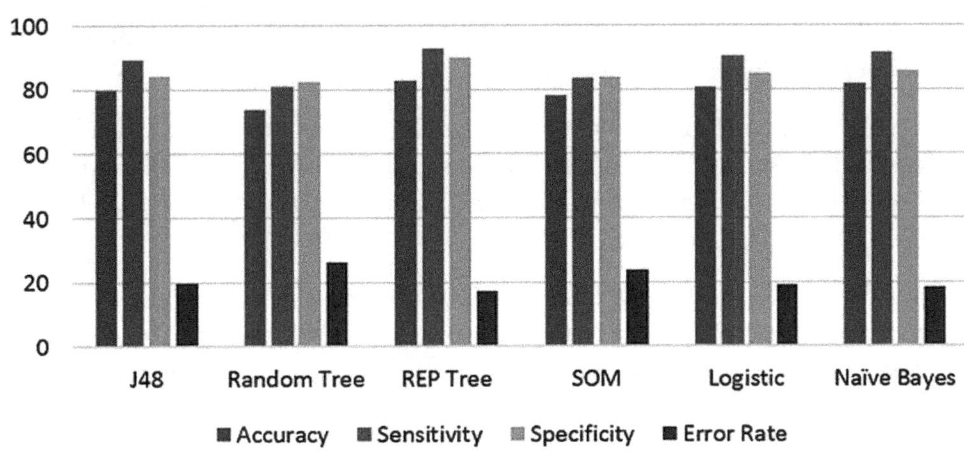

area.Final dataset consists of information of 110 patients suffering from Dengue fever and other fevers and this dataset is split into two classes i.e. Dengue positive and Dengue negative. Further, it is observed that eighty five patients are reported dengue positive and the restis dengue negative. On final dataset, some machine learning approaches such J48, Random Tree, REP tree, SOM,Logistic Regression and Naïve Bayesare applied for earlier detection and diagnosis of Dengue disease. The executions of these approaches are evaluated using Accuracy, Sensitivity, Specificity and Error parameters.From experimental results, it can be reasoned that the REP tree approach provides more beneficial results than other approaches.

REFERENCES

Albinati, J., Meira, W., & Pappa, G. L. (2016). An Accurate Gaussian Process-Based Early Warning System for Dengue Fever. In Intelligent Systems (BRACIS) (pp. 43-48). IEEE.

Althouse, B. M., Ng, Y. Y., & Cummings, D. A. (2011). Prediction of dengue incidence using search query surveillance. *PLoS Neglected Tropical Diseases*, *5*(8), e1258. doi:10.1371/journal.pntd.0001258 PMID:21829744

Andreeva, P. (2006). Data modelling and specific rule generation via data mining techniques, *Proc. International Conference on Computer Systems and Technologies,* 17–23.

Austin, P. C., Lee, D. S., Steyerberg, E. W., & Tu, J. V. (2012). Regression trees for predicting mortality in patients with cardiovascular disease: What improvement is achieved by using ensemble-based methods? *Biometrical Journal. Biometrische Zeitschrift*, *54*(5), 657–673. doi:10.1002/bimj.201100251 PMID:22777999

Breiman, L., Friedman, J., Stone, C. J., & Olshen, R. A. (1984). *Classification and regression trees*. Chapman and Hall/CRC.

Bujlow, T., Riaz, M. T., & Pedersen, J. M. (2012). A method for classification of network traffic based on C5.0 machine learning algorithm. *Proc. of the International Conference on Computing, Networking and Communications (ICNC)*, 237–241. 10.1109/ICCNC.2012.6167418

Cheong, Y. L., Leitão, P. J., & Lakes, T. (2014). Assessment of land use factors associated with dengue cases in Malaysia using Boosted Regression Trees. *Spatial and Spatio-temporal Epidemiology*, *10*, 75–84. doi:10.1016/j.sste.2014.05.002 PMID:25113593

Chopra, A., Saluja, M., & Venugopalan, A. (2014). Effectiveness of chloroquine and inflammatory cytokine response in patients with early persistent musculoskeletal pain and arthritis following chikungunya virus infection. *Arthritis & Rheumatology (Hoboken, N.J.)*, *66*(2), 319–326. doi:10.1002/art.38221 PMID:24504804

Chung-Ho, Lu, Lee, Wen, Min-Huei, & Li. (2011). Novel solutions for an old disease: Diagnosis of acute appendicitis with random forest, support vector machines, and artificial neural networks. *Surgery*, *149*(1). PMID:20466403

Das, R., Turkoglu, I., & Sengur, A. (2009). Effective diagnosis of heart disease through neural networks ensembles. *Expert Systems with Applications*, *36*(4), 7675–7680. doi:10.1016/j.eswa.2008.09.013

Dengue Guidelines for Diagnosis, Treatment, Prevention, and Control in Subsaharan Africa and 1 Countries in South America. (2009). Geneva: World Health Organization.

Er, O., Temurtas, F., & Tanrıkulu, A. Ç. (2010). Tuberculosis disease diagnosis using artificial neural networks. *Journal of Medical Systems*, *34*(3), 299–302. doi:10.100710916-008-9241-x PMID:20503614

Faisal, T., Ibrahim, F., & Taib, M. N. (2010). A noninvasive intelligent approach for predicting the risk in dengue patients. *Expert Systems with Applications*, *37*(3), 2175–2181. doi:10.1016/j.eswa.2009.07.060

Gambhir, S., Malik, S. K., & Kumar, Y. (2016). Role of Soft Computing Approaches in HealthCare Domain: A Mini Review. *Journal of Medical Systems*, *40*(12), 287. doi:10.100710916-016-0651-x PMID:27796841

Gambhir, S., Malik, S. K., & Kumar, Y. (2017). PSO-ANN based diagnostic model for the early detection of dengue disease. *New Horizons in Translational Medicine*, *4*(1-4), 1–8. doi:10.1016/j.nhtm.2017.10.001

Hongmei, Y., Yingtao, J., Jun, Z., Chenglin, P., & Li, Q. (2006). A multilayer perceptron-based medical decision support system for heart disease diagnosis. *Expert Systems with Applications*, *30*(2), 272–281. doi:10.1016/j.eswa.2005.07.022

Jonsson, P., & Wohlin, C. (2004), An evaluation of k-nearest neighbour imputation using likert data. *Proc. software metrics, 10th international, symposium*, 108–118.

Karabatak, M., & Ince, M. C. (2009). An expert system for detection of breast cancer based on association rules and neural network. *Expert Systems with Applications*, *36*(2), 3465–3469. doi:10.1016/j.eswa.2008.02.064

Kobayashi, D., Takahashi, O., Arioka, H., Koga, S., & Fukui, T. (2013). A prediction rule for the development of delirium among patients in medical wards: Chi-Square Automatic Interaction Detector (CHAID) decision tree analysis model. *The American Journal of Geriatric Psychiatry*, *21*(10), 957–962. doi:10.1016/j.jagp.2012.08.009 PMID:23567433

Kumar, Y., & Sahoo, G. (2013). Prediction of different types of liver diseases using rule based classification model. *Technology and Health Care*, *21*(5), 417–432. PMID:23963359

Loh, W. Y., & Shih, X. (1997). Split selection methods for classification tree. *Statistica Sinica*, *7*, 815–840.

Mulyani, Y., Rahman, E. F., & Riza, L. S. (2016). A new approach on prediction of fever disease by using a combination of Dempster Shafer and Naïve bayes. In Science in Information Technology (ICSITech) (pp. 367-371). IEEE.

Muniaraj, M. (2014). Fading chikungunya fever from India: Beginning of the end of another episode? *The Indian Journal of Medical Research*, *139*(3), 468. PMID:24820844

Orhan, E., Yumusak, N., & Temurtas, F. (2012). Diagnosis of chest diseases using artificial immune system. *Expert Systems with Applications*, *39*(2), 1862–1868. doi:10.1016/j.eswa.2011.08.064

Ozcift, A. (2011). Random forests ensemble classifier trained with data resampling strategy to improve cardiac arrhythmia diagnosis. *Computers in Biology and Medicine*, *41*(5), 265–271. doi:10.1016/j.compbiomed.2011.03.001 PMID:21419401

Palaniappan, S., & Awang, R. (2008), Intelligent heart disease prediction system using data mining techniques. *Proc. 2008 IEEE/ACS International Conference on Computer Systems and Applications,* 108–11.

Quinlan, J. R. (1986). Induction of decision tree. *Machine Learning*, *1*(1), 81–106. doi:10.1007/BF00116251

Quinlan, J. R. (1993). *C4.5: Programs for machine learning*. Morgan Kaufman Publishers Inc.

Rahmawati, D., & Huang, Y. P. (2016). Using C-support vector classification to forecast dengue fever epidemics in Taiwan. In System Science and Engineering (ICSSE) (pp. 1-4). IEEE.

Safavian, S. R., & Landgrebe, D. (1991). A survey of decision tree classifier methodology. *IEEE Transactions on Systems, Man, and Cybernetics*, *21*(3), 660–674. doi:10.1109/21.97458

Sahoo, G., Anoop, J., & Kumar, Y. (2014). Seminal quality prediction using data mining methods. *Technology and Health Care*, *22*(4), 531–545. PMID:24898862

Santosh Kumar, P. S. (2017). *Malaria, dengue and chikungunya in India – An update*. Indian J Med Spec. doi:10.1016/j.injms.2017.12.001

Shaukat, K., Masood, N., Mehreen, S., & Azmeen, U. (2015). Dengue Fever Prediction: A Data Mining Problem. *Journal of Data Mining in Genomics & Proteomics*.

Siriyasatien, P., Phumee, A., Ongruk, P., Jampachaisri, K., & Kesorn, K. (2016). Analysis of significant factors for dengue fever incidence prediction. *BMC Bioinformatics*, *17*(1), 166. doi:10.118612859-016-1034-5 PMID:27083696

Tu, M. C. (2009). A comparative study of medical data classification methods based on decision tree and bagging algorithms. *Proc. IEEE 8th international conference on dependable, autonomic and secure, computing*, 183–187. 10.1109/DASC.2009.40

Turney, D. (1995). Cost-sensitive classification: Empirical evaluation of a hybrid genetic decision tree induction algorithm. *Journal of Artificial Intelligence Research*, 369–409.

Utgoff, P. E. (1988). ID5: An incremental ID3. *Proc. of the fifth National Conference on Machine Learning*, 107–120.

Utgoff, P. E. (1989). Incremental induction of decision trees. *Machine Learning*, *4*(2), 161–186. doi:10.1023/A:1022699900025

World Health Organization. (2007). *Anopheline Species Complexes in South and South-East Asia*. SEARO Technical Publication No. 57.

Yadav, G., Kumar, Y., & Sahoo, G. (2012). Predication of Parkinson's disease using data mining methods: A comparative analysis of tree, statistical and support vector machine classifiers. *Proceedings of National Conference on Computing and Communication Systems (NCCCS)*, 1–8. 10.1109/NCCCS.2012.6413034

Yong, M., Xin, H., & Yu, K. (2008). Metabonomic analysis of hepatitis B virus-induced liver failure: Identification of potential diagnostic biomarkers by fuzzy support vector machine. *Journal of Zhejiang University. Science. B.*, *9*(6), 474–481. doi:10.1631/jzus.B0820044 PMID:18543401

Chapter 4
Innovative Approaches for Pre-Screening and Sensing of Diseases

Dharmpal Singh
JIS College of Engineering, India

Gopal Purkait
Pailan College of Management and Technology, India

Abhishek Banerjee
Pailan College of Management and Technology, India

Parag Chatterjee
Pailan College of Management and Technology, India

ABSTRACT

Prescreening and sensing of diseases offers a number of benefits that can help in prevention of major diseases. The aim of disease pre-screening is to detect possible disorders or diseases in people who do not have any symptoms. Earlier screening methods for the detection of diseases was invasive, complicated, and would require extensive tests. Some conventional methods used in clinical diagnoses include many invasive and potentially hazardous biopsy procedures, endoscopy, computed tomography; numerous innovative approaches have evolved to overcome the limitations of traditional techniques. Non-invasive biomedical sensor, genomics, electronic nose, nano-material, plasmonicsensor devices, microfabrication-based technologies, flat-panel detectors, digital breast object models, endomicroscopy, breath biopsy, and wavelet-based enhancement methods are some of the emerging frontiers in prescreening and sensing of diseases. This chapter will provide an in-depth discussion of the abovementioned innovative techniques related to prescreening and sensing of diseases.

DOI: 10.4018/978-1-5225-7131-5.ch004

INTRODUCTION

Today early diagnosis of deadly diseases can save precious human life. Proper pre-screening and sensing of diseases are very important for administering right treatment. In this book chapter we will discuss about different innovative pre-screening and sensing technology of different diseases. The goal of disease pre-screening is to detect potential health disorders or diseases in people who do not have any symptoms of disease. Numerous innovative approaches have evolved over the years which aim to overcome the limitations of traditional techniques for pre-screening and sensing different diseases. The recently evolved methods are Non-invasive biomedical sensor, Genomics, electronic nose, Nano-materials, plasmonic sensor devices, micro fabrication-based technologies with cell biology, flat-panel detectors (FPDs), digital breast object models, endomicroscopy, breath biopsy and wavelet-based enhancement methods. Non-invasive Biomedical sensor devices offer a variety of benefits such as early detection and also provide prevention of the risk of infection.

Carole Foy et al., (2012) used the new generations of technologies, such as ultra-high throughput sequencing to identify the outbreaks of food borne disease as compared to other previous technologies to reduce the risk of the disease. Electronic nose devices were used by Wilson (2015) to analyze the human breath profiles and opined that diagnosis will be much faster than earlier detection of human diseases and disorders. Few of the authors also used the volatile organic compounds (VOCs) (Broza & Haick, 2013) by using Nano-material-based sensors, Surface Plasmon Resonance (SPR) and Localized Surface Plasmon Resonance (LSPR) (Barizuddin, Bok & Gangopadhyay, 2016) to provide earlier detection of diseases and suggest the applications of medical diagnostics, environmental monitoring and food safety.

Moreover, Ertl, et al., (2014) presented a micro-fabrication-based technology based on cell biology for the development of advanced in-vitro diagnostic system which will be capable of analyzing cell cultures under physiologically relevant conditions. O'Connor et al. (2010) have proposed the techniques called digital breast object models for investigation of emerging tomographic breast imaging and opined that it has outperformed the previous mammographic screening technique. Jabbour et. al., (2012) discussed about Confocal endomicroscopy; high resolution and non-invasive imaging technology to evaluate the microscopy of cellular and sub-cellular features in tissues. Therefore, the authors have opined that it can detect any disorder; and may be provide significant advantages over conventional wide-field microscopic imaging.

Breath Biopsy is an innovative technology which can detect the presence of lung and colorectal cancer from breath samples by measuring levels of molecules called volatile organic compounds (VOCs). Z¨ohrer et al., (2010) proposed Interactive Multi-scale Contrast Enhancement for Previously Processed Digital Mammograms based on wavelet-based enhancement method. This will automatically and interactively adjust the contrast of previously processed mammograms and provides better identification of breast cancer. The diversified authors have used different techniques for Pre-Screening and Sensing of diseases but the summary of new innovative approaches has not been stated by most of authors.

Novel biomarkers have evolved that has been found to be useful in pre-screening of diseases. Specifically Biomarkers can be used for patient selection in clinical trials. Biomarkers (Elrakshy& Fayed, 2014) such as high sensitivity cardiac troponin T or B-type natriuretic peptide can be used for screening and thus identifying patients with silent cardiac target organ damage (TOD). This can help in early detection of abnormal cardiovascular problems in human heart. Biomarkers (Abdollah, et al., 2015) has been used for diagnosing asymptomatic prostate cancer (PCa), using Prostate-specific antigen (PSA) testing and also reduce the need for unnecessary biopsies. Therefore, in this chapter an effort has been made to provide an idea of innovative approaches for pre-screening and sensing of diseases along with their implication.

Prescreening of Diseases

The purpose of disease prescreening is to sense physical condition of person who does not have any symptoms of disease. Non-invasive biomedical sensor devices offer a diversity of benefits such as early discovery and thus hindrance of the risk of infection, ease of use and suitability for long-term monitoring.

Significance of Prescreening of Disease

The concepts of pre-screening tests are present but it is not obvious which tests are considered as good and which are not. The concept of diagnostic tests is mainly used to detect the cause of certain symptoms whereas pre-screening tests are done for people who do not have illness feeling. Pre-screening tests can detect diseases at beginning stage, prior to any noticeable symptoms. This gives an advantage in treating the diseases much earlier which also improve a better health outcome at early stage.

Many tests used in medical for pre-screening purposes are not suitable for making an ending diagnosis to sense any abnormalities of direct tests. Screening tests are not done for all time to gaze for a disease but it can also detect risk factors for certain diseases. The concept of pre-screening is based on the logic "prevention is better than cure". People also think that pre-screening is "prevention," from the disease but screening tests cannot protect people from the disease but it takes "preventive" measures to determine risk factors that could afterward culminate into a disease, for example endoscopy of the bowel can be used to sense and eliminate intestinal polyps which could later develop into cancer.

It has been observed that if people have effective pre-screening test, they would have lived longer than without effective pre-screening test. Moreover, screening may enhance quality of life as shown in figure 1a and 1b (cPubMed Health, 2016) respectively.

Impact of Prescreening for Diseases

Many researchers have used various types of scientific methods to perform and evaluate the screening tests. For example, in the beginning analysis was made to find out how trustworthy the test is and furthermore see how a patient benefits from early starting treatment rather than later. Moreover, it is also necessary to see which groups of people benefit from early diagnosis and treatment and how the benefits compare to the risks.

Generally, pre-screening followed two steps. In the first step, it looks for a signs of the disease and test is considered to be "positive" if signs of the disease is found

Figure 1. a) Illustration: Survival rate without screening; b) Illustration: Survival rate with screening

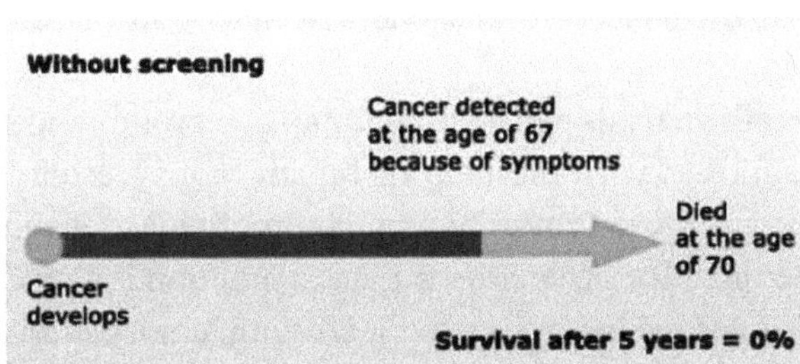

Survival rate without screening

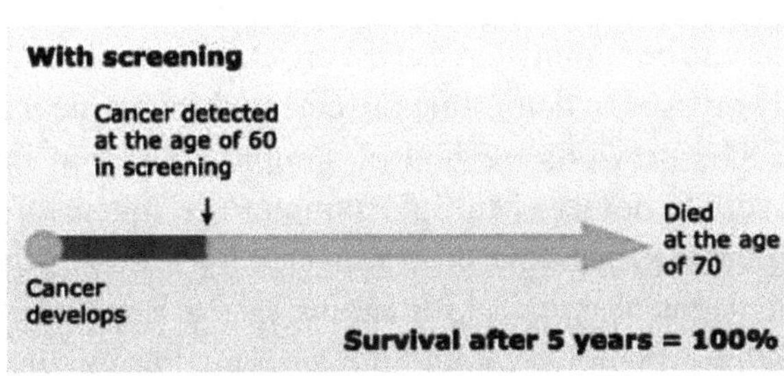

Survival rate with screening

and "negative" if no signs of the disease are present. In the second step, further tests need to be done for more accurate diagnosis and this step is performed only if a positive confirmation from previous step is made.

In technical terms, pre-screening test can be used to recognize disease in people hat whether the disease is "true positive" with high "sensitivity." It means that people who are ill will not missed. A test can also be used to classify the disease in people who do not have the disease as "true negative" with high "specificity." This means that the examination can be used to precisely catch people who already have the disease.

INNOVATIVE TECHNIQUES FORPRE-SCREENING AND SENSING OF DISEASES

Breath Biopsy

Breath is a combination of nitrogen, oxygen, carbon dioxide, and water vapor and trace amounts of volatile organic compounds (VOCs). These trace amounts of VOC can be used to assess state of person's health. Breath biopsy (Phillips et al., 2003; Pereira et al., 2015) is a non-invasive approach that relies upon volatile composition of the exhaled breath (EB) to determine volatile composition of bloodstream and airways which in turn can lead to analysis and detection of status of a person's health and well being.

Furthermore breath analysis can be used for all age groups and sex. Today breast cancers can be diagnosed with the help of breath biopsy. Breast cancer leads to increase in oxidative stress & polymorphic cytochrome oxidase enzymes (CYP). These factors enhance the quantity of volatile organic compounds (VOCs) in the breath. Once the breath samples are taken from patients with abnormal mammograms they are tested for sensitivity & specificity to verify the occurrence of breast cancer. Such breath tests are employed as a primary screen for breast cancer. In addition to breast cancer detection breath analysis can be employed for respiratory, renal etc diseases.

Breath analysis can be used as a detecting biomarker for classification of disease so that correct treatment can be administered at the onset. The presence and concentration of VOC can directly be used to determine the current biochemical activity and state of cells & tissues. The previous method of sample collection in breath analysis was exhaling to a sensor device. Multiple samples are taken for effectiveness of diagnosis from patients. It has now been replaced by a more advanced high end analytical Instruments such as gas chromatograph mass spectrometers (GC-MS) that are capable of detecting VOCs with high analytical accuracy.

Plasmonic Sensors

Plasmonic sensing (Elshorbagy, Cuadrado, & Alda, 2017) can detect nano-scale light after it interacts with the surface of the device. Light is efficiently channeled as the surrounding refractive index changes. Plasmonics can be used to increase the intensity of electromagnetic fields for better sensing. Every human carries some amount of CEA which can be detected by plasmonic sensors for early sensing of cancers and other diseases. Plasmonic sensing can be used for high frequency targets, measurement of PH, can be used for cells and tissues of human body. SurfacePlasmon resonance sensors can be integrated with micro fluidics, photonic circuits, which can be used to build comprehensive sensing systems for single chip lab. A label-free bio-sensing technique is known as Localized surface Plasmon resonance (LSPR) which provides robust and facile detection. Surface Plasmon resonance technologies are now widely used to measure bio-molecular interactions whereas Traditional LSPR-based bio-sensing utilizes the sensitivity of the Plasmon frequency to changes in local index of refraction at the nano-particle surface.

Micro Fabrication

Bio-sensors for prescreening and sensing of diseases can be designed using micro-nano fabrication technologies (Maheshwari, Chatterjee, & Rao, Sept. 2014). Micro-electro-mechanical systems (MEMS) technology was conceived to fabricate complex mechanical structures on a micro level. MEM's devices can be designed using organic, inorganic and biomaterials. Micro fabrication reduces production costs, size of devices making them highly portable. Some of the types of micro fabricated biosensors are given below:

- Micro fabricated biosensor can be used for measuring glucose levels in blood.
- Enzyme bio-sensors are easily available commercially and can be used for a variety of purposes including enzyme isolation and purification.
- Affinity biosensors are popular, since they provide information about binding of antibodies to antigens, cell receptors to their ligands,DNA/RNA to complementary sequences of nucleic acids that can be used for screening of gene products.
- Immunosensors are based on the high selectivity of the antibody–antigen reaction. Measurements can be made directly and results can be obtained in a couple of minutes.

The sensors may operate either as director as indirect sensors often referred to homogeneous and heterogeneous immunosensors, respectively. Bio-sensors also can be designed for optical sensing.

Flat Panel Detector

Flat Panel Detector (Kim, Cunningham, Yin, & Cho, 2008; Iovea et al., 2015) is suitable for a wide range of examination applications. Advantages of flat panel detectors includes high resolution images in digital format which reduces processing and thereby diagnosis times. Another characteristic of FPD is wide field of view which allows better scan of the area under diagnosis. Flat panel detectors are nowadays commonly being employed by speech therapists to perform Video Fluoroscopy VF examinations and endoscopic procedures. 14*17 FPD are very effective for orthopedic and gastrointestinal examinations. FPD are different from image intensifiers since images taken don't have any missing edges thereby rendering a complete and a realistic view of affected areas. VF examinations are also convenient for wheelchair patients. Examinations can be done from the front by adjusting the X-Ray tube as per requirements. This allows reduction in the amount of time taken for examining a patient. Also FPD can be reoriented in a transverse manner for examination of pelvis and also convenient for taking images of elbows and back of hands. Re-imaging may not be required when we are using FPD in VF is for general radiography.

Digital Breast Object Models

Enhancing breast cancer detection capabilities results in reduction of mortality rates. X-ray breast imaging systems are complex and require large number of clinical trials wherein a number of repeated images are taken and then quality parameters are compared. Risk is present in such trials due to exposure from ionizing radiation. A better alternative is to use digital breast imaging chain object models. Digital models (Catanuto, et al., 2006) provide better contrast and resolution than traditional methods. Simulation pipeline is used to perform virtual clinical trials (VCT). Simulation of the image formation process by which the virtual phantom in object space is processed by each component of the imaging system, resulting in the detected data (synthetic images) is a necessary procedure in breast imaging VCTs. The last stage of a breast imaging VCT pipeline models the performance of a particular, relevant clinical task (e.g., lesion detection or the detection of micro calcification clusters), making use of the synthesized imaging data in either the projected data domain or following image reconstruction.

CT Breast Imaging (CTBI) and Breast Tomosynthesis (BT) (Bakic, Ringer, Kuo, Ng, & Maidment, 2010) imaging systems are currently being developed and studied by a number of researchers and commercial vendors. Preliminary evidence suggests that these tomographic breast imaging systems have potential for improving visualization of breast masses at approximately equivalent dose to mammography. Digital Breast Tomosynthesis (DBT) (Yang, Hipwell, Hawkes, & Arridge, 2012) provides information regarding fibroglandular tissues and abnormal lesions by reconstructing a pseudo-3D image of the breast. Digital Breast Tomosynthesis (DBT) involves acquiring a small number of low dose X-ray images, over a limited angle, and reconstructing this data into a pseudo-3D image of the breast. Increased sensitivity relates to early detection of diseases while increased specificity reduces patient anxiety and clinical costs. Optical image analysis (Attia, Blackledge, Abood, & Agool, 2012) for detection of breast cancer is also being employed. Such methods employ feature vectors and require calculation of statistical values such as mean, mode, median. All components of feature vector are calculated to understand characteristics and geometric structure of imaged cells. The recognition process employs a segmentation algorithm called the adaptive imaging threshold procedure that operates using pixel intensity values.

Endomicroscopy

Endomicroscopy (Crowe, Liao, & Curtin, 2015) can be used for obtaining real images from the human body in a relatively short amount of time. Endomicroscopes have higher resolution and a good field of view. Endomicroscopes uses laser light for the imaging process. The uses of Endomicroscopes are in imaging of gastrointestinal tract, pancreatic cysts and lesions. It can be used for characterization of Barrett's Esophagus. Traditional wide field microscopy cannot be used for properly imaging thick tissues due to out of background signal whereas in confocal method a laser is used to obtain a point by point construction of image. Galvanometers and scanning mirrors are used in confocal microscopes to facilitate the scanning process. Today Endomicroscopes have typically a scanning head over an imaging probe and fiber wires are used to transfer the scan signals to a system.

Confocal laser endomicroscopy (Chauhan, 2014) is a newer endomicroscopy method that can be used to obtain high resolution images of living tissues using optics. The accuracy of CLE is high when we are diagnosing intestinal metaplasia, problems in esophagus and problems in peripheral nerves. A new method for diagnosing the upper GI tract disease is called as capsule endomicroscopy wherein microscopy optics is inserted in a capsule which is swallowed by the patient. A thin strand containing optical fiber is used as a connection to the capsule. Rapid images are taken while the capsule travels to the esophagus and it is being pulled back at constant velocity. Multiple iterations are done to get a clearer set of images from which final diagnosis can be made. Advantages include cheap cost of the pill and the ease of administering it to the patient. Also it does not require the patient to be sedated.

Wavelet-Based Enhancements

Breast cancer is one kind of cancer which is developed from breast tissue. It is public health problem in our world. Wavelet transform and homomorphism filtering technique (Gorgel, Sertbas, & Ucan, 6 June 2009) is a new approach for mammographic image enhancement. Wavelet transform of the mammogram is obtained and the approximation coefficients are filtered by homomorphic filter. After that detail coefficients of thewavelet associated with noise and edges are modeled by Gaussian and Laplacian variables. Then coefficients are compressed by the variables with shrinkage function. Then adjusted approximation and other details are thresholded using which objects can be separated from the background. Finally inverse wavelet transform applied for getting the processed image. Another kind of Wavelet-based enhancements (Namdeo & Bhadoriya, 2016) is used for speech enhancement. Different kinds of thresholds are used for different wavelet bands. Then pause detection algorithm is used for estimating the noise profile and after those thresholds are adapted which enables the modified enhancement system to handle colored and non-stationary noises. A wavelet-based voiced/unvoiced classification is implemented which improves the performance of the enhancement system.

Non-Invasive Biomedical Sensor Devices

The term non invasive is related with medical science. It is a technique that does not involve puncturing the skin or entering a body cavity. Non-Invasive Sensor Technology(Lin, Gal, Mayzel, Horman, & Bahartan, July 2017) is used for pre-screening and sensing of diseases. Glucose monitoring system is one kind of non invasive bio-medical sensor devices. Some non invasive biomedical sensor devices are discussed below: -

- **Gluco Watch:** It is a wristwatch-type device that provided real-time measurements of interstitial glucose concentrations at 10-minutes intervals.
- **OrSense NBM-200G:** It is a non-invasive optical measurement platform which combined with a finger attached ring-shaped sensor probe that contains light sources and detectors operating in the red/near-infrared RNIR spectral region.

- **C8 MediSensors:** It measures continuous glucose in every 5 minutes. It was the lack of the need for calibration against blood glucose values.
- **GlucoTrack:** It consists of a main unit MU and a personal ear clip PEC and sensors. These sensors measure specific ultrasonic, electromagnetic and thermal parameters of the earlobe tissue.
- **Combo Glucometer:** It is based on four light emitting diodes LEDs. Due to the absorption, when the light passes by the fingertip, the spectrum that is detected also changes. The processor analyzes the signal and extracts the bio parameters from the signal. The device must be calibrated before use.
- **Sugar BEAT:** It measures the amount of glucose present at 5-minute intervals.
- **Gluco Wise:** It transmits radio waves of low power through a section of the human body, such as the area between the thumb and forefinger or the earlobe to extract glucose levels.

Another kind of non-invasive sensor device (Costanzo,2017) has been implemented for measuring the glucose of a human body. This technology is based on microwave sensors. To improve accuracy different kinds of imaginary part of permittivity is incorporated in the simulation model. The design process of the microwave sensor is improved by adopting analytical models which assumes the biological material as lossy radiation medium. On the other side, further developments are also performed to investigate dielectric models for inhomogeneous biomaterials, thus improving the accuracy of future implementation of microwave biosensors.

Other kind of non invasive wireless sensor devices (Behara & Das, 2017) are implemented for children and infants in Pre-hospital and Acute hospital Environments. Actually it is a prototype which consists of Arduino based multi-input sensor system with wireless transmission. Software used for this hardware device is based on sensor platform developed on the Arduino system and also for database. Another kind of non-invasive biomedical sensor devices are applicable for measuring the Pulse rate (Heart rate), Blood Oxygen, Body heat (body temperature), height, weight and BMI. Different kinds of hardware are implemented for measuring the above mentioned features. Some techniques are the following:

- **Blood Oxygen and Pulse Rate Measurement Using PPG:** It consists of two light sources and a photo-detector. They are connected to a signal processing unit to measure the light intensity of the received light at the photo-detector.
- **Non Contact Body Temperature Measurement:** It is used to measure the body temperature.
- **Anthropometric Measurements:** It is used to measure the height of a person with accuracy 0.3 cm.

Autism Spectrum Disorder (ASD)

Autism Spectrum Disorder (Brentani, et al., 2013; Fuentes, et al., 2012) is a group of neuro-developmental disorders. Here "Spectrum" refers to symptoms, skills, and levels of disability. Autism occurs due to hereditary factor and differences in the development of certain brain functions. Weak communication and interpersonal skills, stereotype eye contact and not understanding another person's feelings are symptoms of Autism. Understanding of child's developmental conditions and arrangement of appropriate assessment and training are the solution of Autism. For initial assessment there are some pre-screening criteria. They are:

1. The Childhood Autism Rating Scale (CARS)
2. Determination of social abilities and adaptive skills.
3. Screening for maladaptive behaviours and comorbid problems
4. Screening for medical comorbidities (history of elimination disorders, seizures, gastrointestinal problems, growth abnormalities.
5. Screening for indicators of genetic syndromes associated with autism.
6. Parent Report Measures: - It measures some clinical observation of behaviours. The instruments may be used as a supplement to the parent report measures.
7. Referral of a Child with Possible ASD: - It is a resource directory which consists of geographic location, individual contact within the team, an explanation of the referral process, accepted insurance plans and rendered services.

Screening Instruments for ASD

There are four categories for pre-screening of Autism.

1. **General Developmental Measures**: These are designed to gather and track developmental progress in young children. Development varies with respect to their reliability, validity and ability
2. **Screening Tools Specific to ASD:** Within the past few years, a variety of screening tools specific to ASD have been developed. They are:-
   a. **The Stage 2—Pervasive Developmental Disorders Screening Test (PDDST-II):** It is a parent report measurement which is designed to indicate the likelihood of global and pervasive developmental disorders in children from birth through 3 years of age.
   b. **The Modified Checklist for Autism in Toddlers (M-CHAT):** It is a 23-item checklist designed as a screen for ASD at 2 years of age.

c. **The Checklist for Autism in Toddlers (CHAT):** It is a psychological questionnaire designed to evaluate risk for autism spectrum disorder in children ages 18–24 months.

d. **The Screening Tool for Autism in Two-Year-Olds (STAT):** These properties were improved when the sample was limited to children 14 months and older.

Other kind of pre-screening and diagnostic tools are listed below:

1. **ADI-R:** It is a Standardized, semi-structured interview for parents and effective under below 4 years of age.
2. **ADOS:** It's use depends on expressive language level and chronological age of child. It is useful for its moderate sensitivity and good specificity for autism.
3. **CARS:** It's diagnostic observation applicable for above 2 years of age.
4. **GARS:** It is one kind of Diagnostic parental interview which is applicable for 3-22 years of age.
5. **PIA:** It is one kind of Diagnostic parental interview process which is applicable for less than three years.
6. **PDDST-II:** It is applicable for its moderate sensitivity and good specificity for birth to 18 months.
7. **STAT:** Trained professional use this tool for 24-36months of child. It is famous for moderate sensitivity and good specificity for autism
8. **Charlie:** Another technology i.e. "Charlie" (Laura, 2014) is a new robot prototype used for developing the performance of children with autism. It is a new single-point infrared sensor technique for detecting breathing and heart rate remotely. It has a head and two arms. Each has two degrees of freedom and a camera. Human hands classifier and face classifier are jointly used for creating two autonomous interactive single player games.

Sniffphone (Smart Phone for Disease Detection From Exhaled Breath)

Breath analysis is a very powerful tool for clinical diagnostics because it is painless. We know that human breath contains a number of volatile organic compounds (VOCs). Accurate detection of specific VOCs in exhaled breath is known as biomarkers which can provide essential information for the diagnosis of specific diseases. Different kinds of techniques are used for detection of exhaled breath.

- **GC-MS:** It is an analysis technique used to identify traces of VOCs in exhaled breath.

- **PTR-MS:** It measures the ionized VOCs produced by reaction with precursor hydronium ions (H3O+) in a drift-tube reactor.
- **SIFT-MS:** It analyzes ions which is produced by the reaction of analyses and precursor ions (H3O+, NO+ or O2+) by quadruple MS.
- **SMO-Based Chemiresistive-Type Sensor:** It measures resistivity changes based on the thinning or thickening the depletion layer of n-type SMOs and hole accumulation layer of p-type SMOs around the surface when exposed to oxidizing or reducing gas ambient.

SNIFFPHONE is a smart phone combining heterogeneous micro and nano technologies used to analyze disease markers from exhaled breath. By nature it is an interaction between samples breath and miniature array of highly sensitive nonmaterial based chemical sensors. Sample breath is recorded, stored and preprocessed by integrated small on-chip micro fluids and electronics. After that relevant electrical signals are transferred via internet to an external server. Then statistical pattern recognition methods are applied on the received data. After that result of clinical report is generated and received by the receiver like specialist or doctor. SNIFFPHONE combine functionalities which are relevant to the health screening applications with decreased size and cost, increased predictive and cognitive functions and full autonomy with energy management and operations.

REVIEW OF NEW APPROACHES

Implication of Innovative Approaches

A disease is one or more abnormal condition that affects parts or whole body which is not caused by external injury. There are different kinds of devices for prescreening of diseases like Non-invasive biomedical sensor, electronic nose, Nano-material, plasmonicsensor devices, micro-fabrication-based technologies, flat-panel detectors (FPDs), digital breast object models, endomicroscopy, breath biopsy and wavelet-based enhancement method and SNIFFPHONE. Besides their advantages there are so many disadvantages. Non active sensors emit radiation and may cause problems to the user. Problems with non invasive sensors are the delay between the blood collection and its analysis, which doesn't permit a real-time patient monitoring in critical situations.

Nano materials are thermodynamically stable and lie in the region of high-energy local-minima. but it has some disadvantages like impurity, instability of particles and it is also biologically harmful. Nano particles are highly reactive. They inherently interact with impurities as well. It is usually considered harmful as they become transparent to the cell-dermis. There are no hard-and-fast safe disposal policies for nano-materials. Results of exposure experiments are also not available. Surface Plasmon resonance sensors can be integrated easily with micro fluidics, photonic circuits, which can be used to build comprehensive sensing systems for single chip lab. A label-free bio-sensing technique is known as Localized surface Plasmon resonance (LSPR) which provides robust and facile detection.

Quality assurance and training for Digital breast object models is a critical factor in its widespread implementation. Interval cancers represent a limitation of breast screening that should prompt further research for optimization. Evaluation of over diagnosis is a highly debated topic in the literature. According to most realistic available calculations, over diagnosis is acceptable as it is compensated by the potential mortality reduction. Nonetheless, this potential side effect warrants optimal adjustment of therapy to the patient's individual risk. The mortality reduction seen in randomized studies was confirmed by results from national screening programs. Another popular device is the Electronic Nose which is an important part of E-sensing system which can be used to detect a variety of flavours artificially. Electronic nose typically includes sensor arrays and pattern recognition systems. The major parts of electronic nose systems are a delivery system, a detection system, a computing system. The delivery system enables the generation of the volatile compounds of a sample, which is the fraction analyzed. The detection system, which consists of a sensor set, is the "reactive" part of the instrument. A specific response is recorded by the electronic interface transforming the signal into a digital value which is measured by the computing process. Electronic nose can be conveniently programmed to detect smells artificially which in turn can be used for effective pre-screening of diseases.

Limitation of Prescreening and Sensing Approaches

A major limitation of modern techniques in prescreening and pre-sensing of disease is in Promoting the development of innovative ICT tools to increase patient's adherence to screening programs and the creation of less invasive tools. A disadvantage of object based image analysis (OBIA) is that its accuracy depends on Segmentation process. A significant point in such image analysis process is the scaling of segmentation. Compared to pixel based techniques the computational cost of object based analysis of images is higher. In the case of micro-fabricated devices the transition from design to reality and implementation has been few in the case of biosensors for example biosensors for measuring glucose levels are commonly available. Problems to be overcome may include sample preparation and system integration. In breath biopsy techniques the main limitation of exhaled breath analysis is the lack of recommended guidelines in the sampling of exhaled breath. Also technical limitations prevented viable implementations of the idea using confocal microscopes for endomicroscopy.

4. CASE STUDY AND IMPLICATION'S SOLUTION OF NEW APPROACHES

Case Study on PneumONIA

A case of Pneumonia has been presented by Zafar et. al. (2016) Pneumonia is a serious infection in lower respiratory tract commonly caused by inhaled bacteria and viruses. The symptoms of pneumonia are high fever, breathing problem, chest pain, and productive thick cough.

Case Presentation

A boy 3 months old was suffering from cough, fever, dyspnoea, vomiting and diarrhoea for the period of last 5 days had been admitted to the hospital. His body temperature, respiratory rate was 102°F and 28 beats /min respectively.

Diagnosis

Complete blood count, Chest X-Ray, Electrolyte count tests were performed. From the Complete blood count doctors found that his Total leukocytes count and lymphocytes concentrations had increased, neutrophils decreased. From the Chest X-Ray doctors detected a white patch on left side upper lobe and they confirmed pneumonia.

Treatment

After confirmation of pneumonia the doctor's started treatment. They prescribed injection Cefotaxime 250 mg intravenous B.D, injection Ampicillin 125 mg intravenous after 6 hours, given Nebolization with ventoline, Oxygen now SOS, and 10 drops of Panadol. The patient fully recovered after 5 days and doctor's discharged the patient.

A Case Study on Breast Cancer

PritishIyer, et. al presented a case study on Breast Cancer. The details of the case study are given below.

Case Presentation

In July 2003, a 40-year-old man went for routine check up to the physician and was found to have a palpable right axillary lymph node.

Diagnosis

The doctors made Excisional biopsy and CT scan for the patient. After analysing the CT scan image they found Widespread Metastatic Disease and confirmed Breast Cancer.

Treatment

The doctors started a course of chemo radiation for unknown primary. Later new left supraclavicular and mediastinal adenopathy was developed, and then doctors gave him chemotherapy with carboplatin and paclitaxel. Biopsy was performed and a PALB 2(Partner and localizer of breast cancer 2) truncating mutation was reported. Then the doctor's suggested for genetic counselling and germline testing for him.

A Case Study on Mixed Connective Tissue Disorder

It is a disease with many connective tissue disorders and the presence of anti-U1RNP (U1 rib nucleoprotein). Katewa et al. (2014) present a case with dyspnea and generalized swelling led to the diagnosis of mixed connective tissue disorder.

Case Presentation

A 60-year-old female admitted with problems was suffering from progressive dyspnea limiting, palpitations, generalized body swelling since 15 days and fever since one week.

Diagnosis

The doctors suggested radiography and Pulmonary function tests for the patient. After analysing the report they found that the patient was suffering from mixed connective tissue disorder.

Treatment

The doctors prescribed for injection amoxicillin/clavulinic acid 1.2 g 1-1-1(three times a day) and paracetamol SOS for fever.

CONCLUSION

In this book chapter an effort has been made to discuss about prescreening and sensing of diseases for earlier detection of deadly diseases. We also present modern available technologies and their implication to detect diseases more accurately. The technologies are non-invasive biomedical sensor, genomics, electronic nose, nano-material, plasmonic sensor devices, micro fabrication-based technologies with cell biology, flat-panel detectors (FPDs), digital breast object models, endomicroscopy, breath biopsy and wavelet-based enhancement method. Novel biomarkers have emerged as a strong candidate in the field of pre-screening since they provide superior diagnostic capability and identification of patient for clinical trials. Popular devices such as electronic nose have been successfully used to detect variety of smells which in turn can be used to identify diseases of the patient. In this book chapter we have also discussed about the limitation of the above technologies. Finally we have presented few case studies of different diseases with diagnosis and treatments.

REFERENCES

Abdollah, F., Dalela, D., Dalela, D., Haffner, M. C., Culig, Z., & Schalken, J. (2015). *The Role of Biomarkers and Genetics in the Diagnosis of Prostate Cancer*. doi:10.1016/j.euf.2015.08.001

Attia, S. J., Blackledge, J. M., Abood, Z. M., & Agool, I. R. (2012). *Diagnosis of Breast Cancer by Optical Image Analysis*. ISSC. doi:10.1049/ic.2012.0198

Bakic, P. R., Ringer, P., Kuo, J., Ng, S., & Maidment, A. D. (2010). Analysis of Geometric Accuracy in Digital Breast Tomosynthesis Reconstruction. *IWDM, 2010*, 62–69.

Barizuddin, S., Bok, S., & Gangopadhyay, S. (2016). Plasmonic Sensors for Disease Detection - A Review [Abstract]. *Journal of Nanomedicine & Nanotechnology, 7*, 373. doi:10.4172/2157-7439.1000373

Behara, S. K., & Das, S. (2017.). Integrated Non-Invasive Biomedical Sensor Module for Measurement of Vital Signs of Human Body for Remote Health Monitoring. *International Journal of Advanced Research in Electrical, Electronics and Instrumentation Engineering, 6*(7). Retrieved July, 2017, from www.ijareeie.com

Brentani, H., Paula, C. S., Bordini, D., Rolim, D., Sato, F., Portolese, J., & McCracken, J. T. (2013). Autism spectrum disorders: An overview on diagnosis and treatment. *RevistaBrasileira De Psiquiatria*. doi:. doi:10.1590/1516-4446-2013-S104

Broza, Y.Y., & Haick, H. (2013). Nanomaterial-based sensors for detection of disease by volatile organic compounds. *Nanomedicine,* (8), 785-806. doi:10.2217/nnm.13.64

Catanuto, G., Spano, A., Pennati, A., Riggio, E., Farinella, G. M., Impoco, G., & Nava, M. B. (2006). *Experimental methodology for digital breast shape analysis and objective surgical outcome evaluation. Journal of Plastic, Reconstructive, & Aesthetic Surgery.* doi:10.1016/j.bjps.2006.11.016

Chauhan, S. (2014). *Confocal laser endomicroscopy.* The American Society for Gastrointestinal Endoscopy; doi:10.1016/j.gie.2014.06.021

Costanzo, S. (2017). *Non-Invasive Microwave Sensors for Biomedical Applications: New Design Perspectives.* Academic Press. doi:10.13164/re.2017.0406

Crowe, C. S., Liao, J. C., & Curtin, C. M. (2015). Optical Biopsy of Peripheral Nerve Using Confocal Laser Endomicroscopy: A New Tool for Nerve Surgeons. *Archives of Plastice Surgery,* 626-629. .2015.42.5.626 doi:10.5999/aps

Elrakshy, Y. M., & Fayed, A. M. (2014, March). Role of biomarkers to identify individuals with silent cardiac disease to help improve primary prevention. *The Egyptian Heart Journal, 66*(1), 22. doi:10.1016/j.ehj.2013.12.062

Elshorbagy, M. H., Cuadrado, A., & Alda, J. (2017). High-sensitivity integrated devices based on surface plasmon resonance for sensing applications. *Photonics Research, 5*(6), 654–661. doi:10.1364/PRJ.5.000654

Ertl, P., Sticker, D., Charwat, V., Kasper, C., & Lepperdinger, G. (2014). *Lab-on-a-chip technologies for stem cell analysis.* Academic Press.

Foy, C., O'Sullivan, D., & O'Brien, S. (2012). Assessing the Potential of Novel Molecular Microbiological Approaches for Managing Food-borne Disease Outbreaks. The Food Standards Agency.

Fuentes, J., Bakare, M., Munir, K., Aguayo, P., Gaddour, N., Öner, Ö., & Mercadante, M. (2012). *Autism Spectrum Disorders.* Academic Press.

Gorgel, P., Sertbas, A., & Ucan, O. N. (2009). *AWavelet-Based Mammographic Image Denoising and Enhancement with Homomorphic Filtering.* Springer Science Business Media, LLC.

Iovea, M., Neagu, M., Stefanescu, B., Mateiasi, G., Porosnicu, I., & Angheluta, E. (2015). Portable low-cost flat panel detectors for real-time digital radiography. *International Symposium on NDT in Aerospace.*

Iyer, P., Jasem, J., Springer, M. A., Klein, C. E., & Kabos, P. (2017). PALB2-Positive Breast Cancer in a 40-Year-Old Man. *Oncology (Williston Park, N.Y.)*, *31*(1), 50–52. PMID:28090623

Jabbour, J., Saluda, M.A., Bixler, J.N., & Maitland, K.C. (2012). Confocal Endomicroscopy: Instrumentation and Medical Applications. *Annals of Biomedical Engineering,* (40), 378-397. doi:10.100710439-011-0426-y

Katewa, R., Jakhar, R. S., & Barala, G. L. (2014). Mixed connective tissue disorder: A case report. *International Journal of Case Reports and Images*, *5*(9), 650–655. doi:10.5348/ijcri-2014116-CR-10427

Kim, H. K., Cunningham, I. A., Yin, Z., & Cho, G. (n.d.). On the Development of Digital Radiography Detectors: A Review. *International Journal of Precision Engineering and Manufacturing, 9*(4), 86-100.

Laura B. (2014). *CHARLIE: a new robot prototype for improving communication and social skills in children with autism and a new single-point infrared sensor technique for detecting breathing and heart rate remotely* (PhD dissertation). University of South Carolina.

Lin, T., Gal, A., Mayzel, Y., Horman, K., & Bahartan, K. (2017). Non-Invasive Glucose Monitoring: A Review of Challenges and Recent Advances. *Current Trends in Biomedical Engineering and Biosciences, 6*(5). DOI:.2017.06.555696 doi:10.19080/CTBEB

Maheshwari, N., Chatterjee, G., & Rao, V. R. (2014, September). A Technology Overview and Applications of Bio-MEMS. *J. ISSS*, *3*(2), 39–59.

Namdeo, A., & Bhadoriya, S. S. (2016). A Review on Image Enhancement Techniques with its Advantages and Disadvantages. *International Journal for Science and Advance Research & Development*, *2*(5).

O'Connor, J. M., Das, M., Didier, C., Mah'd, M., & Glick, S. J. (2010). Development of an Ensemble of Digital Breast ObjectModels. *IWDM*, *2010*, 54–61.

Pereira, J., Porto-Figueira, P., Cavaco, C., Taunk, K., & Camara, J.S. (2015). Breath Analysis as a Potential and Non-Invasive Frontier in Disease Diagnosis: An Overview. *Metabolites, 5*(1), 3–55. doi:10.3390/metabo5010003

Phillips, M., Cataneo, R. N., Ditkoff, B. A., Fisher, P., Greenberg, J., Gunawardena, Rahbari-Oskoui, F., & Wong, C. (2003). *Volatile Markers of Breast Cancer in the Breath.* Blackwell Publishing. doi:1075-122X/03/$15.00/0

PubMed Health. (2016). *Benefits and risks of Screening Tests*. Retrieved from https://www.ncbi.nlm.nih.gov/pubmedhealth/PMH0072602/

Wilson, A. D. (2015). Advances in Electronic-Nose Technologies for the Detection of Volatile Biomarker Metabolites in the Human Breath. *Metabolites,* (5), 140-163. doi:10.3390/metabo5010140

Yang, G., Hipwell, J. H., Hawkes, D. J., & Arridge, S. R. (2012). Numerical Methods for Coupled Reconstruction and Registration inDigital Breast Tomosynthesis. *Annals of the BMVA,* 1-29.

Zafar, M. Z. (2016). A Case Study: Pneumonia. *Occupational Medicine & Health Affairs*, *4*, 242. doi:10.4172/2329-6879.1000242

Z¨ohrer, F., Harz, M. T., B¨odicker, A., Seyffarth, H., Schilling, K. J., Tab´ar, L., & Hahn, H. K. (2010). *Interactive Multi-scale Contrast Enhancement of Previously Processed Digital Mammograms.* Springer-Verlag Berlin Heidelberg.

Chapter 5
Clinical Decision Support System for Early Disease Detection and Management:
Statistics-Based Early Disease Detection

Likewin Thomas
PESITM, India

Manoj Kumar M. V.
NITTE Meenakshi, India

Annappa B.
National Institute of Technology Karnataka, India

ABSTRACT

Medical error is an adverse event of a failure in healthcare management, causing unintended injuries. Proper clinical care can be provided by employing a suitable clinical decision support system (CDSS) for healthcare management. CDSS assists the clinicians in identifying the severity of disease at the time of admission and predicting its progression. In this chapter, CDSS was developed with the help of statistical techniques. Modified cascade neural network (ModCNN) was built upon the architecture of cascade-correlation neural network (CCNN). ModCNN first identifies the independent factors associated with disease and using that factor; it predicts its progression. A case progressing towards severity can be given better care, avoiding later stage complications. Performance of ModCNN was evaluated and compared with artificial neural network (ANN) and CCNN. ModCNN showed better accuracy than other statistical techniques. Thus, CDSS developed in this chapter is aimed at providing better treatment planning by reducing medical error.

DOI: 10.4018/978-1-5225-7131-5.ch005

INTRODUCTION

Nearly every patient hospitalized have a life threat at some point in time during their stay. (Pronovost & Vohr, 2010)

Medical error is a serious threat to the patient's safety. It is being studied that the one of the common causes of a medical error is a faulty health care system. This could be overcome or prevented by providing proper attention towards improving the health care system (Donaldson et al., 2000).

In this section, the authors will introduce a health care system, types, and causes of medical error, along with their statistics. The authors will also introduce an approach to reduce this medical error by using statistical techniques.

Medical Error: Its Cause and Its Types

In the studies conducted during the 1950s regarding patient safety, a medical error was defined as *disease of medical progress* (Moser, 1956). Later in the 1990s, three most important studies on medical error: the "Harvard Medical Practice Study" (Leape et al., 1991), the "Quality in Australian Health Study" (Wilson et al., 1999) and the "Utah and Colorado Medical Practice Study" (Thomas et al., 2000), defined it as an *adverse event*. An adverse event is a failure in medical management, causing unintended injury. As a result of this, the patients may suffer from a disability or longer hospital stay, sometimes even both. But later studies showed that the outcome of an adverse event was a subset of medical error. It is understood that, a safer health care system could be built only by proper design of the processes involved in it. Hence, according to Donaldson et al. (2000) medical error is a *failure in completing the planned action in a pre-defined way or application of an alternative plan (can also be called as the wrong plan)*. The focus of hospitals in a comprehensive health care system is to reduce medical error.

Health care process is compiled by series of clinical and non-clinical activities. Proper treatment management would align these activities and reduce the medical error. For this, it is vital to provide appropriate treatment management from the time of admission. Any failure in this management would lead to an adverse event which is known as medical error.

Statistical Approach for Reducing Medical Errors

Recently, medical error and its consequences were recorded for statistical analysis, and the result has astonished both, the doctors as-well-as a common man (Quaglini, 2009). As a solution for this, an approach was needed that could identify the possible error in the health care system and provide a smoother and safer execution of the treatment process: *care-flow*. Motivated by this, the authors aimed at investigating statistical analysis to assist in reducing this medical error. Thereby, providing proper care to the patients.

The medical community started recording each activity in-order to build a better health care system. Such recorded data is known as Electronic Health Record (EHR). A health care system built using EHR assists the clinicians in taking the critical clinical decision with less medical error (Davidoff et al., 1995). This awareness of medical error and EHR in the medical community was due to clinical pathways proposed by the principles of Evidence-Based Medicine (EBM). The clinical pathways are the protocols written by the multidisciplinary team, who timely intervened and examined the health care system. These protocols aimed to avoid any medical negligence, assist in taking critical clinical decisions and avoid any unseen errors in clinical treatment.

Deployment of Electronic Health Record

With the intention of digitization, deployment of clinical pathways and reducing the medical error, Lary Weed introduced the concept of a problem-oriented medical record in 1960 and named it as EHR (Weed, 2017). EHR assists in retrieving the patient-centric records having information about the treatment plan, medical history and medications of the patients. It also provides access to clinical data and assists in taking appropriate clinical decisions by streamlining the workflow. It aggregates the data of large population and classify them. This aggregation would help the patients in identifying the potential adverse effects that could occur with the new treatment. The illustration of EHR is shown in Figure 1.

Renner (2009) studied that 73% of the health care system with EHR do not correctly use it and in 2013 the statistics remain same. With such a little advancement in deploying EHR in a health care system, implementing a Clinical Decision Support System (CDSS) was a challenge. CDSS is needed for assisting clinicians in taking appropriate clinical decisions and recommending a treatment pathway.

Implementation of EHR in health care promises quality service to the clinical community. But the challenge of this is, there will be a substantial decrease in productivity due to change in traditionally followed the workflow execution, very little knowledge about EHR to the staffs operating this and maintaining both electronic and paper records, at least during the initial transition phase. This delay in process execution was overcome by the application of the California Network for EHR Adoption (CNEA) initiative (Kushinka, 2011). CNEA assist in identifying the data to be recorded, excluding unwanted data. Following information was recorded using CNEA chart abstraction in the current work:

Figure 1. Example structure of EHR system

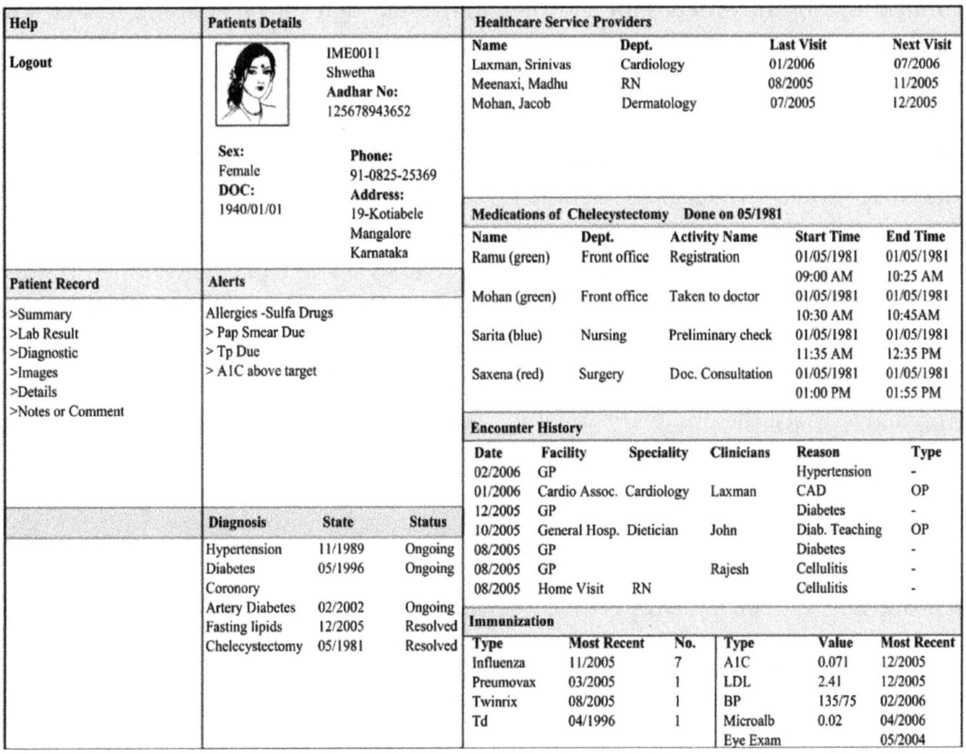

1. The past treatment history, surgeries and consultation.
2. Any allergies and allergies towards drugs.
3. Latest repeat consultation notes.
4. Current and past used medicines.
5. Any immunizations
6. Health maintenance and disease management indicators
7. Alcohol, tobacco or any other bad habits.

The primary chart abstraction methods were:

1. Scanning the already manually recorded documents and then converting them into electronic format.
2. Electronically or automatically recording the data.
3. Manually entering the data.

As the current study is a retrospective analysis, the authors of this paper have scanned already recorded data and then converted that into electronic format for further analysis. Here there was a need of conversion of freely typed clinical note without any structure to structured vocabulary format. The structured vocabulary format was created by using drop-down, checkboxes, radio-button and other data entering tools. Using these tools properly structured data was established. The benefit of structured surgical, treatment, diagnosis, pharmacological and clinical observation is in researching its behaviour and in evidence-based medicine for building Clinical Decision Support System (CDSS). The CDSS developed in this work assists the clinicians in taking clinical decisions and is shown in Figure 2. It is an information system, which extracts the knowledge of the clinical inputs by running the computer-based algorithms and provides an inference from the knowledge extracted to assist the clinicians in taking critical decisions. It also allows the users to study the benefit of the treatment

Proposed System

In proposing system, a CDSS is developed for assisting clinicians in taking clinical decisions. For this, CDSS needed to analyse the recorded clinical data, and build an information model. Developing an information model for a structured and non-

Figure 2. Model of Clinical Decision Support System.

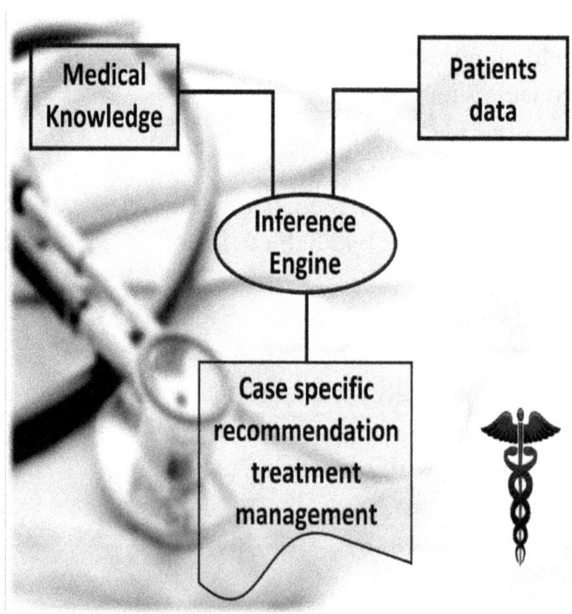

linear representation of clinical data is a challenge. The proposed CDSS works in three phases. In the *first* phase it identifies the risk factors using feature ranking criterion proposed by Yang et al., in 2008. In *a second phase* identify the suitable model using MIPSS. And in *the third phase*, predict the disease progression to identify the critical cases at the time of admission itself.

Identifies the Risk Factors

In this work, the authors in assistance with medical experts re-defined the health care information by first identifying the statistical model best suitable for the input clinical data. In doing this, a statistical comparator: Meta-Model Information and Prognostic Scoring System (MIPSS) using EHR is built. MIPSS compares and selects the useful statistical tool for analysing the EHR and identifying the risk factors associated with them. These risk factors are used as predictors for the prediction of critical cases that may need emergency intervention. Feature ranking criterion proposed by Yang et al., in 2008, measures the importance of any feature by computing its aggregate difference over the feature space. The aggregate difference is the changes in probabilistic output with and without that j^{th} feature. If irrelevant feature is fed into the system, then the prediction goes wrong. So, it is important to identify the right set of risk factors.

Identify the Suitable Model Using MIPSS

Many comparative studies have shown that, Artificial Neural Network (ANN) outperforms regression model. It is known that, ANN mimics the human brain and are composed of a non-linear combination of computational elements known as neurons. Neurons are interconnected using the synaptic connections and are stimulated to process the output. But due to its slow learning and moving target problem (Ohno-Machado, 1996), performance of ANN is unstable. To overcome these limitations of ANN, Fahlman and Lebiere, proposed a Cascade Correlation Neural Network (CCNN) in 1990. It is learned that though CCNN performs better than ANN, it needed further modification/ optimization for showing better performance. In this proposed work, the author modified architecture of CCNN (ModCNN). In ModCNN, the neurons and hidden units are adapted automatically/ dynamically for giving better accuracy.

The MIPSS architecture is shown in Figure 3. Here in the figure, data collected from the retrospective study is fed into Committee of Machines (CoM). ANN, CCNN, and ModCNN are optimized and included in CoM. Each statistical tool finds their significant factors, which are fed back to the system to predict the disease progression eliminating all those features, which are not significant. The accuracy of prediction is measured using the concept of area under the receiver operating characteristic curve (A_Z). Thus, the system first finds the best suitable tool and then using that predicts progression of the disease.

Predicting the Disease Progression

On identifying the risk factors associated with each spectrum of disease, and also by identifying the best suitable statistical model, accurate prediction could be made. The comparison result showed that ModCNN performed better to some extend the data set. Its performance, decreased when the feature set size was increased more than 100. This was overcome using the master - slave model. ModCNN assisted in identifying the independent factors, which were fed to predict and identify the cases which may need an ERCP in later stages of treatment. The experimental comparison of the proposed study with ANN and CCNN showed that ModCNN was better than later techniques.

BACKGROUND

In this section analysis of different statistical techniques for predicting the disease progression is made. As an outcome of this analysis, the authors could find and understand the performance of well-established statistical tools and techniques, for managing the critical cases.

In literature, a lot of regression related studies were found in many diversified areas. But at the same time, many comparative studies were performed between ANN and regression model, and it was observed that ANN had outperformed the regression model. ANN mimics the human brain and are composed of a non-linear combination of computational elements known as neurons. Neurons formed by the biologically non-decomposable units is a mathematical function in ANN. Its task is to receive the inputs, perform some mathematical processing and produce the calculated output. The output is processed through the processing units simulating the neurons. For this, neurons are interconnected using the synaptic connections as in human brains. This synaptic connection allows the signal to pass through the network. The signals are processed elements in ANN which are processed through the interconnecting weights.

ANNs are well-established models for classifying the disease severity and pattern recognition. But, with its high processing units and limited room for computational combinations, it was not only slow in identifying the infrequent patterns, but also failed (Ohno-Machado, 1996). The performance of ANN is unstable due to the presence of local minimum in backpropagation and its convergence is very slow that

Figure 3. The design structure of MIPPS for identifying the efficient model

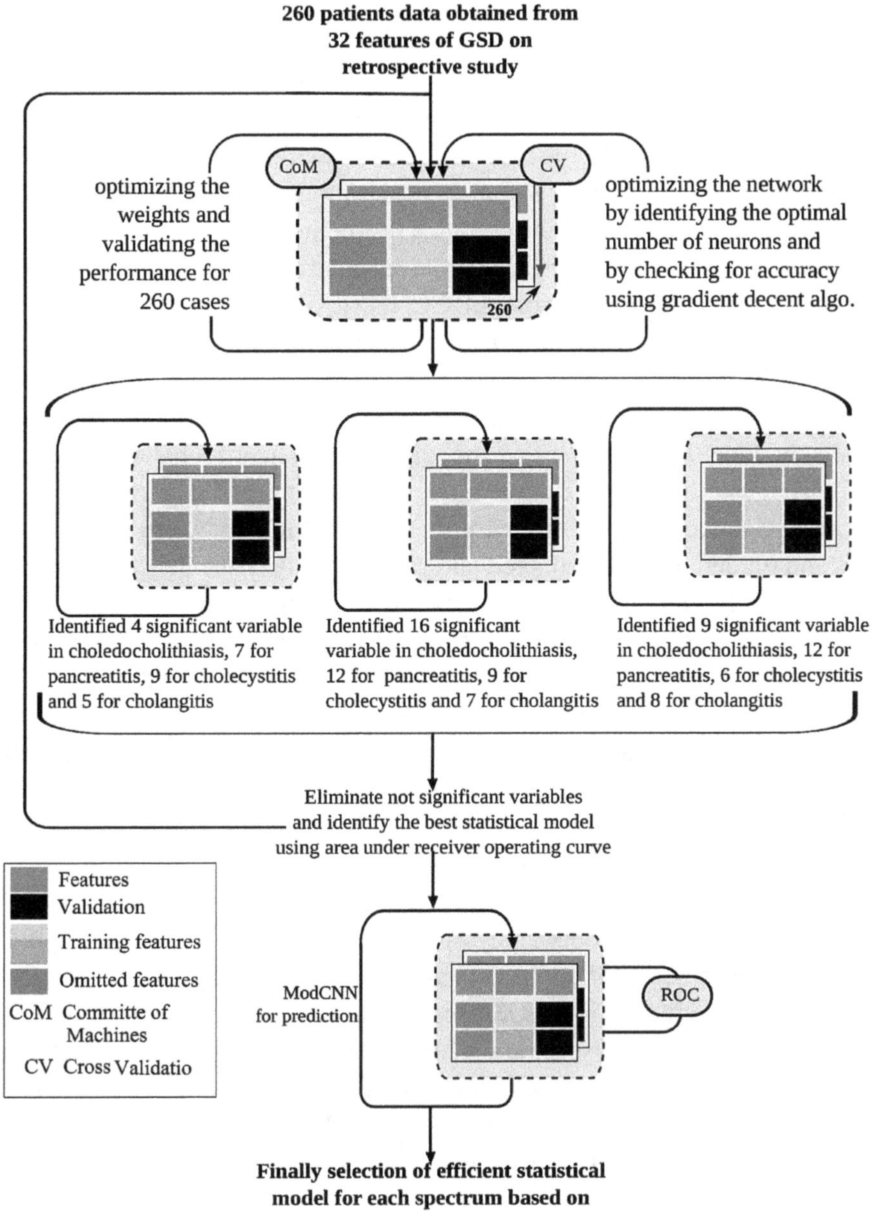

is never ending learning process. Further, backpropagation requires functions in a networked structure and has a high impact on learning capabilities. This limitation of the ANN was widely reported by Cunningham et al. (2000).

To overcome these limitations of ANN, Fahlman and Lebiere (1990), proposed a Cascade Correlation Neural Network (CCNN). In CCNN, the weights are frozen as the hidden units are added to the network. CCNN works on two key architectures: First during the training phase, if the network demands that the addition of new neurons would assist in solving the complex problem more accurately, than CCNN would add new neurons and, secondly addition and training are sequential. Though we found very limited applications of CCNN, it outperformed ANN and other statistical techniques. However, CCNN had a challenge of identifying where to add new neuron Traditionally, it was studied that the neurons were added sequentially. The other challenge was to find, when to add a new node and develop the connection of these new node. It is learned that though CCNN performs better than ANN, it needed further modification/ optimization for showing better performance. This paper presents a modified architecture of CCNN (ModCNN). In ModCNN, the neurons and hidden units are adapted automatically/ dynamically for giving better accuracy. ModCNN assisted in identifying the independent factors, which were fed to predict and identify the cases which may need ERCP in later stages of treatment. The experimental comparison of the proposed study with ANN and CCNN showed that ModCNN was better than later techniques.

This section explains application of regression, ANN and CCNN in the field of medicine and shows the reason for modifying CCNN architecture.

Regression

Due to the limitation of a meta-analysis of being non-operable on a single large experiment, researchers started statistical analysis using regression. Regression application in the epidemiology of GSD is relatively recent. Regression model builds a relationship between the disease and identified risk factors. Historically, the main advantage of a regression model is its computational and theoretical simplicity. This allows the statisticians to have a closer view towards the data behaviour. Following observation were made on studying the performance of regression:

- Regression models assume that all the identified significant risk factors are available in all the test cases. But their absence in the test cases is one of the limitations in applying heterogeneity in regression analysis. Such a restriction of regression is known as data dredging (Marshall, 2001).

- The associative relationship observed by the regression models are less interpreted when compared to the casual relationship. With these restrictions, regression models could be recommended only with pre-analysed significant factors.
- With the restricted samples, discovering the right interpretation is always a challenge in regression.
- Regression models were built with an unrealistic assumption of data and error distributions. Due to which there was a demographic shift from regression analysis to ANN.
- Thus, the authors continued their interest to find the utilization and application of ANN in the field of medicine.

Artificial Neural Network (ANN) Outperforming Regression

In literature, many comparative studies between ANN and regression model were performed, and it was observed that ANN outperforms the regression models. Jovanovic et al. (2014) compared their work on regression (Jovanovic et al., 2011) with ANN for selecting the patients with higher risk towards Endoscopic Retrograde Cholangio-Pancreatography (ERCP). They could find that ANN showed better accuracy with $A_Z = 0{:}884$ when compared to regression model $A_Z = 0{:}787$. Similar kind of comparative study revealed that ANN is better than regression.

Though, it is studied that ANN is a well-established model but, with its high processing units and limited room for computational combinations, it was not only slow for identifying the infrequent patterns, but also failed (Ohno-Machado, 1996). Halonen et al. (2003) compared the performance of regression with ANN for predicting the fatal outcome of severe AP. But, surprisingly the earlier one showed better accuracy of Az=0.862 than the later Az=0.847. The performance of ANN is unstable due to the presence of local minimum in back propagation (Akande et al., 2014). The convergence towards the local minimum is done by backpropagation and is very slow and is the objective of ANN and is a never-ending learning process. Further, backpropagation requires functions in a networked structure and has a high impact on learning capabilities.

Slow-learning nature of ANN prompted the authors to think and research further on constructive training algorithms: CCNN (Fahlman Lebiere, 1990). CCNN automatically adapts the model based on the training process and takes lesser computation, addressing the problems as mentioned earlier of backpropagation. So, the authors continued their research interest to understand CCNN and their suitability in the field of medicine.

Cascade-Correlation Neural Network (CCNN)

Fahlman and Lebiere (1990) introduced a CCNN architecture with cascade correlation of network which learns by experience. Here the weights are frozen as the hidden units are added to the network. The model could solve the classification task more efficiently than the existing models through supervised learning. Itchhaporia et al. (1996) compared the performance with ANN by applying in cardiology for diagnosis of coronary artery disease and myocardial infarction. They found that ANN was too complicated and complex in training process, which made it too slow to get modelled. Doering et al. (1997) modified CCNN and built an optimal CCNN which converged faster than the existing techniques. But on further investigation, it was observed that the existing CCNN needed different training and retraining techniques to improve its performance. Song et al. (2011) regularized the correlation method and reduced complexity of CCNN. This improved the efficiency of CCNN and helped in faster convergence.

Following observations were made on studying performance of CCNN:

- CCNN addressed the limitations of ANN and gave better accuracy.
- However, CCNN had a challenge of identifying when and where to add new neuron.
- On evaluating the ability of CCNN, it was understood that, the model needed training and retraining for further optimization. For this reason, CCNN was modified and named as ModCNN.
- In ModCNN the neurons and hidden units are adapted automatically/ dynamically for giving better accuracy. ModCNN assisted in identifying the independent factors, to predict and identify the cases which may need emergency interventions in later stages of treatment. The experimental comparison of the proposed study with ANN and CCNN showed that ModCNN was better than later techniques.

Assistance of EHR in Clinical Decision Support System (CDSS)

Kim et al. (2008) developed an independent as well as inter-operable and extensible CDSS using EHR. The interoperability was between the CDSS and knowledge engine. Knowledge engine is the key to understanding EHR and assisting in taking appropriate clinical decisions. Focsa (2010) re-engineered EHR for assistance in taking a clinical decision. CDSS that could identify a positive correlation between prior study and EHR about a case was highly needed in an emergency department (Grana & Jackwoski, 2015). From the study of Jalloh and Waitman (2006), it was understood that EHR was the best data source for reducing the medical error.

Using a well-established and adopted EHR process model,

- The best treatment process could be identified.
- The communication about the treatment among the clinical staffs could be made.
- Provide best possible care to the patients.
- Health care resources could be used in a best possible way.

Adoption of EHR in India

Karthikeyan and Sukanesh (2012) observed that the hospitals which have successfully implemented EHR are more efficient and consistent. Most of the health care industry is trying to implement EHR based system. This is achieved by encouraging the conversion of paper-based application to EHR-based. Very soon it can be seen becoming a default health care application in India, marking the beginning of digital India. Sharma and Aggarwal (2016) in their study could find around twenty hospitals where EHR system has been successfully implemented. The medical error in those hospitals are exponentially low, and patients' satisfaction is very high. In a report on "Electronic Health Record standards for India" by Ministry of Health & Family Welfare, Government of India (2013), EHR vendors were classified based on their new scientific creation and workflow processes.

FRAMEWORK AND STUDY MATERIAL

GSD was considered as the case study due to its increasing prevalence in India since last one decade. This study is a retrospective analysis of 260 complicated cases of GSD from the tertiary care centre in North Malabar, Kerala, India, from 2014 to 2015. The pie chart in the Figure 4 shows the classification of different spectrum of GSD. The treatment procedure of these patients was recorded using EHR system for management of GSD.

GSD is a heterogeneous disease and the most common biliary pathology. Due to its unpredictability in progressive organ failure, the mortality rate has been observed from one-third to one-half during the first week of diagnosis. The previous study conducted by Hong et al. (2013) showed that most of the death occurred after admission was due to local complication such as pancreatic necrosis, with the symptoms of sepsis and multi-organ failure. GSD is also studied to be a significant risk factor for gallbladder cancer (Kapoor, 2006). Early detection and timely management of GSD would prevent the progression towards an adverse complication. Thus, there is a need for an optimal classification technique for identifying the spectrum of GSD and significant factors/ predictors associated with each class. These significant factors help in predicting the disease progression from which any unseen complications could be avoided. Significant factors are identified from the features detected by investigations and observations.

GSD leads to a serious complication if neglected and may cause death. The first week of admission is considered as the high-risk period. But, as the disease progresses, there are later stage complications. If not properly treated, it may grow to become cancer. Due to its heterogeneity, predicting its progression is highly difficult and challenging. Hence there was a need for a technique that could categorize the study material, identify the risk factors and predict the disease progression using the identified risk factors. The pie chart in Figure 4 shows the classification of different spectrum of GSD. The treatment procedure of these patients was recorded using EHR system for management of GSD.

In the current study, 32 features associated with GSD were recorded and is shown in Figure 5, 6, 7, 8 and 9 showing each feature distribution. In these figures different attributes along with their prevalence percentage is shown on the top of the bar. The percentage of each observation of these investigations in the current study is represented as stack bar in the Figures 5 to 9 (Clinical readings observed through lab investigation and USG). In these figures, the length of the stacked bar shows the percentage of observation and is shown on top of the bar.

Figure 4. Classification result of GSD patients

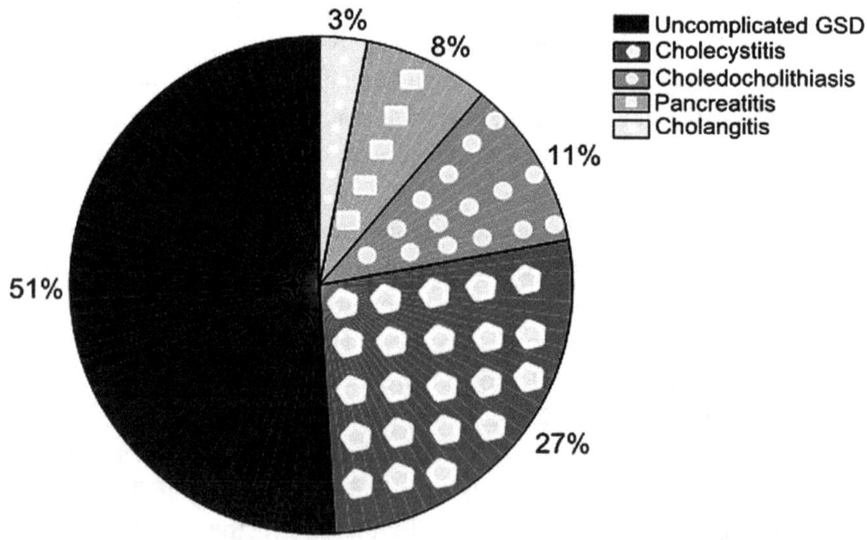

Figure 5. Clinical readings showing SYMPTOMS

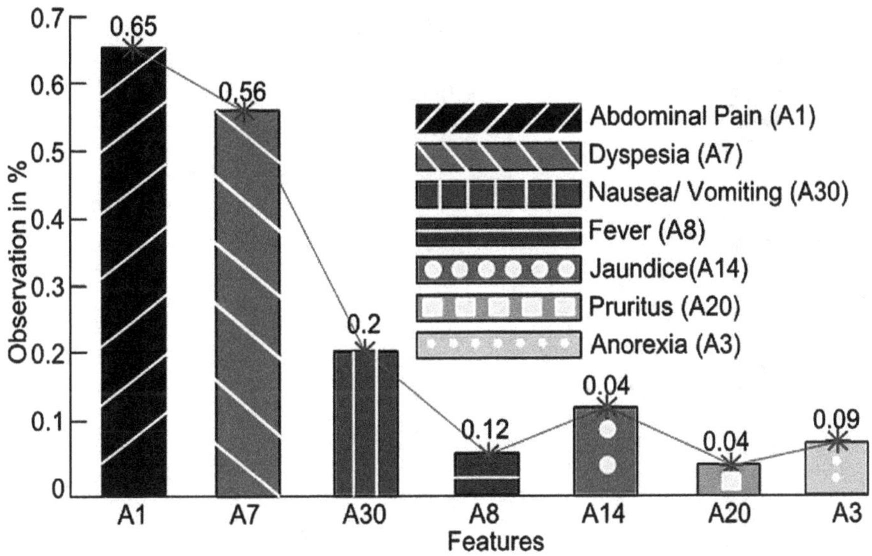

Figure 6. Clinical readings showing SIGNS

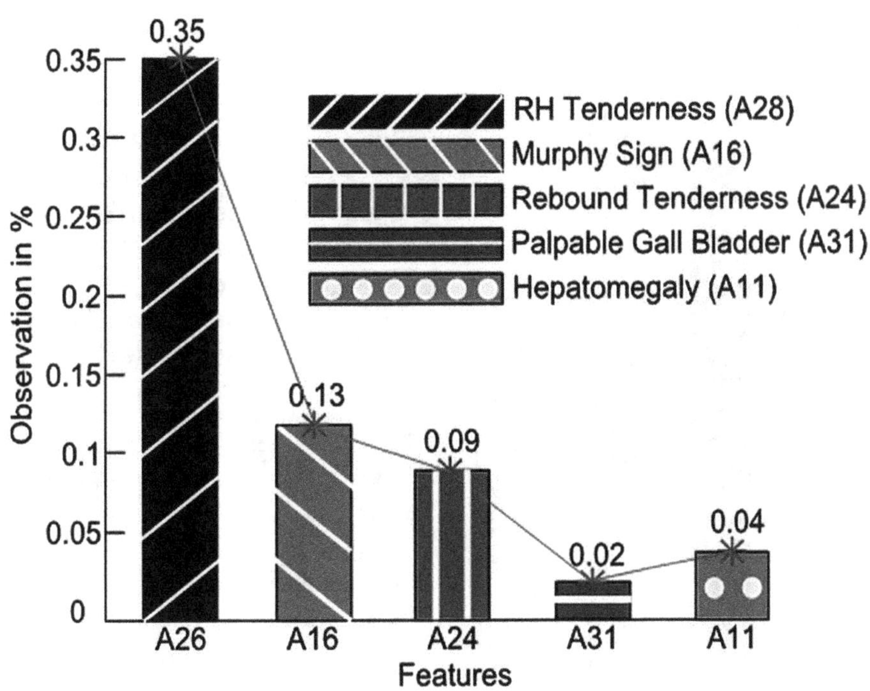

Figure 7. Clinical readings showing COMORBID condition

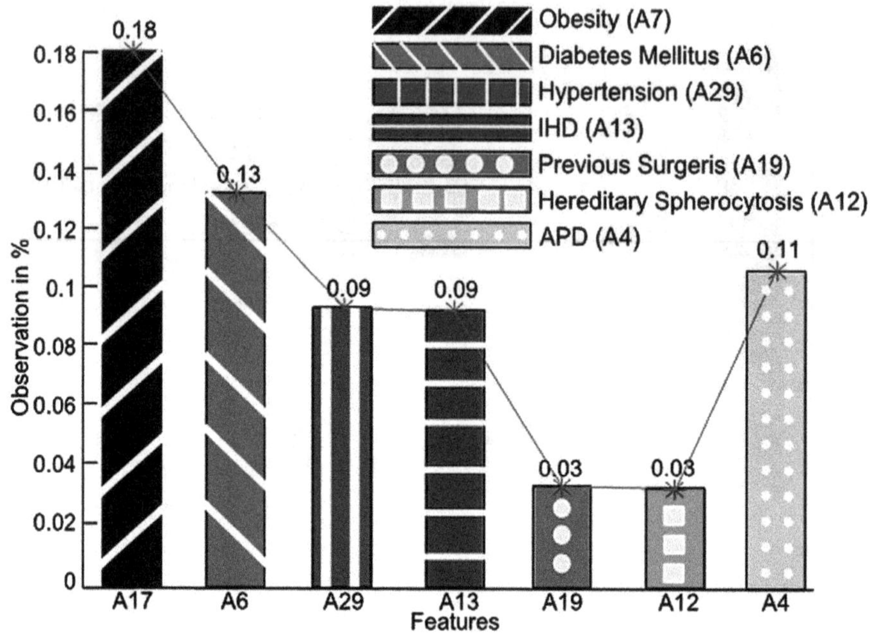

Figure 8. Clinical readings showing TESTS conducted

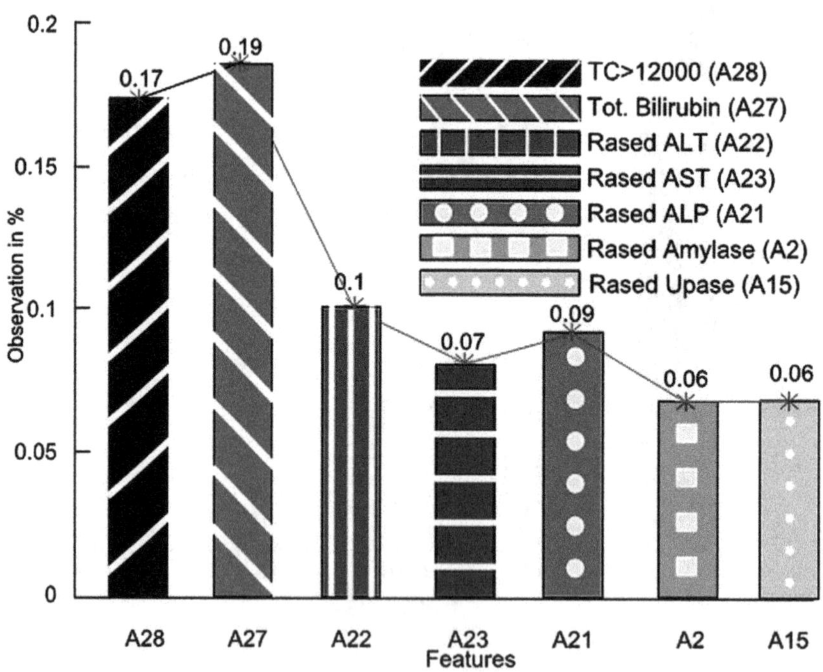

Figure 9. Clinical readings showing USG findings

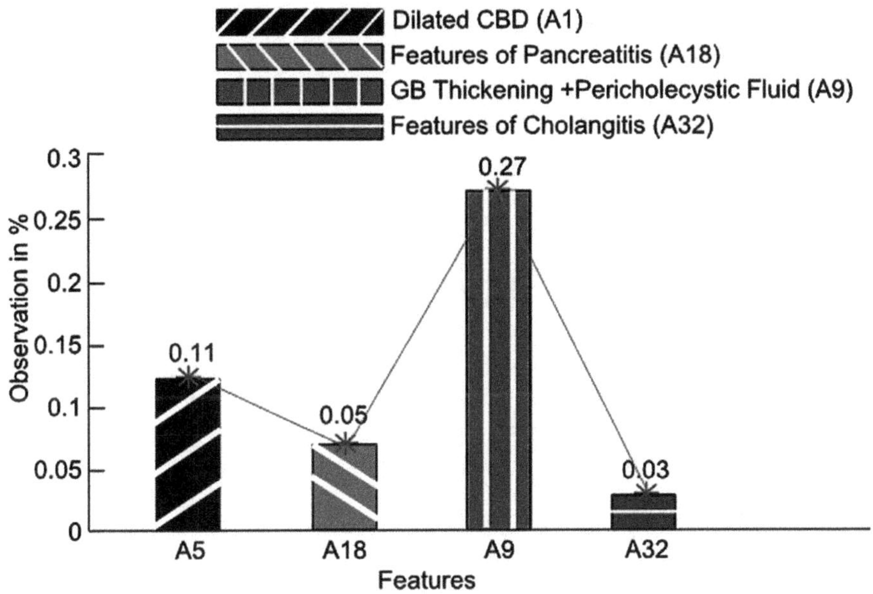

Feature Selection Using Feature Ranking Criterion

Feature selection of the above attribute is needed in order to identify the significant factors from the feature space. This is done to reduce the amount of computation and remove irrelevant feature which reduces the accuracy of prediction. Feature ranking criterion proposed by Yang et al. (2008), was selected after comparing it with Fishers Score *(FisherS)* (Guyon et al., 2003), Mutual Information *(MutualI)* (Peng et al., 2005) and Maximum Output Information *(MOI)* (Sindhwani et al., 2004).

Fishers Score (FisherS)

It is a ratio of "*between variance*" ($\mu_k^j - \mu^j$) and "*within variance*" ($x_i^j - \mu_k^j$) of each feature. Here μ_k^j is the mean of jth feature belonging to k^{th} class and is defined as $\frac{1}{N_k}\sum_{x_i \in w_k} x_i^j$, where N_k is the number of sample $\in$ class w_k. And, $\mu^j = \sum_{k=1}^{c} N_k \mu_k^j / N$ is defined as a mean of μ_k^j overall class *N*. Thus, the *FisherS* is calculated using equation (1).

$$FisherS(j) = \frac{\sum_{k=1}^{c} N_k(\mu_k^j - \mu^j)^2}{\sum_{k=1}^{c}\sum_{x_i \in w_k}(x_i^j - \mu_k^j)^2} \tag{1}$$

Mutual Information (MutualI)

Here feature is selected by combing the mutual information between input and output, and within input variables. Let $A = \{a, b, c, d....m\}$ feature set, then p features among m feature set where $p<m$ can be selected using *MutualI* equation shown in (2).

$$MutualI = \left[I(x^j; y) - \frac{1}{m-1}\sum_{i \in A_{m-1}} I(x^j; x^i) \right] \tag{2}$$

Where, x is the input set and y are the expected output set. I (;) is the mutual information defined in equation (3)

$$I(a;b) = \sum_{a,b} p(a,b)\log\frac{p(a,b)}{p(a)p(b)} \tag{3}$$

Here, *p(a)* and *p(b)* is the distribution function of *a* and *b*, whereas, *p(a, b)* is its joint distribution.

Maximum Output Information (MOI)

MOI is a feature selection process which identifies the feature subset *P* among the *Q* features specified by the user. It increases the mutual information between input (*X*) and output (*Y*) and is defined in the equation (4).

$$MOI = \max_{P:|P|=Q} I(X,Y) \tag{4}$$

This method starts its iteration randomly with some *P* value, using directed search algorithm that iteratively refined the *P*.

Feature-Based Sensitivity of Posterior Probabilities (FSPP)

This is a feature selection process based on the *Posterior Probabilities* of a feature vector $x \in class(w)$ and is defined in the equation (5).

$$FSPP = \sum_{k=1}^{c} \int \left| p(w_k \mid x) - p(w_k \mid x_{-j}) \right| P(x) dx \tag{5}$$

In the equation (5) x_{-j} is the vector space obtained after filtering j^{th} feature and *p(x)* is the probability density function. FSPP selected the feature based on the absolute difference value $\left| p(w_k \mid x) - p(w_k \mid x_{-j}) \right|$. This is a sensitivity of the posterior probability so it is termed as Feature-based Sensitivity of Posterior Probabilities.

Posterior Probabilities

It is a statistical probability calculating that the condition is true under several relevant observations and is defined in equation (6).

$$P(A \mid B) = \frac{P(A) \times P(B \mid A)}{P(B)} \tag{6}$$

Given the prior probability of *P(A)* and *P(B) and* given the conditional probability P(B|A) the posterior probability in equation (6) could be calculated. Conditional probability is the probability of one event *B* conditional on the occurrence of another event *A: P(B|A)* and is defined in equation (7).

$$P(B \mid A) = \frac{P(A \cdot and \cdot B)}{P(A)} \tag{7}$$

Softmax-Based Probabilistic Output

The Figure 10 shows the inclusion of softmax-based probabilistic output for measuring an importance of a feature. Here the experiment was conducted using 10-fold cross verification technique for recursively eliminate the features.

The outline structure of MLP ModCNN considered in this work is shown in Figure 10. It is a probabilistic ModCNN with activation function. The softmax-

Figure 10. Softmax-based function for finding the probabilistic output

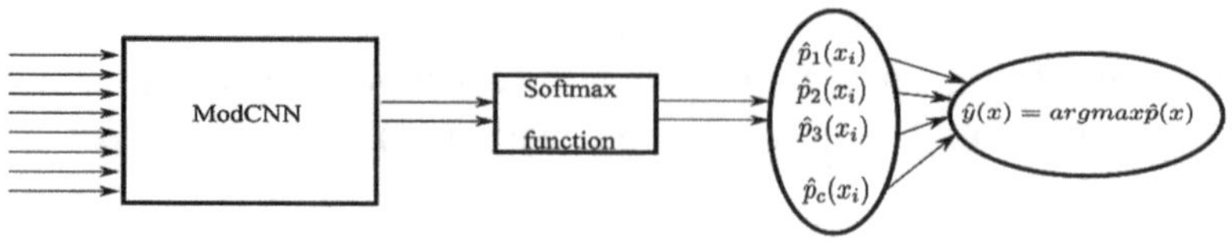

based function is used after output and is shown in equation (8). It provides the probabilistic estimation of the output from ModCNN. The probabilistic estimation determines the probability that the output belong to a particular class.

$$\hat{P}_K(x_i;W) = \frac{e^{\sum Output}}{e^{Output_1} + e^{Output_2} + \ldots\ldots e^{Output_c}} \tag{8}$$

In equation (8), $e^{(\bullet)}$ is an exponential function. FSPP is applied using data $\{x_{-j,i}, y_i\}_{i=1}^{N}$. If there are *d* features retraining of ModCNN has to be carried out *d* times, each time eliminating one feature and checking for the probabilistic output. If there is rise in probability, then it conveys that feature is not important. As in this work 10-fold cross validation technique is applied, the total number of retraining is $d \times 10$.

MODIFIED CASCADE NEURAL NETWORK

ModCNN was built upon the architecture of Cascade-Correlation Neural Network (CCNN). The two key features of CCNN are: neurons are added only when they are needed and if they help in solving the problem: *network on demand* and other feature is, neurons are added sequentially: *one-by-one*.

Artificial Neural Network (ANN)

The synaptic connections in the human brain are unique for every individual and are not entirely inherited. As a learning process, this synaptic connection iteratively trains itself. The Carnegie Mellon University experimented on neurons and studied that every feedback from the different part of human body is purely due to neurons in the brain, which are connected by this synaptic connection. Hence, as a learning process since birth, this feedback system trains the brain to interpret and understand sensory stimuli.

It is impossible by any convention physiological experiment to understand the mechanism of pattern recognition inside the brain. But in 1943, the neurophysiologist Warren and Mc. Cullon, and a mathematician Walter Pitts (McCulloch et al., 1943) understood this mechanism. Using this knowledge of neurons, they introduced its functionality and modelled simple neural network. Since then, a lot of research has been done. The design structure of ANN used to construct ModCNN proposed in this paper is shown in Figure 11.

It consists of a single-layer hidden neuron with a smooth activation function and an output layer with linear activation function. The model was constructed using one hidden layer as it is studied to have sufficient approximating power. The number of hidden neurons is a hyper-parameter with b_1 and b_2 are bias=1 for input and hidden layer respectively. Let w_{ij}^1 denote the weight from j^{th} neuron of *l-1* layer to i^{th} neuron of lth layer and *w* being the set of all weights connecting layer *l-1* to *l*. Then the output $O_k(x_i; w)$ of neural network is shown in equation (9)

$$O_k(x_i;W) = \sum_{u=1}^{m} W_{ku}^{\ 2} \times \phi_u(\sum_{j=1}^{d} W_{uj}^1 \times x_i^j) \qquad (9)$$

Figure 11. Design structure ANN

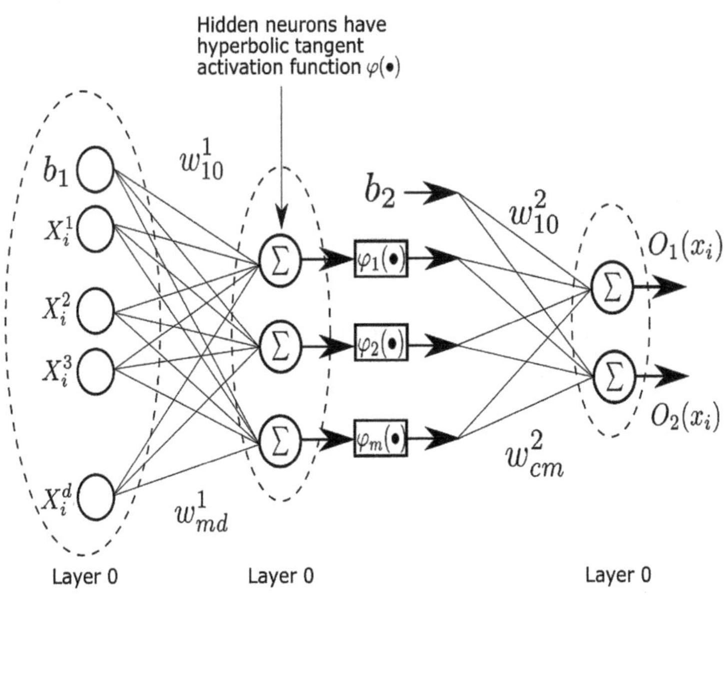

Here ϕ_u is an activation function of uth neuron and is a *sigmoid function*. Optimal weight W_{ij}^1 is discovered using back-propagation rule.

In general, weights in ANN are trained and adjusted using backpropagation algorithm. The technique is said to be *slow learner*, because it uses gradient decent which converges only at local minimum. During this learning, each neurons act as feature detector and they don't communicate with each other. Hence, they learn independently. If the error obtained by selecting a feature has strong signal, then the neuron decides to change its direction by selecting a different feature. Since each neuron are independent, this would significantly slow the learning process and is known as *slow-target problem*. Due to this Fahlman et al., (1990) introduced a new CCNN architecture with cascade correlation of network which learns by experience. Here the weights are frozen as the neurons are added to the network.

Modified Cascade-correlation Neural Network (ModCNN)

Figure 12 shows the design architecture of ModCNN using softmax-based probabilistic function. ModCNN was built upon the architecture of CCNN overcoming the disadvantages of CCNN of not learning when and where to add neurons. In ModCNN, the hidden units are not frozen until an optimal number of neurons are identified, and the hidden units are not added linearly but in parallel. ModCNN was developed for analysing the patterns of the clinical data and predicting the disease progression. The process begins with a minimum number of hidden units and neurons in each hidden unit. After each iteration, error ε is calculated using Least Mean Square (LMS) algorithm also known as Widrow-Hoff or delta algorithm (Windrow et al., 1990). The objective here is to adjust the weights so, the sum S shown in equation (10) is maximized over all output units O. This would give an optimal set of weights for each hidden unit.

$$S = \sum_{o} \left| \sum_{p} \left(V_p - \overline{V}\right)\left(\varepsilon_{p,O} - \overline{\varepsilon_O}\right) \right|. \tag{10}$$

In the equation (10), p is the training pattern, $\overline{V}$ and $\overline{\varepsilon}$ are averaged over V (candidate unit values) and ε respectively. The objective here is to identify the best combinations of hidden units which maximize S. To maximize S the backpropagation rule of taking partial derivation of S concerning each combination of input weights W is applied. As the objective is to maximize the correlation, gradient ascent is used to identify the maximum of S after getting $\frac{\delta S}{\delta W}$ in equation (11).

$$\frac{\delta S}{\delta W} = \sum_{p,O} \sigma_O (E_{p,O} - E_O) f_O^{'} I_{i,p} ......(i = 1,2,3...n) \quad (11)$$

In the equation (11), σ_O is the correlation between candidates values and output O and $f_O^{'}$ is derivative of the pattern p concerning the sum of its inputs.

On obtained MSE, GD was applied to locate the combination of weights which maximizes S minimum ε. Thus, GD converges to discover optimal correlation of neurons to that hidden unit, where the error ε was minimum. On identifying the optimal number of neurons, a new hidden unit is added to the architecture.

Adaline Circuit

ModCNN adopted ADALINE in developing a decision-making model. Bernard Widrow with Marcian E Hoff developed ADALINE and the training algorithm known as LMS in 1959. Since then it has been expanded rapidly. The initial objective using ADALINE is to identify the weights such that cost function J is minimum.

Figure 12. Design structure of ModCNN with softmax-based function

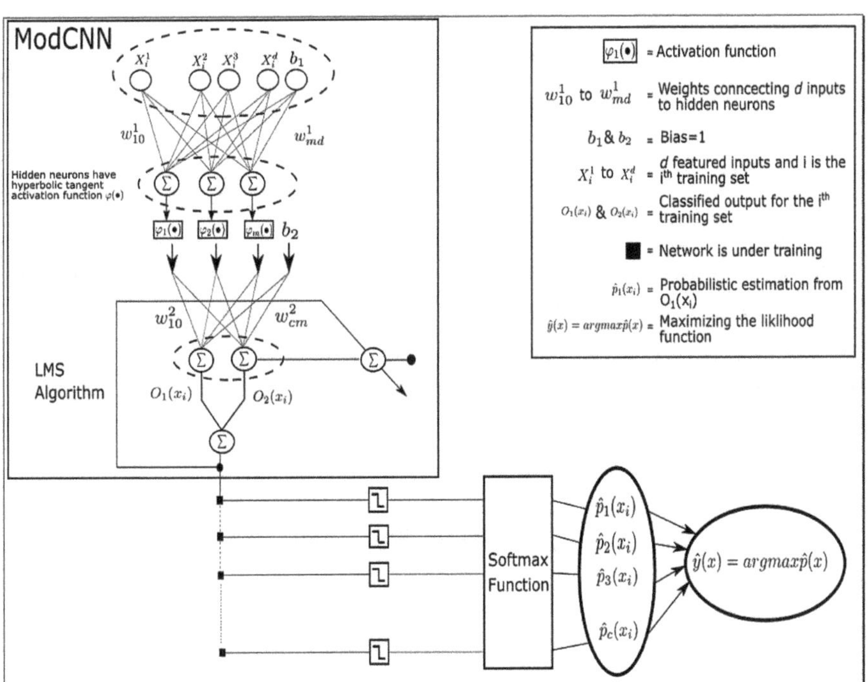

LMS algorithm is applied to identify the set of weights (W) generating MSE and is shown in Figure 13 (Widrow et al., 1994).

t takes different patterns of input x and gives analogue output $h_W(x)$. This analogue output is compared with desired output y to calculate the error $\varepsilon = h_W(x^i) - y^i ...Where,...i = 1, 2, 3...d$ at each iteration, till the minimum error is not achieved.

ADALINE circuit has a hidden unit with multiple combinations of weights. The process of finding error ε is repeated by adjusting the weights till minimum error is obtained. The authors applied the gradient descent technique to identify the optimal weights where the ε .is minimum. This finally resulted in weights (W) with less than a threshold is obtained and they were optimal.

Least Mean Square Algorithm: (LMS Algorithm)

In LMS algorithm each input $X = x_0, x_1, ...x_d$ goes to intermediate weights $W = w_1, w_2, w_3......w_d$ to give the actual output $h_W(x) = X^T \times W$ which is the summation of $\sum_{i=1}^{d} X^T \times W$. For each input pattern, there are *actual output* $h_W(x)$ and *desired output* (y), along with the error ε . The error is used to adjust the weights, so that MSE is minimum. The weight equation is shown in equation 12. In this equation μ is the coefficient of convergence and ∇ is gradient operator. As the minimized error ε is found at the bottom of the slope, there is a subtraction from the current weight w_i and gradient coefficient.

$$w_{i+1} = w_i - \mu \nabla \varepsilon_i \tag{12}$$

$\varepsilon = h_W(x^i) - y^i ...Where,...i = 1, 2, 3...d$ using this the MSE is calculated and is shown in equation (13). On applying

$$h_W(x) = X^T \times W \text{ , } \varepsilon^2 = y^2 - 2yX^T W + W^T X X^T$$

Then

$$\text{MSE} = E[\varepsilon^2] = E[y^2] - 2E[yX^T]W + W^T E[XX^T]W \tag{13}$$

Figure 13. Architecture of ADALINE

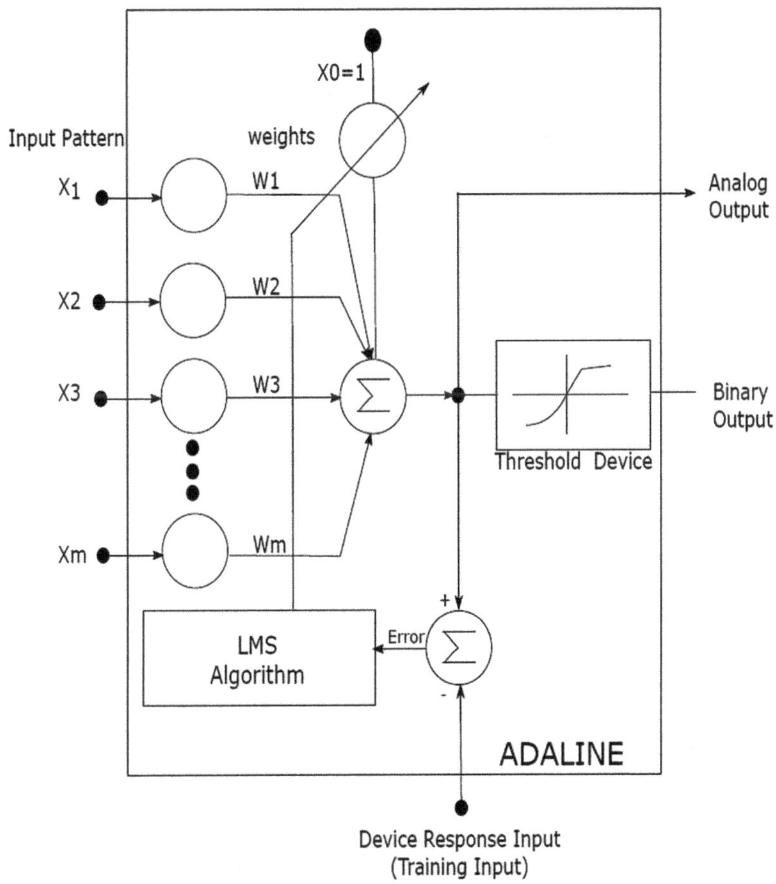

Let $P = E[yX^T]$ be cross-correlation vector and $R = [XX^T]$ be an auto-correlation matrix, then the generalized ADALINE circuit is shown in equation (14).

$$\text{Mean square error} = E[y^2] - 2P^T W + W^T R W \tag{14}$$

This MSE is a quadratic equation and yields a bowl-shaped plane as shown in Figure 14. Here only two weights are considered on the x-axis, y-axis and the MSE on Z-axis. Using gradient descent on this plane of equation (14), optimal set of weights could be identified

Figure 14. Paraboloid of the cost function

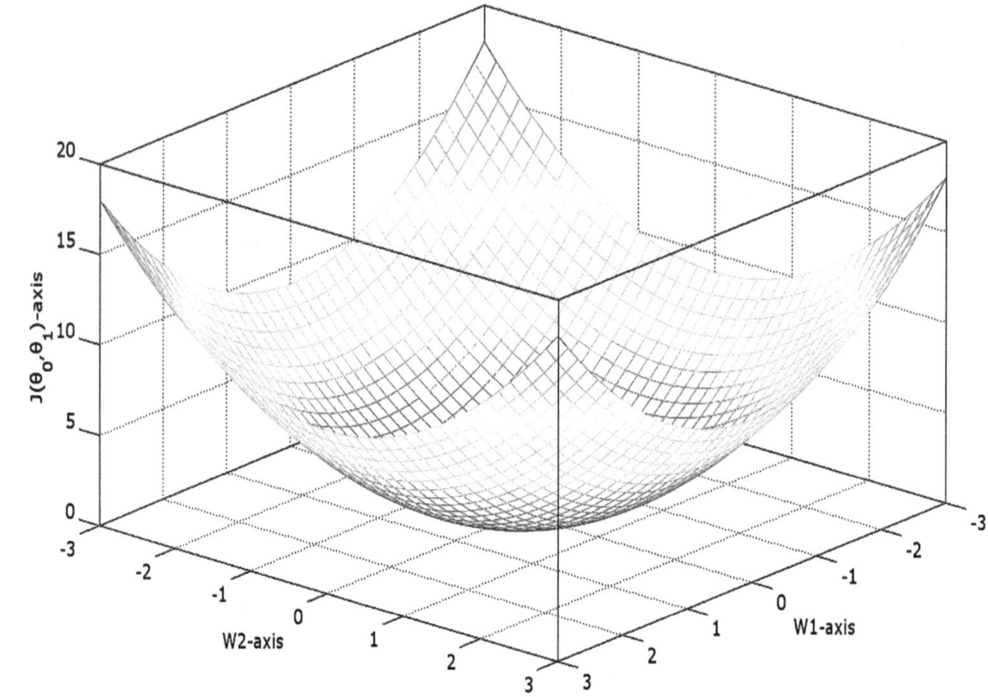

**For a more accurate representation see the electronic version.*

Gradient Descent

The objective of gradient descent is to minimize the cost function *J* for these weights and to identify its global minimum (Burges et al., 2005). Gradient descent algorithm starts the iteration with some initial θ such as $J\left(\theta_0 = 0 \,\&\, \theta_1 = 0\right)$ and iteratively updates θ as shown in equation (15) till the algorithm converges at a local minimum. In the equation (15) α is known as *learning rate.*

$$w_j = w_j - \alpha \frac{\partial}{\partial w_j} J(w) \text{ For all values of J=0,1,2,...n} \quad (15)$$

The objective of gradient algorithm is to minimize the cost function J $(\min_{w_1,w_2,..w_n} J(w_1, w_2....w_n))$. The algorithm starts an iteration by moving with small baby step α in a direction that moves down to reach minimum w. After each iteration, the algorithm will check the direction of movement that converges to a local minimum. The gradient descent repeats the equation (15) until it converges, by updating the

w_j value after every iteration. $\frac{\partial}{\partial w_j}$ is measured by theorem 3. Convergence is the stopping condition: $(\alpha \parallel J \parallel) < \varepsilon$, where $\parallel J \parallel$ is $\sqrt{J(w_1^2) + J(w_2^2) + J(w_3^2) \ldots}$ is the equation of normalization (Zhang, 2004).

Theorem 3

Let $J(w)$ be a cost function whose derivative exists, then $\frac{\partial}{\partial w_j} J(w)$ is a continuous function.

Proof

Let $J(w_0, w_1) = \frac{1}{2d} \sum_{i=1}^{d} (h_w(x^i) - y^i)^2$ ....*d* is the number of input, then

$$\frac{\partial}{\partial w_j} \frac{1}{2d} \sum_{i=1}^{d} (h_w(x^i) - y^i)^2$$

Using product rule

$$\frac{\partial}{\partial w_j} \frac{1}{2d} \sum_{i=1}^{d} 2 \times (h_w(x^i) - y^i) = \frac{\partial}{\partial w_j} \frac{1}{d} \sum_{i=1} (h_w(x^i) - y^i) \times \frac{\partial}{\partial w_j} (h_w(x^i) - y^i) \tag{16}$$

Let

$$\frac{\partial}{\partial w_j} (h_w(x^i) - y^i) = \frac{\partial}{\partial w_j} (h(x^i))$$

where $h_w(x^i) = wx$ if $w_0 = 0$

$$\therefore \frac{\partial}{\partial w_j} (h_w(x^i) - y^i) = x^i \tag{17}$$

Applying result of (17) in (16)

$$\frac{\partial}{\partial w_j} J(w) = (h_w(x) - y) \times x \tag{18}$$

Theorem 4

Let $\frac{\partial}{\partial w_j} J(w) = h_w((x) - y) \times x$ be the partial derivative of the cost function. Using this, gradient descent algorithm for multiple parameters is proved

Proof

Let $w_j = w_j - \alpha \frac{\partial}{\partial w_j} J(w)$ for all values of $j: 0, \ldots, n$ from equation (15), then

where $\frac{\partial}{\partial w_j} J(w) = (h_w(x) - y) \times x$

Then, $w_j = w_j - \alpha(h_w(x) - y) \times x$, Where $h_w(x) = w_0 - w_1 x$

Updating w_0 & w_1

$$temp_0 = w_0 - \alpha \frac{\partial}{\partial w_0} J(w_0, w_1)$$
$$temp_1 = w_1 - \alpha \frac{\partial}{\partial w_1} J(w_0, w_1)$$
$$w_0 = temp_0$$
$$w_1 = temp_1$$

Using theorem 4, the gradient descent for multiple parameters can be achieved as shown in derivation of equation (19) and (20) and the algorithm is shown in algorithm 1

$$\frac{\partial}{\partial w_j} J(w_0, w_1) = \frac{\partial}{\partial w_j} \frac{1}{2d} \sum_{i=1}^{d} (h_w(x^i) - y^i)^2 = \frac{\partial}{\partial w_j} \frac{1}{2d} \sum_{i=1}^{d} (w_0 + w_1 x^i - y^i)^2$$

$$\text{Let } w_0 ie., j = 0 = \frac{\partial}{\partial w_0} J(w_0, w_1) = \frac{1}{d}\sum_{i=1}^{d}(w_0 + w_1 x^i - y^i) \tag{19}$$

$$\text{Let } w_1 ie., j = 1 = \frac{\partial}{\partial w_1} J(w_0, w_1) = \frac{1}{d}\sum_{i=1}^{d}(w_0 + w_1 x^i - y^i) \tag{20}$$

Algorithm 1: Gradient Decent Algorithms

Initialize w_0 & w_1 to random values

While {! converged}

{

$$w_0 = w_0 - \alpha \frac{1}{d}\sum_{i=1}^{d}(w_0 + w_1 x^i - y^i)$$
$$w_1 = w_1 - \alpha \frac{1}{d}\sum_{i=1}^{d}(w_0 + w_1 x^i - y^i) \times x^i$$

}

Feature-Based Sensitivity of Posterior Probabilities (FSPP)

This is a feature selection process based on the *Posterior Probabilities* of a feature vector $x \in class(w)$ and is defined in the equation (21).

$$FSPP = \sum_{k=1}^{c} \int \left| p(w_k \mid x) - p(w_k \mid x_{-j}) \right| P(x) dx \tag{21}$$

The value $p(w_k \mid x_{-j})$ in equation (21), corresponds to the probabilistic output of softmax-based MLP trained using data $\{x_{-j,i}, y_i\}_{i=1}^{N}$. This similar to saying $\{x_i, y_i\}$ - $\{x_{-j}\}$. In this network, suppose there are *m* features in training set, then evaluation of the network will need it to be retrained m times for each $\{x_{-ji}, y_i\}$ but with different j value.

Testing and Validating Using Real World Data Sets

The feature selection in FSPP is done using the posterior probability. FSPP method was selected as it showed better performance when compared to *FisherS*, *MutualI* and *MOI*. The performance of these feature selection model was tested using presentation format presented in Rakotomamonjy(2003). The testing was performed on five real world data stored in UCI machine learning repository (Asuncion et al., 2007), including the GSD data considered in the current work. The description of the data is given in Table (1).

The testing and validation of efficient feature selection model was done by conducting repeated realization on the given data sets. This was carried out by splitting the data sets into training and testing data as shown in Table 1. For example, the heart disease data has 303 instances among which, 227 are considered for training and remaining 76 is considered for testing. Training instances of data set are used to train the ModCNN and identify the optimal number of neurons in each hidden layer and also optimal number of hidden layer. And is this achieved by the help of 10-fold cross-validation technique.

10-Fold Cross-Validation Technique

Cross validation is an evaluation technique for testing the predictive model performance. For this the data set is partitioned into training and testing set for training and testing the model respectively. In *k-fold*, the data set is split in *k*-sample size. Among the *k*-samples, *k-1* samples are used for training and the single sample

Table 1. Description of real world examples along with the GSD data collected in the current work.

	Training D_{set}	Testing D_{set}	No. of Features	No. of Classes	No. Of Hidden Neurons	Features Removed in Each Epoch
Heart Disease	273	30	75	4	2	3
Wisconsin Breast Cancer	512	57	32	2	4	1
Absenteeism at work	666	74	21	21	3	1
Coimbra Breast Cancer	104	12	10	2	2	1
GSD	234	26	32	2	2	1

for testing. In cross-validation, the algorithm is iterated exactly k times, where in each k sub-sample used every time for validation. The k-result is then aggregated, to get single estimated output.

In the current approach, right ModCNN model was obtained by testing five different combinations of architecture with five different real time dataset and 10-fold cross validation technique. Hence, each model was trained using ten repeaters and the result from individual model is tested using the single data sample. Here 10-fold cross validation was used to reduce the data dependency and improve the reliability by creating the random partition of the data samples. Advantage of cross validation is, large portion (90%) of dataset is used to train the model, thus resulting model is highly validated.

In selecting the right model, it requires several key design decisions. The decision includes several topologies and learning process. Topology decision is about building the network architecture with right combination of hidden layer and neurons. In ModCNN we start we no hidden layer in the initial stage. But the process starts with addition of first hidden layer and a neuron on it, establishing synaptic connection with input and output.

Five real world data set were considered for experimenting and building an optimal model. The description of this data set is shown in Table 1. Repeated experiments were conducted out on realizations of the given data set. Splitting of total data set was done using 10-fold cross validation technique for training and testing the model. As shown in Figure 10, softmax-based probabilistic model is used for identifying the significant factors and their optimal number of neurons and hidden layer is discovered by 10-fold cross validation technique. The model that produces highest accuracy is chosen based on test error rate against the selected features. In each test, FSPP is compared with other techniques. Test error rate is the error that is produced when run on the test data set. Figure 15 to 19 shows the comparison of different feature selection method in different data sets mentioned in Table 1. On comparison it is was observed that FSPP model has shown lower error rate when tested with the test data set and when compared with other methods. This test assisted in selecting the best feature selection model, using which the independent risk factors, needed for prediction in identified.

RESULT

GSD was considered here due to its increasing prevalence in last few decades in India. Garg (2013) reported an epidemiological study by a group from All India Institute of Medical Science (AIIMS), Delhi on the prevalence of GSD in Kerala.

Figure 15. Test error on Absenteeism at work

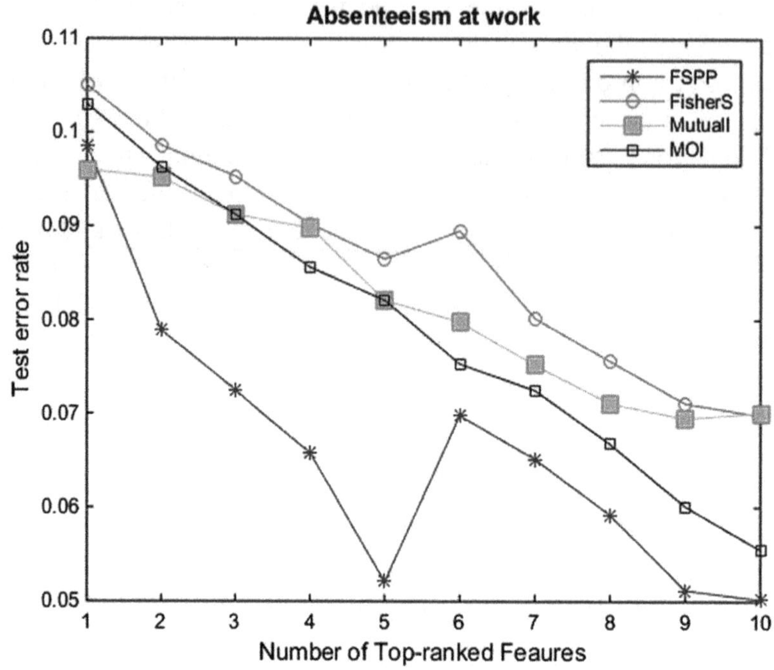

Figure 16. Test error on Coimbra Breast Cancer

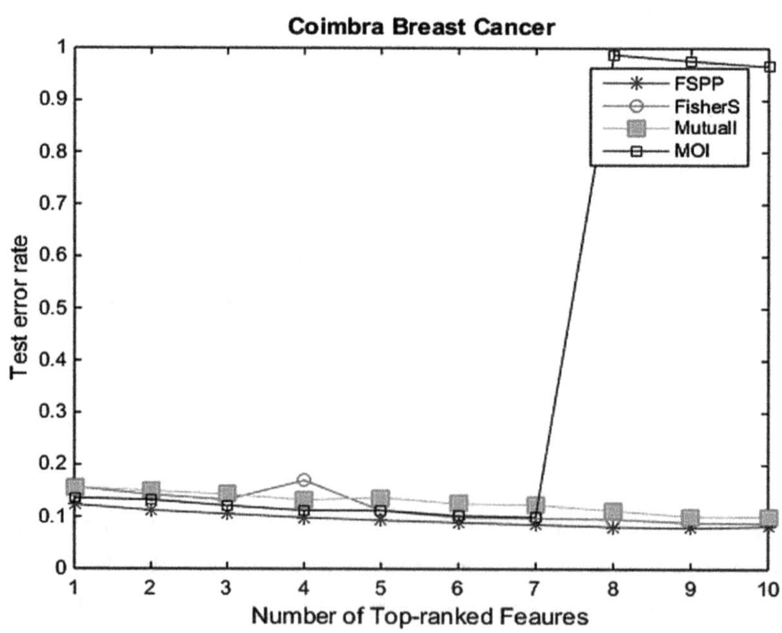

Figure 17. Test error on Wisconsin Breast Cancer

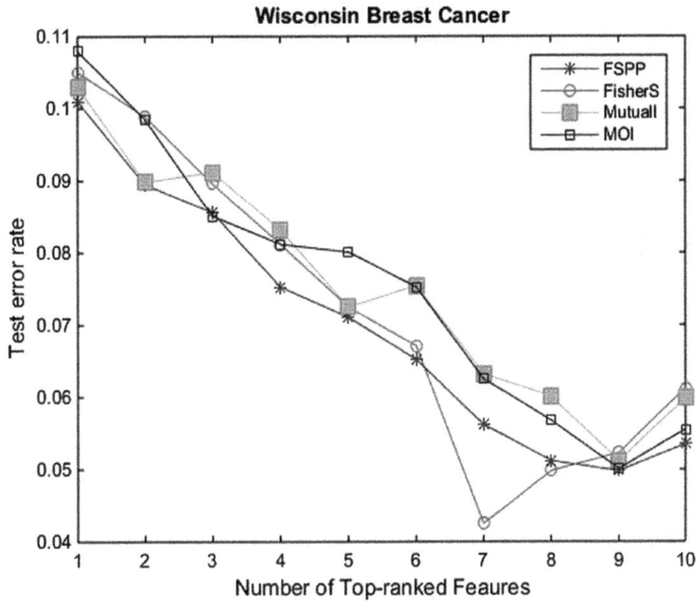

Figure 18. Test error on Heart Disease

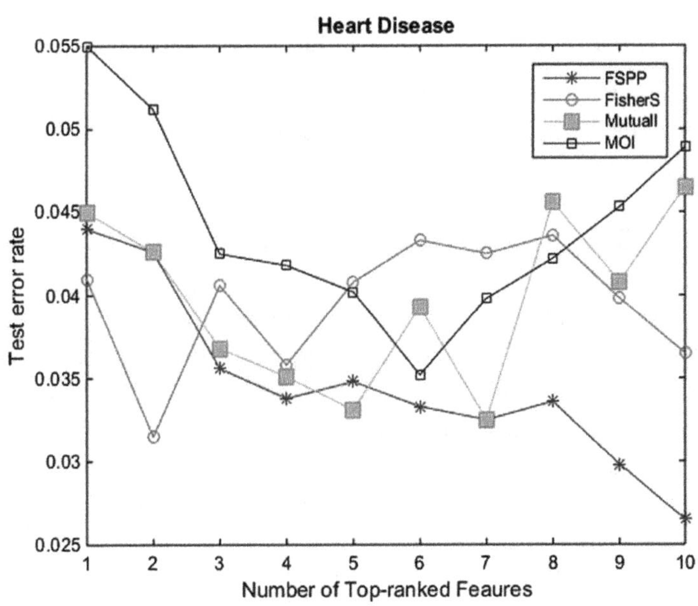

Figure 19. Test error on GSD

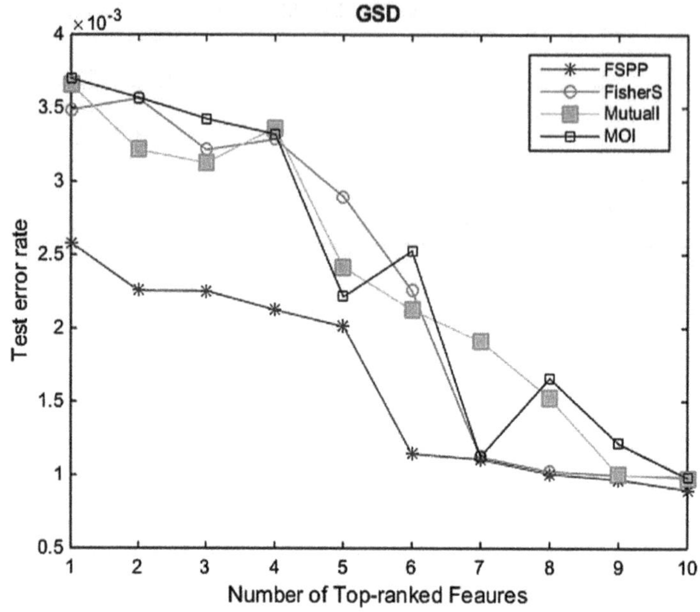

The study showed prevalence of Acute Pancreatitis (AP): $\widetilde{126}\,/\,100,000$ population and calcific pancreatitis: $\widetilde{98}\,/\,100,000$. This observation was very high when compared to $\widetilde{27}\,/\,100,000$ in the western countries. Kumar Sangwan et al., (2016) conducted a retrospective analysis and observed the incidence of GSD is seven times in north India than in the south.

Performance Comparison of ModCNN With ANN and CCNN

This classification accuracy was evaluated by comparing it with ANN and CCNN. The result of this comparison is shown in Figure 20. For illustrating and showing the performance comparison of ModCNN, ANN, and CCNN, the authors have considered ten patients data with equal distribution of the different spectrum of GSD. Here, ten patients' data is considered to show the performance of each model at different epochs, avoid spaghetti-like graphs and give a better explanation.

The inputs are patient's clinical data, and output is the spectrum of GSD ("0" cholecystitis, "1" choledocholithiasis, "2" pancreatitis and "3" cholangitis). It was observed that ModCNN achieved MSE=0.00 (classified output) at 1283 epochs, while CCNN and ANN still needed few more epochs to complete the classification process. Figure 21 shows the rate of error decrease, and it is observed that the convergence of ModCNN was faster than other models.

Figure 20. Performance comparison of ModCNN, CCNN and ANN for classifying spectrum of GSD.

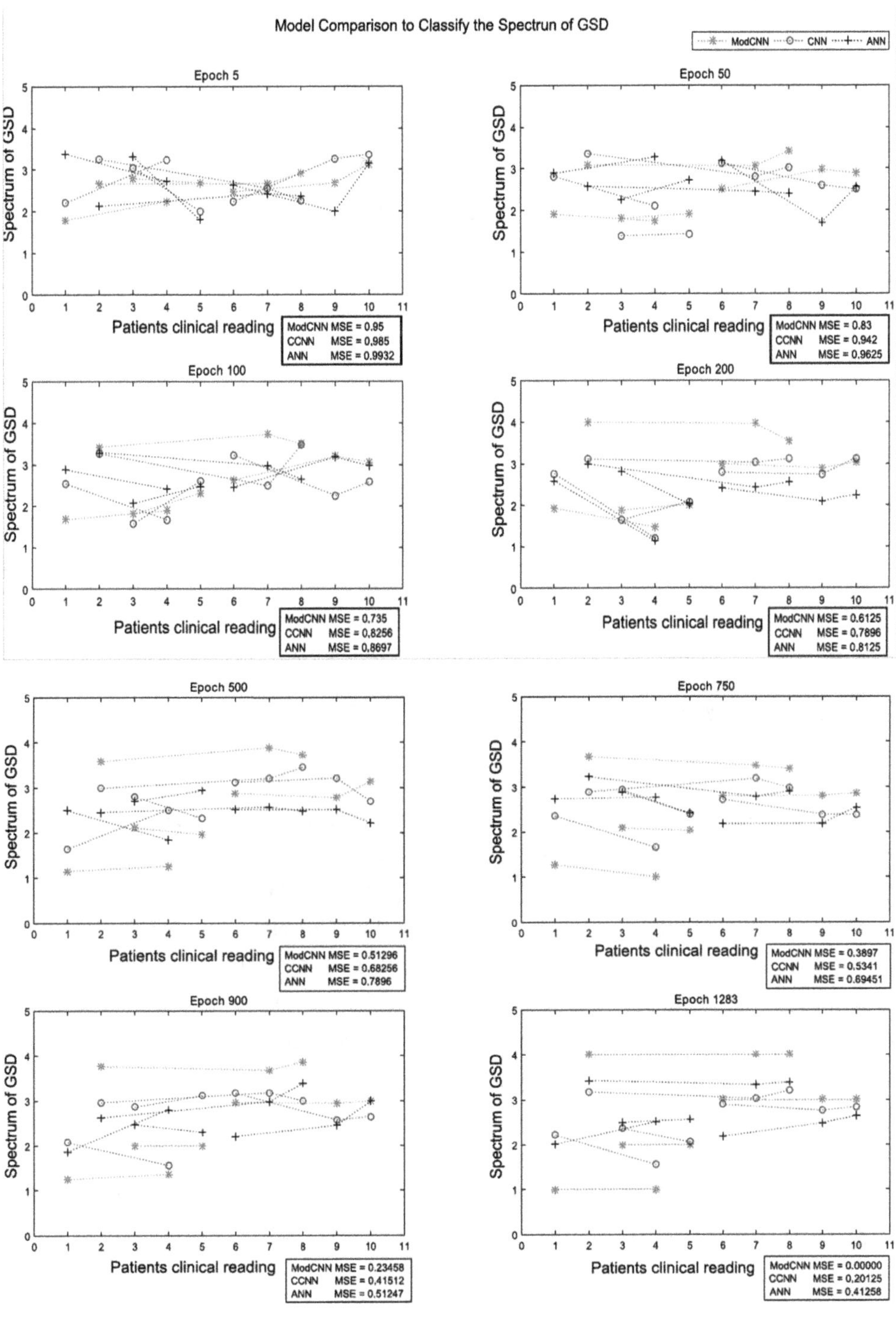

Figure 21. Classification performance of ModCNN, CCNN and ANN.

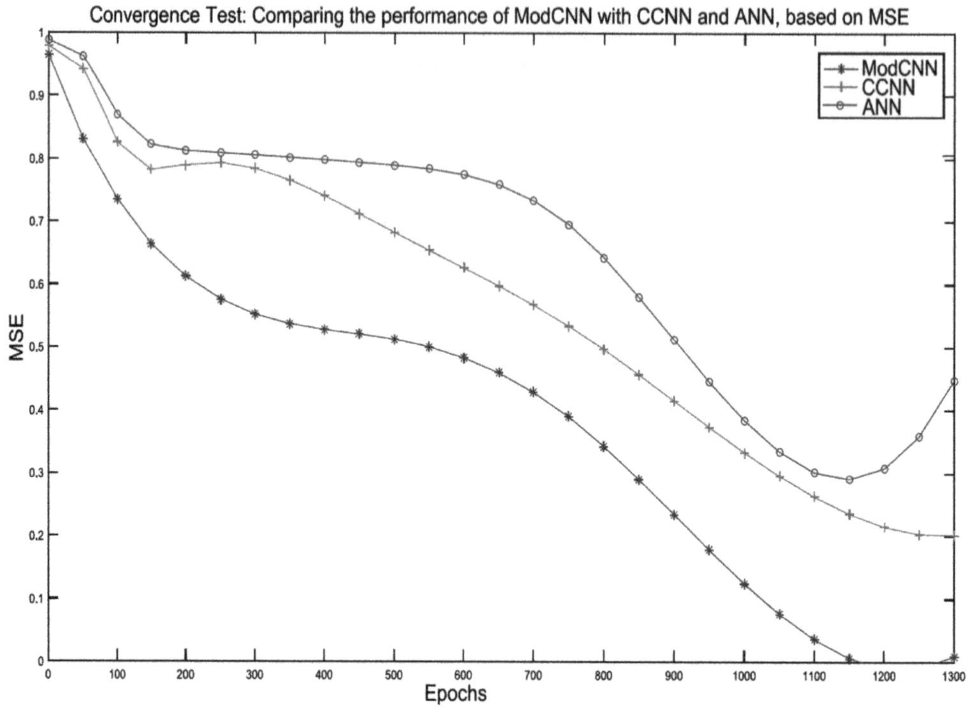

Validation of ModCNN

Along with the statistical analysis for finding the risk factors, authors used ANN, CCNN, and ModCNN for discovering the significant factors associated with each spectrum of GSD. Each model identified a different set of factors. Figure 22 shows the factors identified along with performance comparison using A_z . A1 to A32 are the clinical and USG findings and are shown in the Figures 5 to 9. Each stack in the stacked bar graph is the factor shown as the significant by different techniques. The value on top of the stacked bar is the value of A_z .for that model. Higher the A_z . factors are more significant. On comparison, it was seen that ModCNN outperformed in the accuracy of prediction when compared with ANN and CCNN. The significant factors were validated by testing for accuracy of prediction using the concept of A_z and are tabulated in Table 2. A_z is a ROC curve (plotted with sensitivity versus 1-specificity) that performs the comparison of different tests and chooses the best model? A_z . 1 is known as perfect discrimination, and 0.5 is referred to as absence of discrimination.

Figure 22. Comparison of ANN, CCNN and ModCNN for different spectrum of GSD

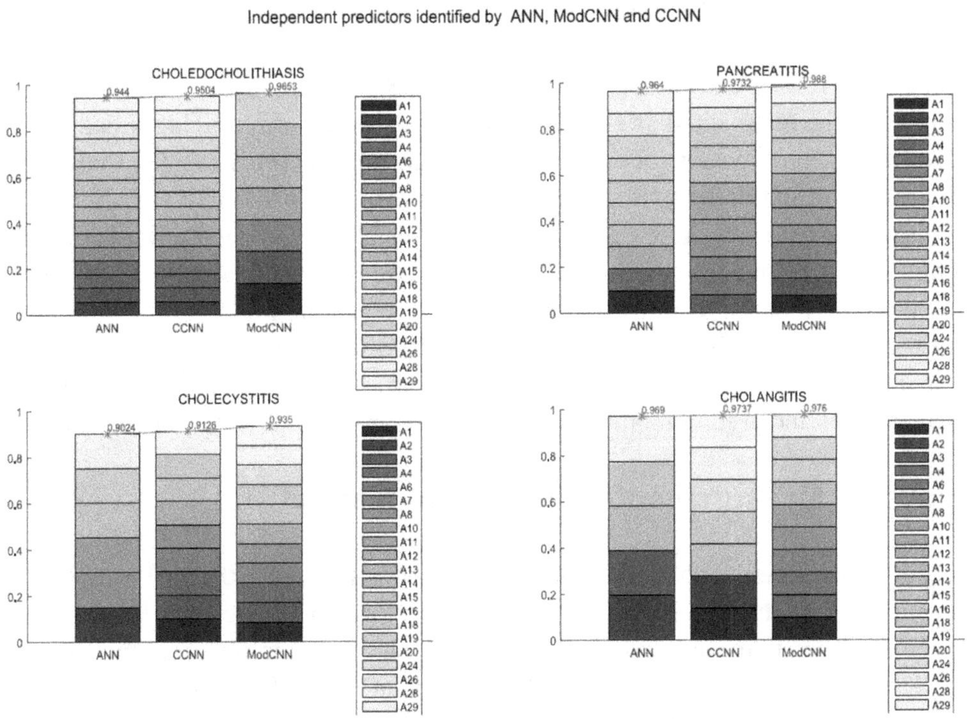

Table 2. Factors associated with each spectrum of GSD and A_Z .of ModCNN. Each factor is parenthesized with its P value.

Spectrum of GSD	Factors Associated	
Cholangitis	A1(P=0.1969), A4(P=0.1190), A7(P<0.001), A8(P=0.2483), A9(P<0.001), A10(P=0.8016), A14(P=0.7571), A19(P=0.2094), A21(P=0.5802), A26(P<0.001)	0.9768
Pancreatitis	A1(P<0.001), A4(P=0.6994), A7(P=0.4563), A8(P<0.001), A9(P<0.001), A10(P<0.001), A12(P=0.6040), A14(P=0.8876), A19(P<0.001), A21(P=0.4855), A22(P=0.6040), A26(P=0.5300), A28(P<0.001).	0.9875
Cholecystitis	A1(P<0.001), A3(P=0.1568), A4(P<0.001), A7(P=0.7350), A8(P<0.001), A11(P<0.001), A16(P<0.001), A17(P=0.2145), A24(P=0.0656), A26(P=0.6537), A29(P=0.9828)	0.9348
Choledocholithiasis	A1(P<0.001), A3(P=0.9179), A7(P<0.001), A11(P=0.2689), A13(P=0.4730), A14(P=0.2689), A19(P=0.5364)	0.9653

Testing Relative Risk of Each Factor for Different Spectrum of GSD

The relative risk of each complicated cases of GSD was analysed and is shown in Figure 23. The relative risk is calculated in a retrospective way and is studied based on the disease progression for every hour, from the time of admission. On analysis, it could be found that all the patients reached normal stage within two days of admission. But it was observed that the thirteen critical cases also descended towards normal as the initial treatment progressed. This would have been the reason the ERCP was conducted on them in the later stage of the disease progression.

On further risk analysis, it was found that those thirteen critical cases had an incline showing high relative risk. The CDSS developed by here aimed at identifying those thirteen cases and predicting the disease progression at the time of admission itself.

Accuracy Measurement Using the Concept of A_z

Area under the receiver operating characteristic curve A_z is one of the well-established statistical technique for evaluating the model performance. Higher the area under the curve more is the accuracy of prediction. The curve is obtained by plotting for *sensitivity* against *(1-specificity)*. Sensitivity and Specificity is obtained using equation (22) and (23) respectively.

$$Sensitivity = \frac{A}{A+B} \tag{22}$$

$$Specificity = \frac{D}{C+D} \tag{23}$$

In the equation (22) and (23), values A, B, C and D is shown in truth Table (3). In this table, TP (True Positive) is when the people with the disease is classified as positive, and FN (False Negative) is when they are classified as negative. TN (True Negative) is when people with no disease are correctly classified as negative, and FP (False Positive) is when they are classified positive. On plotting the obtained values for each feature, we will be able to get A_z. A *true positive* is when the condition is detected and is present. *True negative* is when the condition is not detected and is absent. While, false positive is when the condition is detected when it is absent, and false negative is when condition is not detected and is present. This is illustrated in the Table (4).

Figure 23. Analysing the disease progression and detecting the critical cases.

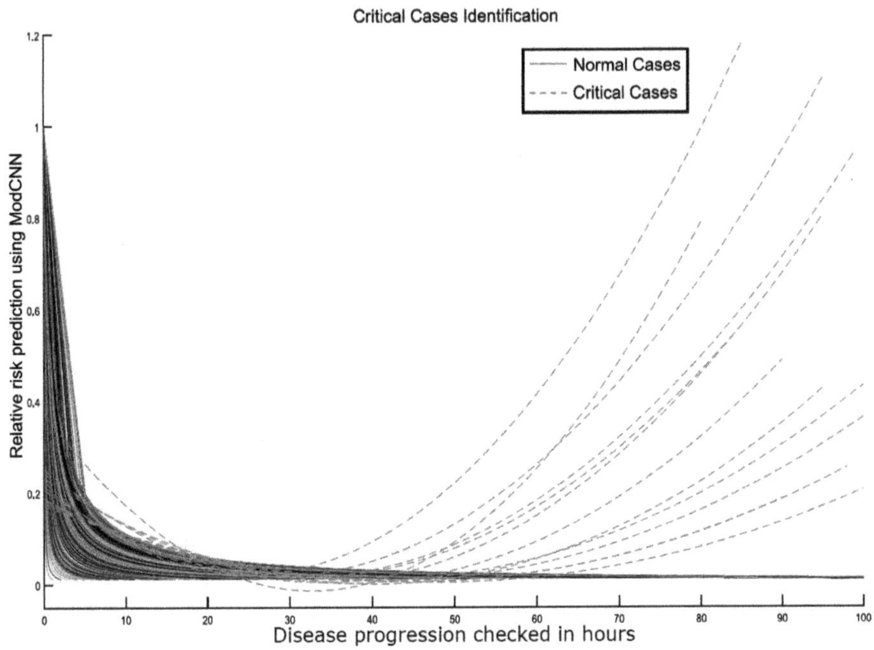

Table 3. Truth Table: Representation of TP, FP, FN and TN

Test	GSD (Yes)	GSD (No)	Row Total
Positive	TP(A)	FP(C)	A+C
Negative	FN(B)	TN(D)	B+D
Total	A+B	C+D	

Table 4. Illustration of truth table

		Condition	
		Present	**Absent**
Test	**Positive**	TP	FP
	Negative	FN	TN

The performance of ModCNN was evaluated and compared with ANN and CCNN. ModCNN showed better accuracy when tested for A_Z with, A_Z=0.9768, 0.9875, 0.9348 and 0.9653 for cholangitis, pancreatitis, cholecystitis, and choledocholithiasis respectively. The independent predictors associated with each spectrum of GSD along with their P-value is tabulated in Table 2, and the comparison of A_Z for each spectrum is shown in Figure 24, 25, 26 and 27. The overall accuracy comparison shows that ModCNN had better accuracy of A_Z .0.9642 when compared to CCNN (A_Z .0.9324) and ANN (A_Z .0.8965). This is shown in Figure 28.

CONCLUSION

The medical error is one of the leading cause of death, hence, it essential to build a CDSS to support the functioning of health care system. A patient can be given proper care-flow in a health care system by analysing the disease progression and their treatment response. The aim of this research work was to provide the quickest treatment and reduce the medical error. ModCNN was built for predicting the disease behaviour and assisting in finding the critical cases. It was designed to discover the optimal combination of hidden units and neurons. The performance of ModCNN

Figure 24. Comparison of accuracy of prediction for cholangitis using A_Z

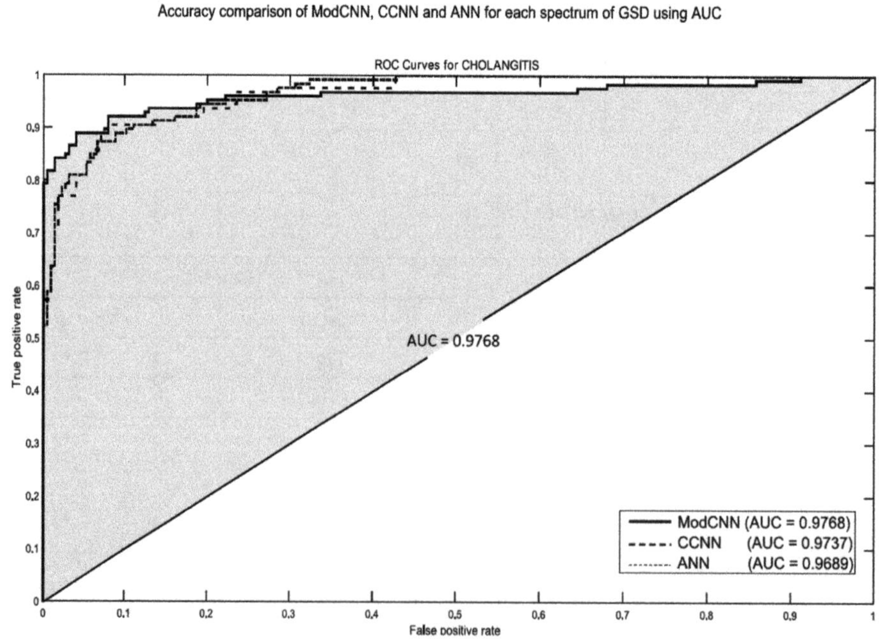

Figure 25. Comparison of accuracy of prediction for pancreatitis using A_Z

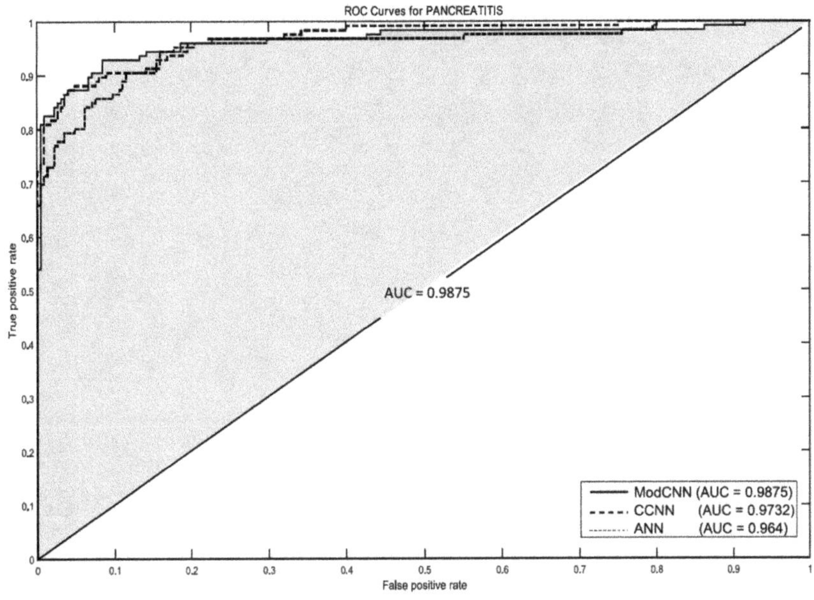

Figure 26. Comparison of accuracy of prediction for cholecystitis using A_Z

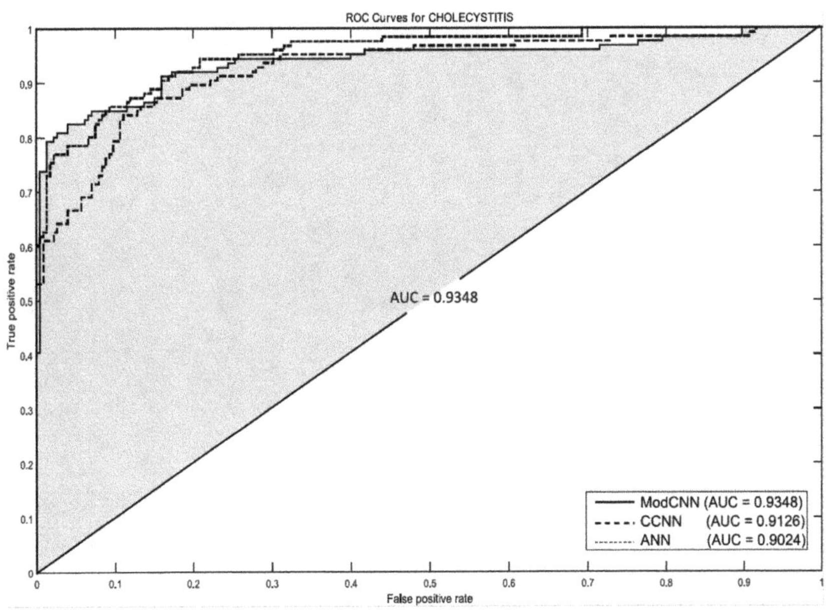

Figure 27. Comparison of accuracy of prediction for choledocholithiasis using A_Z

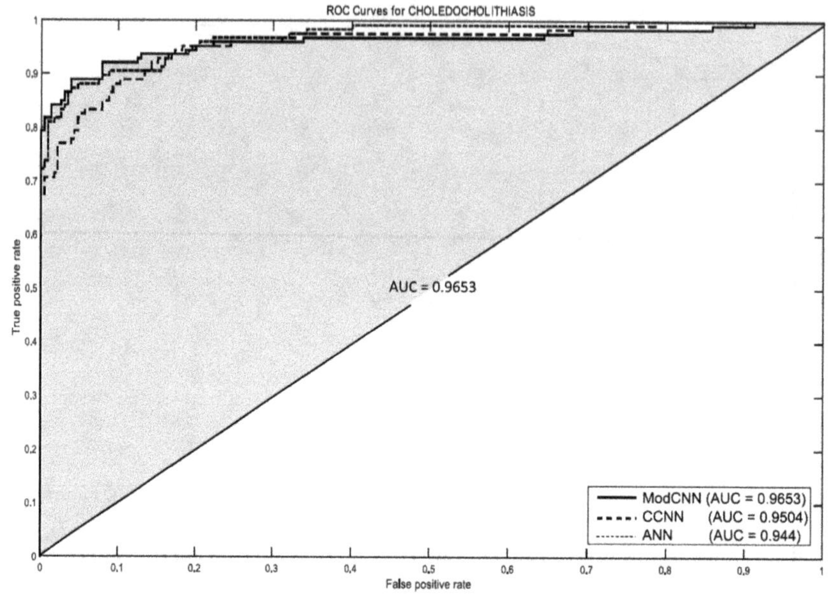

Figure 28. Accuracy comparison of ModCNN with ANN and CCNN using A_Z

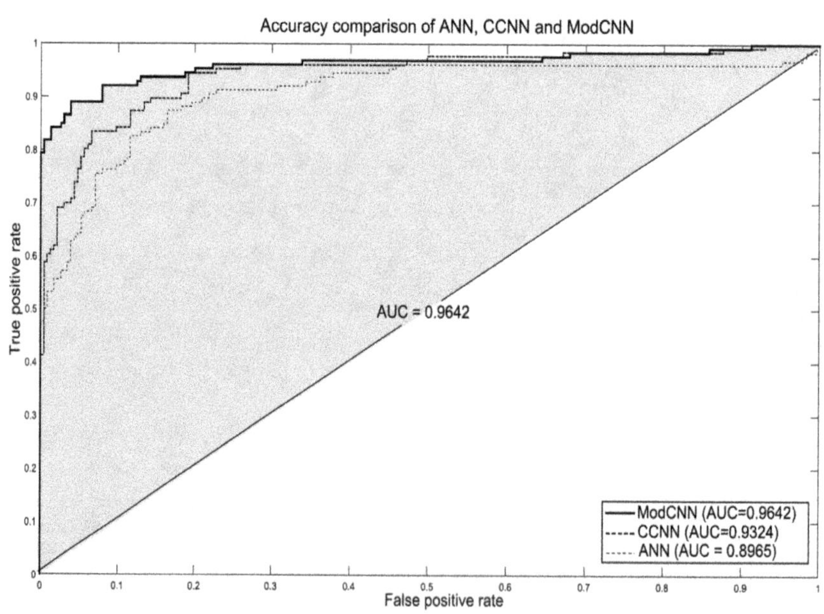

was evaluated by comparing with ANN and CCNN and was validated using A_Z. It was noted that ModCNN outperformed other statistical models in finding the critical cases and showed the highest accuracy.

The study was focused on complicated GSD and was conducted retrospectively from territory care centre in north Malabar, Kerala, India. 260 complicated cases were recorded during the study period, and the spectrum of GSD was comparable with California study conducted by Glasgow et al. (2000). This shows that the prevalence of GSD is increasing in India.

On learning the performance of existing ANN and CCNN models, authors developed ModCNN using the architecture of CCNN. In ModCNN, neurons and hidden units are adapted dynamically for giving better accuracy. ModCNN first identified the significant risk factors associated with each spectrum of GSD which was again fed into the system for predicting the disease progression. As this was a retrospective study, it was noted that ModCNN accurately identified the 13 cases which were critical with an accuracy of $A_Z = 0.9642$.

REFERENCES

Akande, K. O., Owolabi, T. O., Twaha, S., & Olatunji, S. O. (2014). Performance comparison of SVM and ANN in predicting compressive strength of concrete. *IOSR Journal of Computer Engineering*, *16*(5), 88–94. doi:10.9790/0661-16518894

Asuncion, A., & Newman, D. (2007). *UCI machine learning repository*. Academic Press.

Balthazar, E. J., Robinson, D. L., Megibow, A. J., & Ranson, J. (1990). Acute pancreatitis: Value of CT in establishing prognosis. *Radiology*, *174*(2), 331–336. doi:10.1148/radiology.174.2.2296641 PMID:2296641

Burges, C., Shaked, T., Renshaw, E., Lazier, A., Deeds, M., Hamilton, N., & Hullender, G. (2005, August). Learning to rank using gradient descent. In *Proceedings of the 22nd international conference on Machine learning* (pp. 89-96). ACM.

Cunningham, P., Carney, J., & Jacob, S. (2000). Stability problems with artificial neural networks and the ensemble solution. *Artificial Intelligence in Medicine*, *20*(3), 217–225. doi:10.1016/S0933-3657(00)00065-8 PMID:10998588

Davidoff, F., Case, K., & Fried, P. W. (1995). Evidence-based medicine: Why all the fuss? *Annals of Internal Medicine*, *122*(9), 727–727. doi:10.7326/0003-4819-122-9-199505010-00012 PMID:7702236

Donaldson, M. S., Corrigan, J. M., & Kohn, L. T. (Eds.). (2000). *To err is human: building a safer health system* (Vol. 6). National Academies Press.

Fahlman, S. E., & Lebiere, C. (1990). The cascade-correlation learning architecture. In Advances in neural information processing systems (pp. 524-532). Academic Press.

Focsa, M. (2010). Knowledge-based EHR Systems. In *Proceedings of the 31st Romanian National Conference on Medical Informatics "Solution-based Medical Informatics"* (pp. 64-68). Academic Press.

Fukushima, K. (1975). Cognitron: A self-organizing multi-layered neural network. *Biological Cybernetics*, *20*(3-4), 121–136. doi:10.1007/BF00342633 PMID:1203338

Garg, P. K. (Ed.). (2013). *Chronic Pancreatitis-ECAB*. Elsevier Health Sciences.

Glasgow, R. E., Cho, M., Hutter, M. M., & Mulvihill, S. J. (2000). The spectrum and cost of complicated gallstone disease in California. *Archives of Surgery*, *135*(9), 1021–1025. doi:10.1001/archsurg.135.9.1021 PMID:10982504

Grana, M., & Jackwoski, K. (2015, November). Electronic health record: A review. In *Bioinformatics and Biomedicine (BIBM), 2015 IEEE International Conference on* (pp. 1375-1382). IEEE. 10.1109/BIBM.2015.7359879

Guyon, I., & Elisseeff, A. (2003). An introduction to variable and feature selection. *Journal of Machine Learning Research*, *3*(Mar), 1157–1182.

Halonen, K. I., Leppäniemi, A. K., Lundin, J. E., Puolakkainen, P. A., Kemppainen, E. A., & Haapiainen, R. K. (2003). Predicting fatal outcome in the early phase of severe acute pancreatitis by using novel prognostic models. *Pancreatology*, *3*(4), 309–315. doi:10.1159/000071769 PMID:12890993

Hong, W. D., Chen, X. R., Jin, S. Q., Huang, Q. K., Zhu, Q. H., & Pan, J. Y. (2013). Use of an artificial neural network to predict persistent organ failure in patients with acute pancreatitis. *Clinics*, *68*(1), 27–31. doi:10.6061/clinics/2013(01)RC01 PMID:23420153

Imrie, C., Benjamin, I., Ferguson, J., McKay, A., Mackenzie, I., O'neill, J., & Blumgart, L. (1978). A single-centre double-blind trial of trasylol therapy in primary acute pancreatitis. *British Journal of Surgery*, *65*(5), 337–341. doi:10.1002/bjs.1800650514 PMID:348250

Itchhaporia, D., Snow, P. B., Almassy, R. J., & Oetgen, W. J. (1996). Artificial neural networks: Current status in cardiovascular medicine. *Journal of the American College of Cardiology*, *28*(2), 515–521. doi:10.1016/0735-1097(96)00174-X PMID:8800133

Jalloh, O. B., & Waitman, L. R. (2006). Improving Computerized Provider Order Entry (CPOE) usability by data mining users' queries from access logs. *AMIA ... Annual Symposium Proceedings - AMIA Symposium. AMIA Symposium, 2006*, 379. PMID:17238367

Jovanovic, P., Salkic, N. N., & Zerem, E. (2014). Artificial neural network predicts the need for therapeutic ERCP in patients with suspected choledocholithiasis. *Gastrointestinal Endoscopy, 80*(2), 260–268. doi:10.1016/j.gie.2014.01.023 PMID:24593947

Jovanović, P., Salkić, N. N., Zerem, E., & Ljuca, F. (2011). Biochemical and ultrasound parameters may help predict the need for therapeutic endoscopic retrograde cholangiopancreatography (ERCP) in patients with a firm clinical and biochemical suspicion for choledocholithiasis. *European Journal of Internal Medicine, 22*(6), e110–e114. doi:10.1016/j.ejim.2011.02.008 PMID:22075294

Kapoor, V. (2006). Cholecystectomy in patients with asymptomatic gallstones to prevent gall bladder cancer-the case against. *Indian Journal of Gastroenterology, 25*, 152–154. PMID:16877831

Karthikeyan, N., & Sukanesh, R. (2012). Cloud based emergency health care information service in India. *Journal of Medical Systems, 36*(6), 4031–4036. doi:10.100710916-012-9875-6 PMID:22865161

Kim, J. A., Cho, I., & Kim, Y. (2008, August). CDSS (clinical decision support system) architecture in Korea. In *Convergence and Hybrid Information Technology, 2008. ICHIT'08. International Conference on* (pp. 700-703). IEEE.

Knaus, W. A., Draper, E. A., Wagner, D. P., & Zimmerman, J. E. (1985). APACHE II: A severity of disease classification system. *Critical Care Medicine, 13*(10), 818–829. doi:10.1097/00003246-198510000-00009 PMID:3928249

Kumar Sangwan, M., & Sangwan, V., Kumar Garg, M., Singla, D., Thami, G., & Malik, P. (2016). Gallstone disease menacing rural population in north India: A retrospective study of 576 cases in a rural hospital. *International Surgery Journal, 2*(4), 487–491.

Kushinka, S. A. (2011). *Electronic health record deployment techniques*. Retrieved from https://www.chcf.org/publication/electronic-health-record-deployment-techniques/

Leape, L. L., Brennan, T. A., Laird, N., Lawthers, A. G., Localio, A. R., Barnes, B. A., & Hiatt, H. (1991). The nature of adverse events in hospitalized patients: Results of the Harvard Medical Practice Study II. *The New England Journal of Medicine*, *324*(6), 377–384. doi:10.1056/NEJM199102073240605 PMID:1824793

LeLorier, J., Gregoire, G., Benhaddad, A., Lapierre, J., & Derderian, F. (1997). Discrepancies between meta-analyses and subsequent large randomized, controlled trials. *The New England Journal of Medicine*, *337*(8), 536–542. doi:10.1056/NEJM199708213370806 PMID:9262498

Marshall, J. C., Cook, D. J., Christou, N. V., Bernard, G. R., Sprung, C. L., & Sibbald, W. J. (1995). Multiple organ dysfunction score: A reliable descriptor of a complex clinical outcome. *Critical Care Medicine*, *23*(10), 1638–1652. doi:10.1097/00003246-199510000-00007 PMID:7587228

Marshall, R. J. (2001). The use of classification and regression trees in clinical epidemiology. *Journal of Clinical Epidemiology*, *54*(6), 603–609. doi:10.1016/S0895-4356(00)00344-9 PMID:11377121

McCulloch, W. S., & Pitts, W. (1943). A logical calculus of the ideas immanent in nervous activity. *The Bulletin of Mathematical Biophysics*, *5*(4), 115–133. doi:10.1007/BF02478259

Moser, R. H. (1956). Diseases of medical progress. *The New England Journal of Medicine*, *255*(13), 606–614. doi:10.1056/NEJM195609272551306 PMID:13369682

Ohno-Machado, L. (1996). *Medical applications of artificial neural networks: connectionist models of survival* (Doctoral dissertation). Stanford University.

Peng, H., Long, F., & Ding, C. (2005). Feature selection based on mutual information criteria of max-dependency, max-relevance, and min-redundancy. *IEEE Transactions on Pattern Analysis and Machine Intelligence*, *27*(8), 1226–1238. doi:10.1109/TPAMI.2005.159 PMID:16119262

Pronovost, P., & Vohr, E. (2010). *Safe patients, smart hospitals: how one doctor's checklist can help us change health care from the inside out*. Penguin.

Quaglini, S. (2008, September). Process mining in healthcare: a contribution to change the culture of blame. In *International Conference on Business Process Management* (pp. 308-311). Springer.

Rakotomamonjy, A. (2003). Variable selection using SVM-based criteria. *Journal of Machine Learning Research*, *3*(Mar), 1357–1370.

Ranson, J. H. C. (1974). Prognostic signs and the role of operative management in acute pancreatitis. *Surgery, Gynecology & Obstetrics*, *139*, 69–81. PMID:4834279

Renner, P. (2009). *Why most EMR implementations fail: How to protect your practice and enjoy successfully implementation*. Retrieved from http://www.emrindustry.com/wpcontent/ uploads/2014/04/StreamlineMD_WhitePaper_1B.pdf

Sharma, M., & Aggarwal, H. (2016). EHR adoption in India: Potential and the challenges. *Indian Journal of Science and Technology*, *9*(34). doi:10.17485/ijst/2016/v9i34/100211

Simpson, R. J. S., & Pearson, K. (1904). Report on certain enteric fever inoculation statistics. *British Medical Journal*, 1243–1246. PMID:20761760

Sindhwani, V., Rakshit, S., Deodhare, D., Erdogmus, D., Principe, J. C., & Niyogi, P. (2004). Feature selection in MLPs and SVMs based on maximum output information. *IEEE Transactions on Neural Networks*, *15*(4), 937–948. doi:10.1109/TNN.2004.828772 PMID:15461085

Slavin, R. E. (1986). Best-evidence synthesis: An alternative to meta-analytic and traditional reviews. *Educational Researcher*, *15*(9), 5–11. doi:10.3102/0013189X015009005

Song, J. G., Zeng, W. H., Xu, Y., & Xu, W. X. (2011, May). The Improvement of Neural Network Cascade-correlation Algorithm and its Application in Picking Seismic First Break. *73rd EAGE Conference and Exhibition incorporating SPE EUROPEC 2011*. 10.3997/2214-4609.20149418

Thomas, E. J., Studdert, D. M., Burstin, H. R., Orav, E. J., Zeena, T., Williams, E. J., & Brennan, T. A. (2000). Incidence and types of adverse events and negligent care in Utah and Colorado. *Medical Care*, *38*(3), 261–271. doi:10.1097/00005650-200003000-00003 PMID:10718351

Vincent, J. L., Moreno, R., Takala, J., Willatts, S., De Mendonça, A., Bruining, H., … Thijs, L. G. (1996). *The SOFA (Sepsis-related Organ Failure Assessment) score to describe organ dysfunction/failure*. Academic Press.

Weed, L. (2017). *History of EHR*. Retrieved from http://v2020eresource.org/home/newsletter/SM116

Widrow, B., & Hoff, M. E. (1960). *Adaptive switching circuits (No. TR-1553-1)*. Stanford Univ.

Widrow, B., Rumelhart, D. E., & Lehr, M. A. (1994). Neural networks: Applications in industry, business and science. *Communications of the ACM, 37*(3), 93–106. doi:10.1145/175247.175257

Wilson, R. M., Harrison, B. T., Gibberd, R. W., & Hamilton, J. D. (1999). An analysis of the causes of adverse events from the Quality in Australian Health Care Study. *The Medical Journal of Australia, 170*(9), 411–415. PMID:10341771

Yang, J. B., Shen, K. Q., Ong, C. J., & Li, X. P. (2008, October). Feature selection via sensitivity analysis of MLP probabilistic outputs. In *Systems, Man and Cybernetics, 2008. SMC 2008. IEEE International Conference on* (pp. 774-779). IEEE. 10.1109/ICSMC.2008.4811372

Zhang, T. (2004, July). Solving large scale linear prediction problems using stochastic gradient descent algorithms. In *Proceedings of the twenty-first international conference on Machine learning* (p. 116). ACM. 10.1145/1015330.1015332

ADDITIONAL READING

Berner, E. S. (2007). Clinical decision support systems (Vol. 233). New York: Springer Science+ Business Media, LLC.

Bountris, P., Haritou, M., Pouliakis, A., Margari, N., Kyrgiou, M., Spathis, A., ... Koutsouris, D. D. (2014). An intelligent clinical decision support system for patient-specific predictions to improve cervical intraepithelial neoplasia detection. *BioMed Research International*, 2014. PMID:24812614

Kong, G., Xu, D. L., & Yang, J. B. (2008). Clinical decision support systems: A review on knowledge representation and inference under uncertainties. *International Journal of Computational Intelligence Systems, 1*(2), 159–167.

Laske, C., Sohrabi, H. R., Frost, S. M., López-de-Ipiña, K., Garrard, P., Buscema, M., & Bridenbaugh, S. A. (2015). Innovative diagnostic tools for early detection of Alzheimer's disease. *Alzheimer's & dementia: the journal of the Alzheimer's Association, 11*(5), 561-578.

Lobach, D., & Kawamoto, K. (2007). *U.S. Patent Application No. 11/515,556.*

Miller, R. A. (1994). Medical diagnostic decision support systems—past, present, and future: A threaded bibliography and brief commentary. *Journal of the American Medical Informatics Association, 1*(1), 8–27. doi:10.1136/jamia.1994.95236141 PMID:7719792

Musen, M. A., Middleton, B., & Greenes, R. A. (2014). Clinical decision-support systems. In *Biomedical informatics* (pp. 643–674). London: Springer. doi:10.1007/978-1-4471-4474-8_22

Shin, H., & Markey, M. K. (2006). A machine learning perspective on the development of clinical decision support systems utilizing mass spectra of blood samples. *Journal of Biomedical Informatics*, *39*(2), 227–248. doi:10.1016/j.jbi.2005.04.002 PMID:15963765

Chapter 6
Impact of Patient Health Education on the Screening for Disease Test-Outcomes:
The Case of Using Educational Materials From the Internet and Online Health Communities

Thierry O. C. Edoh
Technical University of Munich, Germany

ABSTRACT

Screening for diseases is a medical process to predict, prevent, detect, and cure a disease in people at high risk. However, it is limited in the quality and accuracy of the outcomes. The reason for this is the lack of long-term data about the health condition of the patient. Launching modern information and communication technology in the screening process has shown promise of improving the screening outcomes. A previous study has shown that patient education can positively impact the patient behavior face to a disease and can empower the patient to adopt a healthy lifestyle and thus avoid certain diseases. Offering medical education to the patient can positively impact screening outcomes since educated and empowered patients are more aware of certain diseases and can collect significant information. This can minimize the rate of false positive as well as false negative screening results. This chapter analyzes how medical education can contribute to improving screening outcomes.

DOI: 10.4018/978-1-5225-7131-5.ch006

INTRODUCTION

The screening for diseases is a medical test procedure to predict, prevent, early detect a disease of concern, and cure people at high risk to develop the said diseases. However, a screening for diseases has limitations. These limitations include the quality and accuracy of the screening-test-outcomes that can be assessed based on the level of the test sensitivity and specificity which in turn can be measured based on the number of false-positive and false-negative test-outcomes. The main reasons underlying these limitations are under others the lack of long-term and accurate data about the health condition of a patient.

Long-term data is data unbrokenly collected over a long period. This implies an appropriate health conditions and/or diseases awareness level. Health conditions awareness level and individual's behavior towards diseases are associated with the patient health education level. Patient education can also empower individuals to adopt a healthy lifestyle. Based on the existing literature, the patient education is supported by the health literacy which in turn influences health outcomes. Since the medical knowledge level is, somehow, associated with the health outcomes, a question arises: can the patient health education and the health literacy impact the screening-test-outcomes? How can this happen?

This chapter has investigated the research questions above and got insight into how the health literacy level influences the health outcomes and analyzes how the patient education can contribute to improving the screening outcomes too. An experiment involving participants with different health literacy level (high, medium, low, poor or inexistent) level had figured out that both the health literacy level combined with patient health education level can contribute to reducing the rate of false-positive and false-negative screening test-results and thus increase the sensitivity and specificity of screening tests.

1. BACKGROUND AND LITERATURE REVIEW

Patient education can empower patient, increase his diseases awareness level, and thus contribute to adopting a healthy lifestyle to prevent disease as far as possible (Edoh, Zogbochi, Pawar, Hounsou, & Alahassa, 2017). Health education is a well-spread process but not sustainable. The existing methods are limited due to financial concerns, education level of the population, especially in developing countries, lack of adequate materials. Furthermore, this limitation is due to infrastructural and structural issues healthcare systems are facing worldwide, but developing countries bear a big burden of this issue.

1.1 Association Patient Health Education, Health Literacy, and Health Outcomes

1.1.1 Health Literacy

Health literacy is the ability to independently look for, find, process, and understand health-related information as well as to use healthcare services for taking appropriate health relevant decisions. Health literacy implies health education which in turn implies health-related information. The health education level is strongly dependent on the quality of the content of materials used, thus, health literacy also depends on health-related information that people receive.

Literacy is also defined as a cognitive ability to read, write, understand written information, effectively communicate, and listen to someone. Thus, Health Literacy is the literacy applied to health (written) information and management (Roberts, 2015). Sørensen et al. (2012) have conducted a review of papers dealing with the term of health literacy in order to *identify the definitions and conceptual framework* of the term. They proposed, based on the results of the review, to integrate the medical and public health views of health literacy for a better understanding of the term.

In Edoh et al., (2017), concrete examples of health literacy have been discussed. The case study has pointed out how the health literacy level can impact individual behavior. Furthermore, it has revealed that health literacy is not only to own knowledge about some medical conditions but also die attitude and individual behavior. This means that high health literacy provides more empowerment to the individual to involve himself in his health concerns. Additionally, the health literacy level can impact one's health, well-being, quality of life, and, hence, increase diseases prevention. The individual is more attentive to a healthy lifestyle. The individual becomes more aware of the power of information and data as well as the power and impact of health education. Generally, people performing diet are known as people who collect data on the course of the diet for an analysis at the end of the diet. We can imagine that the health literacy can bring people to collect data o the health in general. This data and information can be provided to a physician in the scope of screening for diseases and, thus, represent a long-term data basis on which the medical doctor can base his medical examination.

1.1.2 Health Education

Health education is defined as providing an individual with necessary information on given health conditions to make them get informed about health conditions or diseases, the diseases leading causes, and how to prevent developing the disease or to maintain his health.

Health care systems, worldwide, regularly provide information brochures to the population to get educated. The population, despite, further looks for information on the Internet in diverse online health communities for self-education.

The quality of the education depends on the source of the educational materials as well as the quality and the validity of the content of the materials.

1.1.3 Patient- and Health-Outcomes

Patient and health outcomes are variable concepts. The concept includes and reflects individual, healthcare professionals, family, or community state, behavior, or perception rather than expected even defined medical goals. The concept of outcome is measurable using measurement scales like Likert type scale to point out any variability in the patient state (Moorhead, Johnson, Maas, & Swanson, 2018). According to Koroukian et al., (2018), health outcomes are based on patient *self-reported fair/poor health, 2-year self-rated worse health, and 2-year mortality*. The outcome is then classified positive if the patient health status from good to excellent. A recent study (Traczynski & Udalova, 2018) has classified the health-outcomes reported by the patient and found an interesting association between the outcome level and the nurse practitioner independence. The outcomes have been classified using scales from 1 to 5 (1 = poor, 5 = excellent).

Based on the literature review and the performed observation, the patient and health outcomes are the results including medical examinations and patient health status self-report. The patient self-report may confirm the medical examination outcomes and vice-versa.

In the following section, the impacts of health literacy on patient and health outcomes will be discussed.

1.1.4 Impact of Health Literacy Level and Patient Health Education Level on Health Outcomes

Patient Health Education (PHE) is defined as a process where healthcare professionals assist patients to acquire knowledge, build skill, and adopt favorable and appropriate attitudes towards medical conditions. Patient education implies providing an individual with adequate health and medical information. Today, people look by themselves for health-related information on the Internet in several online health communities.

The great benefits of patient education are the empowerment that increases diseases awareness. It ensures that patients have detailed information on their health conditions and thus increases the patient understanding. An educated patient is featured with knowledge and ability to self-manage certain personal health conditions. If the patient has more insight into and understands their health condition, the patient is then more motivated to participate in the improvement of their health.

Recent studies on the topic highlighted the association between the patient education level with the health outcomes. In Linder et al., (2018), the authors collected data from a Swedish esophageal cancer treatment center and investigated the effects of patient-education on the curative outcomes of the disease. They found out an association between the education level and the probability of curative outcomes. Zolezzi et al. (2018) have evaluated the lithium patient education and its impacts. The evaluation revealed an association between the lithium patient education and the safe use of lithium. This study shows the positive impacts of the patient education on the patient attitude towards diseases and how an individual with high health education can contribute to improving the health outcomes. According to the chapter 17 (Patient Education) from the book by Corcos and Przydacz, (2018), patient education is an important principle. The book chapter has investigated the education of the patient suffering from urinary tract dysfunction. It pointed out an important aspect of the patient education. In the special case of patients suffering from urinary tract dysfunction, the authors highlighted the role of the role of the clinician in the patient education. The clinician, involved in training the patient self-Catheterization, should be a well-trained and experienced clinician.

Regarding the results of the literature review, the impact of patient education on the health outcomes is obvious. The curative probability increases when the patient education level also increases. A study conducted in 2010, Demarco and Nystrom, (2010), demonstrated the association between health literacy and patient education. The study recommended adjusting the patient education to their health literacy level. Hence, the readability of educational materials must be adapted to the literacy level of the patient. For example, a picture-based material would be appropriate and comfortable for a patient with very low (health) literacy. Though, how will this happen? Let us first look at the health literacy and its impacts on the health outcomes. A further difference between both patient education and health literacy is the disease awareness. Patient health education is linked to diseases awareness (Edoh et al., 2017). Though, the health literacy is not really related to diseases awareness (Devraj, Borrego, Vilay, Pailden, & Horowitz, 2018).

Individuals with high health literacy have the cognitive capacity to manage and set their health. They further use this skill to access, understand, and analyze health information. Furthermore, they are able to easily access health care services than people with less health literacy (Berkman, Sheridan, Donahue, Halpern, & Crotty, 2011). Demarco and Nystrom, (2010) have pointed out that *low health literacy contributes to inefficiently use of health care services.* A study on chemotherapy education (Parker et al., 2018), revealed that the education does not apply the health literacy principles, and the authors claimed that developing the patient education grounded on the health literacy principles may present multiple benefits like overall comprehension of education and high adherence. Earlier studies have figured out similar results in different health fields; for example, Abiodun, Olu-Abiodun, Sotunsa, and Oluwole, (2014) for cervical cancer patients in Nigeria. Similar works were in done for heart failure (Evangelista et al., 2010).

The literature review, including 30 papers, had figured out the relationship between the health literacy and the health outcome. Beyond this, many works have concluded that the education[1] level influences the health literacy level which in turn impacts the health outcomes. Robert et al. in had investigated how the health literacy level influences the health outcomes. The study revealed that poor health literacy links to poor health behavior like smoking, poor diet, low physical activities, etc. Chesser et al. (2016) had conducted a systematic review on the health literacy among older/elderly adults. They found out that the theme is less investigated. Though, the review of the existing study's outcomes revealed that the education affects the health among the elderly people. They further found out a link to age, income level, and race. An interesting point also pointed out in this study is an association between health literacy and physical as well cognitive health. Though, an important remains open; especially if high education automatically implies high health literacy.

In Fabbri et al., (2018), authors have investigated the relationship between health literacy level, hospitalizations, and death. The investigation reveals an increased risk of hospitalization and death for low health literacy. This study once again has shown the impact of the health literacy on the health outcomes. It further investigated the risk factors leading to high rate of hospitalization and death among the people with low health literacy, for example, poor utilization of health care services. The authors call for evaluating how to address these risks and claim that the mechanism *"whereby low health literacy leads to poor outcomes are only partially understood. "*

In Saeed, Saleem, Naeem, Shahzadi, and Islam, (2018), authors have evaluated the impacts of health literacy on diabetes outcomes and found out that the poor blood glucose level control is associated with a low health literacy. The authors, therefore, recommended to launching *patient education and training to improve the functional health literacy.*

As earlier described, the health literacy level, as well as patient, have shown promise to positively impact the health outcome. People with high literacy better follow the medical recommendation, medication, and can easily search for information about their health. They sufficiently collect information on their health and are more aware of their health condition. For example, people with high health literacy and suffering from diabetes regularly control their blood glucose level and are more aware of the disease. This behavior contributes to the high curability probability in this patient group. Through their diseases awareness level and regularly collected data on the health condition, the healthcare professionals are providing with valuable materials and have more insight into the status of the patient. Due to the diseases awareness, the patient knows when to visit the doctor and which information they need to collect prior to a medical visit. In contrary to people with high health literacy, people with low literacy cannot make a decision by themselves regarding the health conditions (Demarco & Nystrom, 2010).

The following section will discuss diagnostics errors and associated factors. According to World Health Organization (2016), the health literacy level can impact diagnosis outcomes and in the worse case be linked to diagnostics errors. The digest (Table 1) presents a factor associated with diagnostics errors.

1.1.5 Impacts of Health Literacy Level and Patient Health Education Level on Diagnostics Errors Rates

Diagnostics error remains an important issue in the medicine. A medical doctor can be accurate in diagnosing a disease or health condition only if he already has significant experiences with the given disease symptoms. Jerome Groopman wrote the book entitled "What's wrong with doctors" where he criticized the medical doctor's attitudes regarding the decision taking process in the scope of a diseases diagnostics procedure. In early 2007, Richard Horton's review the book of Groopman and highlighted following medical doctor's behaviors during a diagnostics process and decision making. The doctors mostly like to rely on their own experiences only instead of on the available evidence and could, therefore, make wrong decisions. Horton wrote in his review:

.... Patients might be stigmatized if they are thought to have a mental health problem or caricatured if they are judged to have engaged in self-harming behavior, such as alcoholism. This kind of mistake is called "attribution error." "Availability error" occurs when a doctor makes a decision based on an experience that is at the forefront of his mind, but which bears little or no relation to the patient before him. For instance, a specialist in gastroenterology may only think of the gut when evaluating a woman with abdominal pain. He may not think of gynecological causes for her symptoms.

Table 1. Digest (a) of Table 1. Factors that may contribute to diagnostic errors in primary care

Factors	Possible Issues Contributing to Error
Access to high-quality primary care	Limited access due to lack of money, remoteness, illiteracy, travel constraints or a limited number of healthcare facilities.

Source: (World Health Organization, 2016)

The ready availability of his own specialized experience in his assessment of what is wrong with a patient can seriously bias a doctor's judgment.... (Horton, 2007)

Caroline Wellbery, a medical doctor, presents in his commentary on "Flaws in Clinical Reasoning: A Common Cause of Diagnostic Error" a case scenario where a doctor missed a diagnosis and asks himself how he can make his diagnoses more reliable. a striking point in his remarks was his statement saying that *he made some lucky guesses* (Wellbery, 2011). This statement clearly shows that clinical reasoning and doctor's experiences with a given medical condition impact the diagnostics outcomes. Wellbery summarized in a table presented in Wellbery, (2011) the causes associated with diagnostics errors. interesting biases are presented in the table. Two of them retain particularly our attention: (i) Availability and (ii) Premature closure (see the digest below in Table 2).

The World Health Organization (WHO) discusses in its report (World Health Organization, 2016) the factors associated with the diagnostics errors and summarized similar factor in the table (*Table 1. Factors that may contribute to diagnostic errors in primary care*). The second factor cited in the table (see digest below - Table 3 -) clearly underlines the preponderant role of the competence of the healthcare professionals.

Recent works (Murcia-Robayo, Jouanisson, Beauchamp, & Diaw, 2018; Whalen, Maliszewski, Sheinfeld, Gardner, & Baptiste, 2018) have also pointed out the doctor's clinical experience level and information technology as factors that influence the diagnostics outcomes.

The literature review on the factors associated with the diagnostics errors had revealed the preponderant place of the clinical reasoning as the leading source of diagnostics errors. The study (Minue et al., 2014) on the *factors associated with diagnostic errors in primary care* has provided a novel framework to that makes possible to evaluate the impact of the clinical experience and situational factors

Table 2. Digest of Table 1 summarizing the diagnostics Biases

Bias	Description	Example	Corrective Strategy
Availability	Referring to what comes to mind most easily	Making a diagnosis based on a previous patient with similar symptoms	Know baseline prevalence and statistical likelihoods of the condition diagnosed
Premature closure	Failing to seek additional information after reaching a diagnostic conclusion	Failing to note a second fracture after the first has been identified	Review the case, seek other opinions (e.g., radiology backup), and consult objective resources (e.g., an orthopedic review that might include mention of a common concomitant fracture)

Source: (Wellbery, 2011)

Table 3. Digest (b) of Table 1. Factors that may contribute to diagnostic errors in primary care

Availability of healthcare professionals and specialists	Lack of sufficient, competent health care professionals, for example, due to lack of training, outward migration or a poor employment situation. Specialty expertise may not exist or may be limited in number or quality.

Source: (World Health Organization, 2016)

like *overwork, fatigue, and stress on the diagnostic process*. This study has, thus, pointed out that doctor's clinical experience can obviously influence the clinical reasoning, which in turn impacts the diagnostics outcomes.

1.2 Association Health Education, Health Literacy, and Screening-Test-Outcomes

The literature review has clearly shown the relation between the health literacy levels and health outcomes. It also demonstrates the higher the health literacy level, the higher the patient involvement in their health concerns. The study (Oldach & Katz, 2014), on the impact of patient's health literacy on cancer-screening-test-outcomes, have concluded that the patient's health literacy is potentially a contributing factor on the outcomes.

This conclusion does not clearly establish the relationship between the health literacy level and the cancer screening-test-outcomes. The reason for this is following: the authors evaluated 10 articles including 14 comparisons. However, only one article has definitively found a significant association between the terms. All other articles fail to definitively establish the relationship.

In Sentell, Tsoh, Davis, Davis, and Braun, (2015), the authors investigated the association between the *low health literacy and the up-to-date breast and colorectal cancer screening*. The study revealed that the low health literacy combined with limited English proficiency have negatively influenced an up-to-date screening.

Both studies did not clearly investigate the impact of the health level on the screening test-outcomes. The authors of the first study claim that it was not possible to definitively establish the relationship health between literacy and cancer screening.

To our best knowledge, the topic is less investigated since only a few kinds of literature were found dealing with the association between the health literacy level and the screening test-outcomes. Most of the references have only investigated the impact of the health literacy on the cancer screening test-outcomes. We are not able to find articles on how the health literacy level influences the rate of false-positive and false-negative screening outcomes. Furthermore, no article has dealt with the impact of the health literacy level on the sensitivity and specificity of screening tests. No study has especially investigated if the health literacy level can influence a screening test sensitivity and specificity and how this is made. Furthermore, the following questions seem to not be answered by any studies:

1. Does the health literacy impact the rate of false-positive than false-negatives and vice versa?
2. If the questions above are answered by YES, then how does the health literacy impact the screening outcome's quality?

Most reviewed articles have mostly focused their works on the involvement of the individual in the decision-making process and their satisfaction, but not how the acquired knowledge, through the health literacy and health education, helps the individual to influences significant points and steps of the screening procedure like qualitative and quantitative long-term information provision.

Since we did conduct an exhaustive literature review, it possible that works are conducted on the topic somewhere, but we found no paper presenting work on the topic. Our literature dataset consisted of papers from PubMed, Scopus, dlpb, etc.

1.2.1 What is Screening Diseases?

Screening for diseases is defined as medical examination provided to the population (mass screening) or individual with the main objective of early detection, prevent, predict, and/or cure certain diseases. Cf. the chapter 1 for more insight into the term regarding its definition, subcategories, and process. The conventional screening is patient-centered, it means that a part of information and data used in the scope of the screening come from the patient and/or his relatives. The data and information are being collected through a patient-physician discussion or interview. In Australian Institute of Primary Care, (2008) the authors have defined the screening for diseases as:

Screening involves the systematic use of a test or investigatory tool to detect individuals at risk of developing a specific disease that is amenable to prevention or treatment. It is a population-based strategy to identify specific conditions in targeted groups before any symptoms appear and are undertaken in accordance with community-based screening protocols. Screening can also be an effective community engagement strategy that can lead to involvement in other health promotion activities for targeted population groups.

The central point, in screening for diseases, is the early detection or prediction of diseases before the symptoms appear. This point differs the screening for diseases from diseases diagnostics, which is essentially on analyzing the symptoms of the disease. An early study (Gunn et al., 2008) conducted on adults subjects with depressive symptoms revealed a morbidity (co-existence of multiple health conditions) in these subject's group. This study raises the question if the depressive symptoms can be classified as a factor and sign of a risk of being developing a disease? Tendentially, the answer could be yes, since the study of concern was longitudinal and involved 789 female participants (71% of the cohort, statistically significant) respecting the gender criteria, and englobing diverse categories of women (single, married, etc.). The study lasted 3 years (from 2005 to 2008) (Gunn et al., 2008).

The results of screening for diseases relied on analyzing information/data coming from two different sources (i) patient-physician interviews and (ii) medical examination or tests. Data analysis is then performed using exploratory data analysis methodology to find patterns and relationships in data and, thus, detect if the prevalence of developing the given disease is high or not. Figure 1 illustrates the screening process as well as the data sources.

Figure 1. Screening data: sources and process

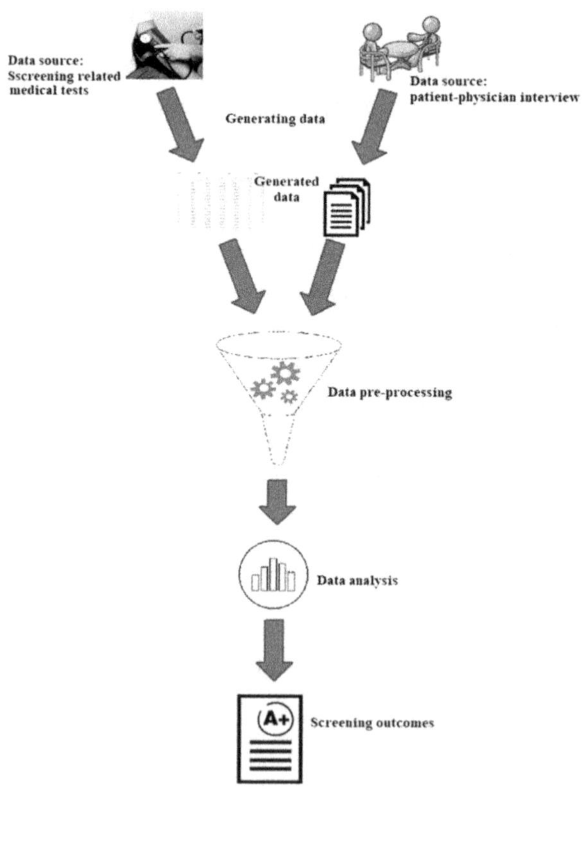

1.3 Health Educational Materials

Health literacy and diagnostics error are discussed in the previous subsections. The two previous subsections have shown the link between both health literacy and health outcomes. Since education implies educational materials, it is judicious to get insight into the materials involved in patient education.

Using patient educational materials from online health communities for building and/or improving health literacy among the population is the main objective as well as the context of the present study. The main hypothesis is defined as follows:

Hypothesis: *High health literacy could be associated with screening-test-outcomes in impacting the test-accuracy, sensitivity, and specificity since health literacy is known as positively impacting the health outcomes.*

It is, therefore, necessary to briefly define the online health communities and to evaluate the impact on health outcomes (diagnostics outcomes).

1.3.1 Online Health Communities as Educational Materials Source

Online health communities present the source of the patient educational materials in the context of the present study. In general, there exist many medical materials sources like a brochure, publications on the Internet, WHO Site, etc. Though, this study focuses on materials from online communities only.

In the age of information and communication, patients are more active on the Internet in seeking for information on diseases, thus, various online health communities are creating or being created day after day on the Internet. "Patient like me" (https://www.patientslikeme.com/) is an example of professional health communities on the Internet with high impact factor. Table 4 summarizes a set of online health communities.

Studies conducted on the impacts of online communities on diseases diagnostics have shown numerous benefits the patient can take from regularly being "visiting" online communities. In Juusola, Quisel, Foschini, and Ladapo (2016), the authors found out that certain online communities mostly help for getting definitive diagnostics especially for those who are lacking one.

In such health online communities, patients can meet diverse patients suffering from similar health condition like themselves as well as medical personnel who will provide a diagnosis. These communities have the advantages that all members of the communities can read the responses to a question and, thus, can react if they think that the response is weak, insufficient, false. Though these communities present the risk of providing not valid information to the patient and, thus, to hazard the patient.

This rise the question of the validity of the material and information available on the online communication and, hence, the need of providing policies for ensuring high quality for the documents and information circulating on the Internet regarding health concerns.

The quality of the information is important. To our best knowledge, there exists no policy as well as a quality metric to measure these documents and information available in the online communities. In Nath, Huh, Adupa, and Jonnalagadda, (2016), the authors have analyzed the content of several documents available on different online communities and found out that the quality of these documents relies more on the trust to and reputation of the publisher than on the quality. The more the site is related to the governmental or renowned institution, the more the consumer trust the content. In comparison, social websites are less trusted. The authors wrote:

The .gov and .edu websites are not found to have accreditations in general, but they might be trusted when associated with institutions with solid reputations. None of the social media websites contained trust codes because they do not have an obligation to validate their health information quality; their primary focus is not necessarily sharing health information. (Nath et al., 2016)

and concluded:

To further develop automated information quality detection, we need to rethink what is high-quality information. (Nath et al., 2016)

Despite the quality issues facing the documents available on the Internet, intended to serve as educational materials, online health communities positively impact the quality of life (QoL). In Rana, Wahlin, Lundborg, and Kabir, (2008), the authors have shown how the health education can impact the QoL. A case study among elderly people shown increasement of the QoL among the elderly people who have adhered to the educational intervention.

There exist communities that provide high-quality documents contents like Netforum of Philips. Is that a kind of policy to be used to high the quality of the document contents and, thus, guarantee patient safety as well as positive impact screening outcomes?

In Hajli, Sims, Featherman, and Love, (2015), the authors conducted a comprehensive study about the credibility of information contents in online communities, but not exhaustive since they analyzed 156 posts. The study revealed that information available in online health communities are credible. Though, this study fails to point out if credible information also a valid on is.

Obviously, information is of a certain quality, though, they contribute to patient empowerment so that patient can involve in his own health concerns. In Australian Institute of Primary Care, (2008) a report carried out by Australian Institute of Primary Care, health information objectives are defined as:

Health information interventions aim to increase people's capacity to make informed choices about their health and wellbeing. This includes providing opportunities for preventive care, by improving their understanding about the causes of health and illness, the services and support available to help maintain or improve health, and personal responsibility for actions affecting their health.

The report, further, presents a policy about how to measure the factor impact of health information.

Overall, health information supported education shows promises to impact patient health, increase his understanding of the disease and their causes. Since screening for diseases (see definition in the chapter entitled: Internet of Things Enabled Pre-Screening for Diseases) is partially based on patient-centered information, understanding diseases and its causes consists already a set of data the patient owns and can provide the medical doctor with that if needed.

This chapter aims at investigating rather the impacts of appropriate health education on screening outcomes than investigating the quality of the document contents in the online communities. It furthers, makes policies to the improvement of the process and outcomes of screening for diseases. The policies presented in this chapters rely on the use of the modern information technology and the research results.

Beyond the issues regarding the quality of the materials available in such online health communities, the readability of those materials poses an additional challenge to be tackled. In early 2017, Betschart et al. conducted a readability assessment of patient education materials written in German. Three European countries have the German language in common: Germany, Swiss, and Austrian. The assessment englobes materials published by the associations of urology from all these three countries and materials issued by the European Association of Urology (EAU). This study (Betschart, Zumstein, Ali, Schmid, & Abt, 2018) found out that materials issued by EAU are easiest to read and, thus, shows that the readability of patient educational materials is also a challenge to be considered. Xie et al. had also assessed online educational materials intended for the education on "velopharyngeal insufficiency" (VPI) and "velopharyngeal dysfunction" (VPD) and found out that the published VPI materials are written in a complex language for the common reader (Xie, Wang, & Chinnadurai, 2018). This study highlighted an important issue regarding the adaptability of online materials to the reader literacy level. Another study (Ghodasra et al., 2018) came to the same conclusion and claimed that additionally to the poor/ low quality of the online documents, the literacy of the reader is overestimated.

It is, however, something difficult for some experts to write down high specific documents in an easier language since they tend to use filed related terminologies that make the document or the language complex. Though, how could the modern technology, like machine learning (ML) and artificial intelligence (AI) help to solve this issue? Today, most online shops are utilizing the machine learning capability to learning from the user preferences and thus adapt accordingly their offers and advertisement to the users. Fiumara et al. have conducted a work (Fiumara, Celesti, Galletta, Carnevale, & Villari, 2018) on similar them and proposed to use AI and ML to automatically analyze patients "posts" available on the diverse online health communities. They presented and discussed the architecture of the proposed system. The system has shown promise to help to improve the quality of the contents of health-related materials on the Internet. The architecture involves medical doctors who can intervene and improve the posts of concern.

1.4 Context

Analphabet people are excluded from the present study. An ambitious project has to be initiated to define the "health literacy" for illiterates in replacing the term "read"

Table 4. Sample Online Health Communities

Community	Description	URLs
SparkPeople	Provides information about dietetics and brings people having body weight issues in common together.	http://sparkpeople.com/
Everyday Health	Every health platform is health community providing his members with information, advises, health materials on various health topics like living healthy, lose weight that contribute to preventing diabetes, for example.	https://www.everydayhealth.com/
Mayo Clinic Connect	This platform is like every Health community platforms. The patient is offered the possibility to follow the discussion and get alerted once new entries about the discussion are available.	https://connect.mayoclinic.org/
Health.MSN.com	This platform is not a common community as the other ones, but it provides exhaustive health information.	https://www.msn.com/en-us/health
WebMD Exchange	This community offers a huge on the online discussion in diverse forums. It, further, interesting material on numerous health topics like cancer, diabetes, etc.	https://exchanges.webmd.com/default.htm
Netforum	This community is owned by Philips for healthcare professionals. It serves to share cases studies outcomes, experiences, etc. The quality of the documents available here is very high.	http://netforum.healthcare.philips.com/global

with "listing to", "write" with "clearly and audibly speak". Educational materials should mostly audio and video based.

The present study is focusing patient health education supporting by educational materials from the diverse online health communities and from the Internet.

1.5 Chapter Structure

The remainder of the chapter includes 5 sections whereas section 2 presents the problems and analysis followed by the research methodology in section 3. Section 4 presents the results of the study. The chapter is concluded in section 5 where the results are further discussed. Section 6 outlines the future works.

2. PROBLEM STATEMENT AND ANALYSIS

This section will present and analyze the main problems facing the screening for diseases. Certain groups of individuals are considered to not take any benefits from screening for diseases, based on diverse data analysis. For example in Maxim, Niebo, and Utell, (2014), the Medicare Evidence Development and Coverage Advisory Committee (MEDCAC) recommends stopping screening women aged from 40 to 49 years, because the data analysis does not show any evidence-based benefits for the group of concern. An early study (Thombs et al., 2008) has evaluated the benefit of screening the depression in a patient with cardiovascular disease as recommended by several practice guidelines. It concluded that the treatment of depression in such patient does not improve the cardiac outcomes. The study has demonstrated that patients with cardiovascular diseases do not take any benefits from the depression screening. The question here is why the practice guidelines recommend the depression screening for such patient despite the lack of improvement of the cardiac outcomes?

In addition to the controversies above, the screening is facing a huge of issues like high rates of false-positive and false-negative test-outcomes. The number of false-positive and false-negative outcomes determine the sensitivity and specificity of a screening test.

A *False-Negative screening test outcome* indicates that an individual, who basically has the pathology for which they are screened for, is identified as not having or not presenting any sign to develop or not at risk to contract the diseases. This type of outcomes is life threating for the individual and facing and can end up in an eventual risk of morbidity and mortality.

A *False-Positive screening test outcome* is, in contrary to a false-negative test-outcome, an individual is unfortunately declared having or is at risk to develop a given disease according to the screening test outcomes. Hence, the individual is exposed to unnecessary and costly medical examinations.

The sensitivity of a screening test = the ratio of true-negative to {true-negative + false positive}

The specificity of a screening test = the ratio of true-positive to {true-positive + false-positive}

The Specificity and sensitivity are interdependent and are used to qualify the screening test outcomes.

The literature review found out a high number of works claiming the high rates of false-negative and false-positive test-outcomes. The set of these articles includes studies like Renshaw and Gould, (2013), Maxim et al., (2014), or recent works like Yang, Zhang, Yao, and Fan, (2018) and Di and Li, (2018). All available studies concluded the same results and pointed also out the same controversies regarding the benefit of the screening procedures for certain groups of individuals. The reasons why the screening is facing those controversies and why the rate of false outcomes is so high is diverse. One reason is the lack of long-term data. The data acquisition relies on 1:1 interview (patient: medical doctor) and on the patient medical records are available. The patient health record and patient-centric data are quasi-inexistent. Thus, the data on which the screening is relying is insufficient and incomplete.

The patient-centered data (not patient-centric data[2]) is often subjective. Furthermore, the patient can omit some important details if their knowledge regarding health concerns is low.

The literature review has highlighted the association between patient health education, health literacy, and health outcomes. It is also demonstrated that the health literacy level influences the patient self-management ability, capacity to search for information, understanding of health condition level (depending on literacy level), diseases awareness, and insight into health concerns.

The main problem to tackle is how to improve patient's medical knowledge so that the patient can collect screening significant and sufficient data to build a long-term data pool to support the screening procedure.

This study aims to verify the unique hypothesis:

Hypothesis: *Since the healthy literacy positively impacts the health outcomes, it will obviously also positively impact the screening test outcomes.*

3. METHODOLOGY

This section presents the research methodology and data. This study is essentially based on literature reviews and a few interviews conducted to control the literature reviews results.

3.1 Sampling Methods and Research Approaches

- **Snowball Sampling Method:** The test period was relatively short. Therefore, the recruitment of patient was challenging. The participants were, therefore, recruited using the snowball approach the first recruited participants were requested to recruit further participants according to the defined criteria.

The literature pool was also build using the snowball technique where recently cited references in an article were added to the pool. The operation was repeated for each article added to the pool.

The pool was in afterward filtered. Only the articles that handle the topic of the present study were retained.

Qualitative Research Approach: The qualitative approach was implemented to measure the quality of the provided answers. Following are measured:

1. The Quality of the Patient's Answers
2. The Patient's Quality of Life
3. The Patient's Diseases Awareness Level
4. The Quality of the Provided Long-term Data4
5. The Accuracy Level of the Screening Test-Outcomes

3.2 Literature Search and Sampling

A comprehensive literature review was conducted following the snowball approach. Additionally, posts available in some online health communities were analyzed. Literature dealing with topics like:

1. Impact of health education on individual health and wellbeing
2. Quality and validity of education material available in online (health) communities
3. Impact of health literacy on diseases prevention, lifestyle, quality of life
4. Health education and screening for diseases
5. Health literacy and screening for diseases

The objective of analyzing posts available in online health communities was to study the impact on the quality of life of communities through the content of their posts, structural quality of posts and the plausibility level of the given answers.

Results of interviews and investigations conducted in were considered in Edoh et al., (2017) the scope of investigating the impact of health education on the level of health literacy.

The main objective of the study is to find out to what extent health education can contribute to improving the accuracy of outcomes of conventional screening for diseases.

3.3 Cohort Sampling

The study involved 45 participants divided into three (03) categories and screened for cardiovascular diseases and malaria:

1. Participants with high health literacy level (Test Cohort): Group 1
2. Participants with low health literacy level (Control Cohort): Group 2
3. Participants without health literacy level (Control Cohort): Group 3

The test foresaw following control strategy (a) test involving group 1 aims at investigating the impact of health literacy on the accuracy and quality of screening for diseases. A control test involved the group 2 to verify if the accuracy depends on the literacy level. The group 3 aims at confirming the results obtained.

3.4 Evaluation of the Impact of Health Literacy on the Screening Test-Outcomes

To investigate the impaction of the health education on the screening for diseases test-outcomes, people with diverse health literacy level (high, medium, and low/poor) as well as healthcare professionals experienced with regular screening people were interviewed.

The impact of health literacy level on the quality and accuracy of the outcomes of screening for diseases was investigated since it determines the health education which in turn implies the diseases awareness and medical knowledge.

Healthcare professionals were asked to evaluate the quality of the information collected in the scope of screening in a patient-physician interview in three different cohorts. One cohort consists of participants with high, medium, and low health literacy level. People with low/poor literacy are illiterate.

Beyond this, the involved healthcare professionals were further asked to evaluate the impact of thus collected data on the screening test-outcomes. For this purpose, the cohort consisted of health semi-literate participants (medium health literacy), was selected as a control-cohort to evaluate the *research hypothesis stating that health literacy can increase the accuracy of screening outcomes.*

Health Literacy Level Classification: As classified in (Edoh et al., 2017) using the Medical Term Recognition Test (METER) to measure the literacy level, the health literacy level is measured using the METER. The classification is as follows:

1. Low Literacy (0 - 15 words)
2. Marginal Literacy (16 - 25 words)
3. Functional Literacy (26 - 32 words)

The metrics used in the study can be mapped as shown in Table 5.

3.5 Data Collection and Analysis

Questionnaires

The medical doctors collect independently from the present study all needed data as the national screening requests using the national standard questionnaire.

The study questionnaire was intended for the healthcare professionals. Five structured interview questions (see Table 6) were sent to the involved healthcare professionals.

Data Gathering

Following data have been collected for the study purpose:

1. Quality of the participant's answer
2. Diseases awareness
3. Lifestyle and quality of life
4. Long-term data/information provided by the participant

Table 5.

Low health literacy		Low Literacy
Medium health literacy	corresponds	Marginal Literacy
High health literacy		Functional Literacy

Table 6. Questionnaire

Pos.	Question	Number of Answers				
		Excellent	Very Good	Good	Satisfactory	Low/Poor
1	What is the quality of the patient's answers?					
2	What is the participant's diseases awareness level?					
3	What is the quality of Life of the patient?					
4	Could the patient provide useful long-term data?					
5	What is the accuracy level of the outcomes?					

5. The accuracy level of the outcomes before any medical tests
6. Outcomes of eventual medical tests
7. Medical tests outcomes/data-drive screening outcomes Ratio

Each collected information is scored on a scalar from 1 to 5 where 5 is the best score. All scores were added together and evaluate according to following indicators defined in Table 7. A score between 20 and 29 is classified as a good key indicator if, additionally to the score, the rate outcomes test/data-driven outcomes ≥ 3 and the data-driven outcomes accuracy > 3 otherwise it is classified as "satisfactory"

Data Analysis

Microsoft Excel was used for the data analysis. We first built an AVG of the scores each reaches. Before building the AVG, the different scores a participant obtains were compared with each other. In the case of strong discrepancy between the scores of the same participant, the scores were classified biased and were not included in the analysis.

3.6 Evaluation and Measurement Metrics

To evaluate the validity and reliability of investigated data, each participant was screened by five different medical doctors. The medical doctors did not know about the health literacy of each examined participant, so we ensure to prevent any subjectivity in the data evaluation and analysis.

Table 7. Scores and Indicators

Scores	Key Indicators	Description
35	Excellent	Fully impact the screening outcomes and ensure high accuracy
30 - 34	Very good	Rate outcomes test/data-driven outcomes ≥ 3 Impact the screening outcomes and ensure very good accuracy
30 – 34	Good	Rate outcomes test/data-driven outcomes < 3 Impact the screening outcomes and ensure good accuracy
20 - 29	Good	Rate outcomes test/data-driven outcomes ≥ 3 Data-driven outcomes accuracy > 3 Lightly impact the screening outcomes and ensure less accuracy
20 - 29	Satisfactory	Rate outcomes test/data-driven outcomes < 3 Data-driven outcomes accuracy ≤ 3 Lightly impact the screening outcomes with sporadic accuracy
< 20	Bad/worst	Do not impact the screening outcomes, No accuracy

Data Validity and Reliability

Validity and reliability are two metrics to assess the quality of the measurement methods. They enable to assess for consistency of a given number of measurement and validity of measured data.

For validity and reliability purposes, data is gathered 3 times in same conditions and compared with each other.

Error Rate

The participants were meticulously sorted regarding their background, literacy level diseases awareness and health education level.

All collected data and information were for plausibility checked. The data and information were double-stored (audio, video, and write) and compared in afterward. This procedure was used to detect any biases in the data provided by medical doctors to us.

The rate of biases and errors were extremely low thus insignificant.

4. EXPERIMENT AND RESULTS

4.1 Test Period

The experiment lasted eight (08) weeks whereas 4 weeks were to recruitment and preparation issues. Information about participants background was collected. The relevant data is defined.

4.2 Test Results

To analyze and point out to what extent health literacy can impact screening outcomes, gathered data were pre-processed. Table 8 indicates which score how many people in each cohort have reached. Participants in the cohort with high literacy level obtained very good and positive results. Participants in the cohort with low literacy level mostly scored less than 30 while participants from the last cohort obtained the worst score.

After recording the scores, a further analysis was performed to understand the score differential between the participant in each group.

G1 - High Health Literacy: 3 people have attained the maximal score. The analysis revealed that these people have a high disease awareness level and continuously get educated on health concerns. They are active in several online health communities and regularly visit the doctors.

10 people obtained a score between 30 and 34. In this subgroup, the diseases awareness level is medium, and people are moderately health educated. They are less active than people in the subgroup whit high score.

2 people obtain a score between 20 and 29. The disease awareness low despite the high health literacy. They are not active in any online communities.

G2 - Medium to Low Health Literacy: 11 people in this group present similar characteristics as the two people with the lowest score in the G1. The analysis revealed that in contrary to people with high literacy level, medium to low diseases awareness level in this subgroup is associated with the low health literacy. People in this subgroup claim facing difficulties in searching for information and understanding the content.

The lowest subgroup obtained a score less than 20. These people were assessed 3 times for validity and reliability purpose. The results remain the same. This subgroup shows a poor diseases awareness.

G3 - Low to Poor Health Literacy: Most people (12 persons) in this group obtain a score less than 20. They claim to face a language barrier since the educational materials are written in the official language (French and English). They request audio materials for the education and the possibility to improve the literacy level.

Scores obtained in each indicator and measurement category were processed for the analysis purposes. It does matter to investigate which factor impact the average scores obtained by each cohort. For this reason, Table 9 summarizes the diverse factor-related outcomes. This table presents only the positive outcomes in percentage.

Table 8. Structure of Cumulative Scores obtained by the involved Participants

Scores	Health Literacy Level		
	High	Low	Poor
35	3	0	0
30 - 34	10	2	0
20 - 29	2	11	3
< 20	0	2	12

Table 9. Structure of the diverse positive Screening Outcomes in each Indicator Category

Categories of the Key Indicators	Percentage of Positive Outcomes		
	G1	G2	G3
Quality of answers to the interviews questions	80%	33%	03%
Level of the Diseases awareness	90%	45%	00%
Lifestyle and quality of life	100%	25%	11%
Long-term data/information provided	60%	02%	00%
Outcomes accuracy level	95%	65%	40%
Outcomes of medical tests	100%	100%	100%
Medical tests outcomes/data-drive screening outcomes ratio	95%	65%	40%

G1 = Participants with high health literacy level
G2 = Participants with low health literacy level
G3 = Participants without health literacy level

4.2.1 Quality of the Participant's Answers

Answers provided by the participants from the cohort with high literacy level were structured, precise. The analysis revealed that this (well-structured and precise answers) is associated with the education level of the interviewees, but not with health literacy. As presented in Table 8 there are people with high literacy level who obtain a low score. Furthermore, there are people with medium health literacy level who have obtained better score than people with high health literacy. *People with high diseases awareness gave detailed answers independently of their health literacy level.* The analysis of interview questions revealed a correlation between the knowledge level and the quality of provided answers. The higher a participant's knowledge in the domain, the more precise and detailed is the answer. The participant's knowledge is related to the level of the diseases awareness. The knowledge level is not associated with the literacy level. The study thus figures out that the health literacy level is a knowledge acquisition facilitator but does not automatically imply a knowledge possession.

The correlation between the education level and the health literacy and patient health education level was not investigated. The answer to this question is not obvious since people with low education level can become autodidact and thus will acquire the ability to read, write, and understand complex things. The point will be investigated in a forthcoming article.

4.2.2 Diseases Awareness

It can be noticed that disease awareness relies on health education. In turn, it seems that diseases awareness level can impact the quality of the answer during a screening interview.

4.2.3 Lifestyle and Quality of Life

The Quality of Life (QoL) among the cohort with high literacy level combined with high health education and knowledge is higher than the QoL in the other cohorts or subgroups. The high health educated participants are more aware of the benefits one can take from having a healthy lifestyle. Furthermore, they know what to do to have a healthy lifestyle while the other cohort members lack this knowledge.

The health literacy level combined with the health and medical knowledge level seem to impact the QoL. "seem" is used because the duration of the present study does not allow us to make a definitive statement on the relation between QoL and health literacy associated with health and medical knowledge. A longitudinal study over several years observing various cohorts is needed for the definitive assertion.

4.2.4 Long-Term Data and Information Provided by the Participants

A deep analysis of the screening protocols has revealed that mostly provided longer-term data came from participants in the cohort with high literacy level. More than 50% of these participants were aware of the importance of long-term data in the screening and which data are needed for successful screening. Based on this knowledge, they collect by themselves relevant data. Since lack of long-term data is a crucial issue facing the screening evaluation and, thus, being impacting the accuracy of the outcomes, providing these data will definitive positive impact the accuracy screening outcomes.

We noticed a significant difference in the degree of details in which the collected long-term data is described. Data provided by people with high diseases awareness is more detailed and contains more screening relevant information. The literacy level plays a significant role here too, but it must be combined with the diseases awareness which implies patient health education.

4.2.5 Accuracy Level of the Test-Outcomes

The level of the outcomes accuracy in screening the cohort with high literacy level is higher than the others. Since long-term information is a matter factor that can significantly impact the accuracy. It is worth noticing that the diseases awareness and patient health education are the important factors that have influenced the outcomes. This study reveals that indirectly the literacy level can impact the quality and accuracy of screening outcomes since it supports or enables the patient health education.

4.2.6 Outcomes of Eventual Medical Tests

This factor is independent of literacy level one has. Though, this factor is constant and is not impacted by the literacy level. It is but somehow a control test to verify the data-driven evaluation outcomes.

4.2.7 Ratio Medical Test-Outcomes/ Data Driven Screening Outcomes

The quality and accuracy of the outcome can be measured by the ratio medical test outcome / evaluation outcomes. The evaluation can be considered accurate and high quality if the ratio strongly approaches one (01).

The ratio of the cohort with high literacy level is the highest and approaches 1 (0,95).

The probability that health education positively the quality and accuracy of screening outcomes is high and thus needs to be deeply investigated in a longitudinal study.

4.2.8 Research Findings

The main findings of this study are:

1. Health literacy is a pre-requisite for patient health education. The educational materials need to be adapted to the health literacy level of the individual. Though, people with poor (health) literacy can be health education if the paradigm is changed, so that more video and audio materials in the native tongue is offered
2. Patient health education underlines the diseases awareness. High Health literacy doe does not automatically imply high diseases awareness level
3. Health literacy, patient health education, and diseases awareness combined in suited proportion can positively influence the screening test-outcomes.

4.3 Resulting Concept

Many works have been done regarding the health literacy level measurement, for ex. Ahmed, Shaikh, Soomro, Qazi, and Soomro, (2018); Merker et al., (2018) and the influences of health literacy on the health outcomes. In a previous study (Edoh et al., 2017) we showed how to assess the diseases awareness level in an individual.

Based on previous works done by several authors and the findings of the present study, we propose a system to improve the health literacy, patient education, and diseases awareness. The main objectives are to decrease the rate of false-positive and false-negative screening test-outcomes and thus increase the test sensitivity and specificity.

1. Regularly assess the health literacy (HL) of the individuals.

This work proposes an AI and ML enabled and questionnaire-based mobile application to verify the individual ability to read, write, and understand a text and thus classify the literacy level. The system will be featured with a self-decision-making ability. Based on the test score propose to the patient a training to improve their literacy.

2. Training the HL ability of the individual in asking them to regularly perform some exercises like read, write, and understand complex tests.

An individual with a minimum of literacy can be trained to increase their level. A training system is proposed to help the patient through this process.

A mobile application using the AI and ML technologies will guide the patient, give them exercises and help them to perform their read, write and understanding ability.

3. Improving the readability and adapted it to the educational materials using AI and ML

The readability of educational materials available on the Internet or in various healthcare units remains challenging. Several studies (see literature review) have pointed out this issue. To tackle this issue, some lexica are needed. These lexica will support the readability in rewording complex phrases used in an educational material.

Beyond rewording the educational using AI and ML technologies, it important to create adapt appropriate materials to the illiterate abilities using pictures for the illustration, audio, or videos

5. CONCLUSION

It is well known that health literacy impacts health outcomes. The literature review conducted has shown the association between health literacy and health outcomes. Furthermore, the study demonstrates that the health literacy alone is not sufficient to impact health outcomes. It is obvious that health literacy does not imply the patient health education and thus the diseases awareness level. The health literacy supports the patient health education. It is the cornerstone of the patient health education. The health literacy just influences the readability and understanding of educational materials. This means that patient with low health literacy level can also be health educated if the educational materials are adapted to the cognitive capability of the patient.

Based on the results of the conducted experiment and the data analysis, this study demonstrates that the patient health education level can positively impact the screening test-outcomes. Though it needs to be supported by an adequate health literacy level.

6. FUTURE WORKS

The health literacy is known as a pre-requisite for the patient health education. This means individuals with poor or no (health) literacy level are excluded from any patient health education program and, hence, cannot any diseases awareness.

Regarding the number of people with poor or no (health) literacy in the developing world. a paradigm change and re-definition of the said terms are therefore needed. The next challenges to tackle are (i) enabling patient health education for the said people and (ii) redefining or extending the term of "health literacy" and hence the measurement paradigm. Our future works would focus on implementing AI and ML-based systems to help illiterates to take part in any patient health education and also attain high health education level and thus appropriate diseases awareness.

Beyond this, it is a need to work on improving the readability and quality of those educational information materials available on the diverse online health communities.

REFERENCES

Abiodun, O. A., Olu-Abiodun, O. O., Sotunsa, J. O., & Oluwole, F. A. (2014). Impact of health education intervention on knowledge and perception of cervical cancer and cervical screening uptake among adult women in rural communities in Nigeria. *BMC Public Health, 14*(814), 1–9. doi:10.1186/1471-2458-14-814 PMID:25103189

Ahmed, W., Shaikh, Z. N., Soomro, J. A., Qazi, H. A., & Soomro, A. K. (2018). Assessment of health literacy in adult population of Karachi: A preliminary investigation for concept-based evidence. *International Journal of Health Promotion and Education, 56*(2), 95–104. doi:10.1080/14635240.2017.1421866

Australian Institute of Primary Care. (2008). Measuring health promotion impacts : A guide to impact evaluation in integrated health promotion. *Community Health.*

Berkman, N. D., Sheridan, S. L., Donahue, K. E., Halpern, D. J., & Crotty, K. (2011). Low health literacy and health outcomes: An updated systematic review. *Annals of Internal Medicine, 155*(2), 97–107. doi:10.7326/0003-4819-155-2-201107190-00005 PMID:21768583

Betschart, P., Zumstein, V., Ali, O. H., Schmid, H. P., & Abt, D. (2018). Readability assessment of patient education material published by German-speaking associations of urology. *Urologia Internationalis, 100*(1), 79–84. doi:10.1159/000480095 PMID:29151111

Chesser, A. K., Keene Woods, N., Smothers, K., & Rogers, N. (2016). Health Literacy and Older Adults. *Gerontology and Geriatric Medicine, 2*, 233372141663049. doi:10.1177/2333721416630492 PMID:28138488

Corcos, J., & Przydacz, M. (2018). Patient education. In *Consultation in Neurourology: A Practical Evidence-Based Guide* (Vol. 17, pp. 285–297). Springer International Publishing AG.

Demarco, J., & Nystrom, M. (2010). The importance of health literacy in patient education. *Journal of Consumer Health on the Internet, 14*(3), 294–301. doi:10.1080/15398285.2010.502021

Devraj, R., Borrego, M. E., Vilay, A. M., Pailden, J., & Horowitz, B. (2018). Awareness, self-management behaviors, health literacy and kidney function relationships in specialty practice. *World Journal of Nephrology, 7*(1), 41–50. doi:10.5527/wjn.v7.i1.41 PMID:29359119

Di, L., & Li, Y. (2018). The risk factor of false-negative and false-positive for T-SPOT.TB in active tuberculosis. *Journal of Clinical Laboratory Analysis, 32*(2), e22273. doi:10.1002/jcla.22273 PMID:28594104

Edoh, T., Zogbochi, V., Pawar, P., Hounsou, J. T., & Alahassa, B. R. (2017). Impact of the Internet on diseases awareness and patient empowerment — A study in Benin (West Africa). In *2017 Fourth International Conference on Advances in Biomedical Engineering (ICABME)* (pp. 1–4). IEEE. 10.1109/ICABME.2017.8167543

Evangelista, L. S., Rasmusson, K. D., Laramee, A. S., Barr, J., Ammon, S. E., Dunbar, S., ... Yancy, C. W. (2010). Health Literacy and the Patient With Heart Failure-Implications for Patient Care and Research: A Consensus Statement of the Heart Failure Society of America. *Journal of Cardiac Failure, 16*(1), 9–16. doi:10.1016/j.cardfail.2009.10.026 PMID:20123313

Fabbri, M., Yost, K., Finney Rutten, L. J., Manemann, S. M., Boyd, C. M., Jensen, D., ... Roger, V. L. (2018). Health Literacy and Outcomes in Patients With Heart Failure: A Prospective Community Study. *Mayo Clinic Proceedings, 93*(1), 9–15. doi:10.1016/j.mayocp.2017.09.018 PMID:29217337

Fiumara, G., Celesti, A., Galletta, A., Carnevale, L., & Villari, M. (2018). Applying Artificial Intelligence in Healthcare Social Networks to Identity Critical Issues in Patients' Posts. In *Proceedings of the 11th International Joint Conference on Biomedical Engineering Systems and Technologies* (pp. 680–687). SCITEPRESS - Science and Technology Publications. 10.5220/0006750606800687

Ghodasra, J. H., Wang, D., Jayakar, R. G., Jensen, A. R., Yamaguchi, K. T., Hegde, V. V., & Jones, K. J. (2018). The Assessment of Quality, Accuracy, and Readability of Online Educational Resources for Platelet-Rich Plasma. *Arthroscopy, 34*(1), 272–278. doi:10.1016/j.arthro.2017.06.023 PMID:28784239

Gunn, J., Gilchrist, G., Chondros, P., Ramp, M., Hegarty, K., Blashki, G., ... Herrman, H. (2008). Who is identified when screening for depression in general practice? Findings from the Diagnosis, Management and Outcomes of Depressive Symptoms Longitudinal (diamond) Study. *The Medical Journal of Australia, 188*(12), S119–S125. PMID:18558911

Hajli, M. N., Sims, J., Featherman, M., & Love, P. E. D. (2015). Credibility of information in online communities. *Journal of Strategic Marketing, 23*(3), 238–253. doi:10.1080/0965254X.2014.920904

Horton, R. (2007). What ' s Wrong with Doctors. *The New York Review of Books, 54*(13), 66. Retrieved from http://www.nybooks.com/articles/2007/05/31/whats-wrong-with-doctors/

Juusola, J. L., Quisel, T. R., Foschini, L., & Ladapo, J. A. (2016). The impact of an online crowdsourcing diagnostic tool on health care utilization: A case study using a novel approach to retrospective claims analysis. *Journal of Medical Internet Research, 18*(6), 1–10. doi:10.2196/jmir.5644 PMID:27251384

Koroukian, S. M., Basu, J., Schiltz, N. K., Navale, S., Bakaki, P. M., Warner, D. F., ... Stange, K. C. (2018). Changes in Case-Mix and Health Outcomes of Medicare Fee-for-Service Beneficiaries and Managed Care Enrollees during the Years 1992-2011. *Medical Care, 56*(1), 39–46. doi:10.1097/MLR.0000000000000847 PMID:29176368

Linder, G., Sandin, F., Johansson, J., Lindblad, M., Lundell, L., & Hedberg, J. (2018). Patient education-level affects treatment allocation and prognosis in esophageal- and gastroesophageal junctional cancer in Sweden. *Cancer Epidemiology, 52*, 91–98. doi:10.1016/j.canep.2017.12.008

Maxim, L. D., Niebo, R., & Utell, M. J. (2014). Screening tests: A review with examples. *Inhalation Toxicology, 26*(13), 811–828. doi:10.3109/08958378.2014.955932 PMID:25264934

Merker, V. L., McDannold, S., Riklin, E., Talaei-Khoei, M., Sheridan, M. R., Jordan, J. T., ... Vranceanu, A. M. (2018). Health literacy assessment in adults with neurofibromatosis: Electronic and short-form measurement using FCCHL and Health LiTT. *Journal of Neuro-Oncology, 136*(2), 335–342. doi:10.100711060-017-2657-8 PMID:29119424

Minue, S., Bermudez-Tamayo, C., Fernandez, A., Martin-Martin, J. J., Benitez, V., Melguizo, M., ... Montoro, R. (2014). Identification of factors associated with diagnostic error in primary care. *BMC Family Practice, 15*(1), 92. doi:10.1186/1471-2296-15-92 PMID:24884984

Moorhead, S., Johnson, M., Maas, M., & Swanson, E. (2018). *Nursing Outcomes Classification (NOC)-E-Book: Measurement of Health Outcomes*. Elsevier. Retrieved from https://books.google.de/books?hl=de&lr=&id=LYlIDwAAQBAJ&oi=fnd&pg=PP1&dq=define+health+outcomes&ots=bOTv_XytcU&sig=hqWEjophQarxuLKuIOw7ea6XdNY#v=onepage&q=definehealthoutcomes&f=false

Murcia-Robayo, R. Y., Jouanisson, E., Beauchamp, G., & Diaw, M. (2018). Effects of staining method and clinician experience on the evaluation of stallion sperm morphology. *Animal Reproduction Science, 188*, 165–169. doi:10.1016/j.anireprosci.2017.11.021

Nath, C., Huh, J., Adupa, A. K., & Jonnalagadda, S. R. (2016). Website Sharing in Online Health Communities: A Descriptive Analysis. *Journal of Medical Internet Research, 18*(1), e11. doi:10.2196/jmir.5237 PMID:26764193

Oldach, B. R., & Katz, M. L. (2014). Health literacy and cancer screening: A systematic review. *Patient Education and Counseling, 94*(2), 149–157. doi:10.1016/j.pec.2013.10.001 PMID:24207115

Parker, P. D., Heiney, S. P., Friedman, D. B., Felder, T. M., Estrada, R. D., Harris, E. H., & Adams, S. A. (2018). How are health literacy principles incorporated into breast cancer chemotherapy education? A review of the literature. *Journal of Nursing Education and Practice, 8*(6), 77. doi:10.5430/jnep.v8n6p77

Rana, A. K. M. M., Wahlin, A., Lundborg, C. S., & Kabir, Z. N. (2008). Impact of health education on health-related quality of life among elderly persons: Results from a community-based intervention study in rural Bangladesh. *Health Promotion International, 24*(1), 36–45. doi:10.1093/heapro/dan042 PMID:19136677

Renshaw, A. A., & Gould, E. W. (2013). Reducing false-negative and false-positive diagnoses in anatomic pathology consultation material. *Archives of Pathology & Laboratory Medicine, 137*(12), 1770–1773. doi:10.5858/arpa.2013-0012-OA PMID:24283857

Roberts, G. (2015). Improving Health Literacy to Reduce Health Inequalities. *UCL Institute for Health Equity*. Retrieved from file:///Users/janereeve/Documents/Janes Documents/EGA Module 4/M4 Documents/Improving Health Literacy to Reduce Health Inequalities.webarchive

Saeed, H., Saleem, Z., Naeem, R., Shahzadi, I., & Islam, M. (2018). Impact of health literacy on diabetes outcomes: A cross-sectional study from Lahore, Pakistan. *Public Health, 156*, 8–14. doi:10.1016/j.puhe.2017.12.005 PMID:29353668

Sentell, T. L., Tsoh, J. Y., Davis, T., Davis, J., & Braun, K. L. (2015). Low health literacy and cancer screening among Chinese Americans in California: A cross-sectional analysis. *BMJ Open*, *5*(1), e006104. doi:10.1136/bmjopen-2014-006104 PMID:25564140

Sørensen, K., Van den Broucke, S., Fullam, J., Doyle, G., Pelikan, J., Slonska, Z., & Brand, H. (2012). Health literacy and public health: A systematic review and integration of definitions and models. *BMC Public Health*, *12*(1), 80. doi:10.1186/1471-2458-12-80 PMID:22276600

Thombs, B. D., de Jonge, P., Coyne, J. C., & Whooley, M. A., Frasure-Smith, N., Mitchell, A. J., … Ziegelstein, R. C. (2008). Clinician's Corner Depression Screening and Patient Outcomes in Cardiovascular Care A. *Systematic Reviews*, *300*(18).

Traczynski, J., & Udalova, V. (2018). Nurse practitioner independence, health care utilization, and health outcomes. *Journal of Health Economics*, *58*, 90–109. doi:10.1016/j.jhealeco.2018.01.001 PMID:29475093

Wellbery, C. (2011). Flaws in Clinical Reasoning: A Common Cause of Diagnostic Error. *American Family Physician*, *84*(9), 1042–1044. PMID:22046946

Whalen, M., Maliszewski, B., Sheinfeld, R., Gardner, H., & Baptiste, D. (2018). Outcomes of an Innovative Evidence-Based Practice Project: Building a Difficult-Access Team in the Emergency Department. *Journal of Emergency Nursing: JEN*, *1–5*. doi:10.1016/j.jen.2018.03.011 PMID:29704977

World Health Organization. (2016). *Diagnostic Errors. Technical Series on Safer Primary Care*. Retrieved from http://apps.who.int/iris

Xie, D. X., Wang, R. Y., & Chinnadurai, S. (2018). Readability of online patient education materials for velopharyngeal insufficiency. *International Journal of Pediatric Otorhinolaryngology*, *104*, 113–119. doi:10.1016/j.ijporl.2017.09.016 PMID:29287850

Yang, C., Zhang, S., Yao, L., & Fan, L. (2018). *Evaluation of risk factors for false-negative results with an antigen-specific peripheral blood-based quantitative cell assay (T -SPOT . TB) in the diagnosis of active tuberculosis: A large-scale retrospective study in China*. Academic Press. doi:10.1177/0300060518757381

Zolezzi, M., Eltorki, Y. H., Almaamoon, M., Fathy, M., & Omar, N. E. (2018). Outcomes of patient education practices to optimize the safe use of lithium: A literature review. *Mental Health Clinician*, *8*(1), 41–48. doi:10.9740/mhc.2018.01.041 PMID:29955544

ENDNOTES

1 School-based education.

2 Patient-centric data is data collected using modern information and communication technology. This data set includes vital parameters, etc., while patient-centered data is data emanated from the patient or their relatives.

Chapter 7
Ubiquitous Wearable Healthcare Monitoring System Architectural Design for Prevention, Detection, and Monitoring of Chronic Diseases

Gaurav Paliwal
R. C. Patel Institute of Technology, India

Aaquil Bunglowala
NMIMS University, India

ABSTRACT

Chronic diseases have become the leading cause of death and disability worldwide. Major chronic diseases currently account for almost 60% of all deaths, and this contribution is expected to rise up to 73% by 2020. An integrated approach is needed for detection, prevention, and monitoring of these diseases. For better and specialized healthcare services, there is a need to develop a technology that should be fast, reliable, secure, accurate, and economical. In this chapter, the authors have presented an architectural design for wearable healthcare monitoring systems. The main motivation behind this architectural design is to improve the efficiency, accuracy, and generosity of WHMS. The architecture design divides the system into three layers or subsystems. The chapter provides a detailed description of subsystems, components, functionalities, requirements, and realization mechanisms along with their merits and demerits. The resolution of design issues like data fusion, data delivery, data processing, security, accuracy, and efficiency are the main points of this architecture design.

DOI: 10.4018/978-1-5225-7131-5.ch007

INTRODUCTION

Currently, world's population is increasing at the rate of 1.1% and so is the number of patients. Disease rates from poor lifestyle choices such as lack of physical activity, poor diet, stress, smoking and overuse of alcohol are accelerating globally, advancing across every region and pervading all socioeconomic classes. To provide impeccable health care services to the society healthcare sector needs a transformation. For better and specialized healthcare services, there is a need to develop a technology that should be fast, reliable, secure, accurate, and economical. Such astonishing expectations can only be contented with Wearable Healthcare Monitoring Systems (WHMS), which will make use of different ICT based technologies to provide continuous healthcare support to the user. A system which will provide complete mobility, privacy, security and it will take care of the patient even in the absence of a physician. A system which will continuously monitor the patient's biosignals along with the physical activities performed. A system designed in such a manner that it will provide complete generosity and delineate the requisites of a broad range of diseases. The system which will make use of different wearable sensors, smartphones, communication, and computation technologies to provide healthcare services. In this chapter, the authors are going to present system architecture for WHMS to envision this expectation in an effective manner. Through this architectural design, the authors are attempting to answer the following question frequently raised by researchers and system designers.

- Which design alternative will be most suitable for system design?
- How to improve the efficiency and accuracy of system?
- How to decrease the cost of wearable monitoring systems?
- How to make the system ubiquitous in nature to take over a broad range of diseases?

The answers to this entire question can be found in a sound architectural design. The architectural design of WHMS presented in this chapter is divided into various sections. The first Section of this chapter briefly describes the basic working of the WHMS and its subsystems. In the second, third, and fourth sections the authors have described the three subsystems of WHMS that includes the body area network, mobile base unit and the back-end server unit. Each of these sections further includes an elaborated discussion about the functionalities, requirements, and architectural alternative available with the subsystems. At the last, the chapter has been ended with some concluding remarks and future scopes.

WEARABLE HEALTHCARE MONITORING SYSTEM ARCHITECTURE

The architectural design of Wearable Healthcare Monitoring System (WHMS) plays a vital role in making them generic in nature. The structure of WHMS is designed in such a manner that it can be modified easily for monitoring of many diseases. The proposed architecture of WHMS consists of many standards and semantics that are necessary to provide interoperability, data sharing and knowledge sharing over various platforms.

The WHMS is architectured using the product line architecture to decrease the designing and developing time and achieve a high quality product with low cost (Paliwal & Kiwelekar, 2015; Paliwal & Bunglowala, 2017). The system will be designed with two different perspectives product and process (Pawar, Jones, Van, & Hermens, 2012; Paliwal, & Kiwelekar, 2013). From the product perspective, the architecture is having three layers, consisting of three different subsystems Wearable Body Area Network (WBAN), Mobile Base Unit (MBU), and Back-End Server (BESys). On the other hand, the process perspective consists of data acquisition, initial data processing and transmission, biosignal interpretation, notification and intervention. Figure 1 shows a basic architectural design for wearable healthcare monitoring system.

The first layer of WHMS includes wearable biosensors to acquire the primary physiological parameters. These sensors in the BAN will be modified according to the patient and disease monitoring needs. The BAN will consist of a central node to monitor and acquire the biosignals from sensors and deliver them to MBU. The BAN will also acquire some contextual data for the identification of low and high-level

Figure 1. Architecture design for wearable healthcare monitoring system

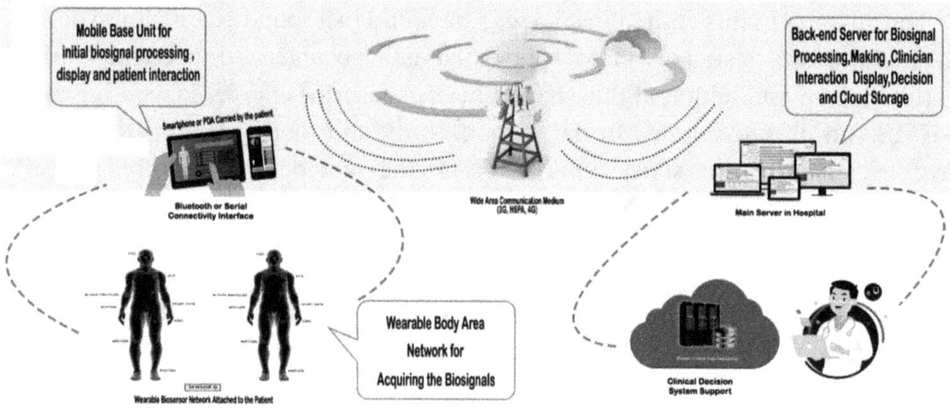

activities along with the physiological parameters. For the formation of the second layer, smartphones will prove to be very effective since they provide excellent data processing capabilities, storage, and easy availability at low cost. The MBU will process the biosignal data on the initial level for any discrepancies and will transfer the data to BESys for further processing. The BESys can be considered as a brain to the WHMS. It will store and mine the data for knowledge abstraction and decision making. It will also assist the physician in making critical decisions regarding the patients' health. The BESys will be provided with most advanced algorithms to process the data and make decisions based on the gathered knowledge. The intra and inter subsystem connectivity is provided using different modes of short and long range communicating media like Bluetooth, Zigbee, mobile data networks and wireless data networks. In the subsequent sections, the authors will focus on the architectural design issues and alternatives of these subsystems for achieving the process perspectives of WHMS.

BODY AREA NETWORK (BAN)

The body area network is the first subsystem of WHMS and forms the 1st logical layer which will be deployed over the patient's body for continuous biosignal processing. Since the subsystem will be mounted on the patient's body it should follow the rules and regulations prescribed by ISO and IEEE along with that, it should be power efficient, easily wearable, easy to use, and should provide hassle-free connectivity (Espina et al., 2014).

The main components of a BAN typically consist of different biological sensors. The sensors or actuators that are most frequently included in the system are blood pressure monitor, respiration monitor, SPO2, blood glucose, motion sensors and ECG. Table 1 shows typical sensors included in the BAN for monitoring of physiological and contextual parameters with their sensitivity and data generation rate (Latré et al., 2011; Cavallari et al., 2014). Some of the advanced sensors like EEG and EMG can also be included in the system but the data generated by these sensors is very hard to interpret and needs specialized systems to process.

These sensors are available with mainly two options to choose from invasive (sensors that are placed inside the skin) or noninvasive (sensors that are deployed on the body) sensors. Invasive sensors provide more accurate data as compared to noninvasive sensors but to achieve easy usability all the proposed sensors in the WHMS will be non-invasive in nature so that it can be used even in the absence of any medical supervision. A trained person can easily connect and deploy these sensors on to the patient's body and since they are non-invasive in nature it will be safer as compared to the invasive sensors. These sensors will connect to a central

Table 1. Biosensors data transfer requirements

Biosensors	Sampling Frequency (Hz)	Sensitivity	Bits per Sample	Data Rate (bps)
Electroencephalography (EEG)	256 (x24 Ch.)	~ 1 s	16	98,304
Electrocardiography (ECG)	200 (x3 Ch.)	~ 1 s	12 – 16	7,200 – 9,600
Motion detection	50 (x9 Ch.)	NO	16	7,200
Glucose monitoring	40 – 200	NO	16	640 – 3,200
Blood oxygen (SpO2)	60 (x2 Ch.)	NO	16	1,920
Blood pressure	120	NO	16	1,920
Cardiac output	40	NO	16	640
Respiration	50	NO	6	300
Body temperature	0.2	NO	12	2.4
Contextual and Activity Data (Latré et al., 2011; Cavallari et al., 2014; Negra, Jemili, & Belghith, 2016)	-	-	-	20000

micro control unit to provide access and control. The connectivity between the central node and the sensors will be provided by the Zigbee/Bluetooth protocol (Negra, Jemili, & Belghith, 2016). Sensors used in the systems will follow the ISO/IEEE standard 11073-20601 (ISO/IEEE 11073-20601, 2016) and HL7 standard (HL7 Version 2.6) for bio signal acquisition and biosignal transfer. Data generated by these standards can be interpreted throughout the world on different platforms.

The BAN design is considered to be very important for many reasons. The design issue like wearability is considered to be a very important factor because if the patient will not feel comfortable with BAN, he/she is not going to wear it continuously. Moreover, it may also cause some negative psychological effects. So the issues with wearability along with other issues like data acquisition, data processing, data fusion and contextual data gathering also need to be addressed. The succeeding subsections of BAN cover these concerns accompanied by their architectural solutions.

Biosignal Data Fusion and Processing

Characteristically, the authors consider the BAN as a single device that monitors the patient's physiological information, but in reality, it is a multi-device constellation of potentially heterogeneous sensors generating vast amount of physiological data that cannot be interpreted independently. Moreover, BAN's relying on a single node or considering node data separately will have many limitations (Elmenreich, 2002) like sensory deprivation, limited spatial coverage, uncertainty and imprecision (Murphy, 1996). Alternatively, multiple sensor fusion data can provide many advantages such as improved signal to noise ratio, reduced ambiguity and uncertainty, increased confidence, enhanced robustness and reliability, robustness against interference, improved resolution, precision and hypothesis discrimination, integration of independent features, and prior knowledge (Thomopoulos, 1990; Bosse, Roy, & Grenier, 1996). Therefore it becomes a trivial task to create an effective fusion of data generated from these sensors to get the desirable perceptions.

The sensor fusion can be achieved through three different models that are competitive, complementary, and cooperative (Yang, Andreu-Perez, Hu, & Thiemjarus, 2014). In competitive fusion, multiple equivalent sources of information are used to obtain the self-calibration and redundancy. It is very uncommon in practice even when we use multiple common sources of information because the sources are placed on different locations of the body so it provides complementary information instead of competitive information. Complementary fusion is used to improve the system's accuracy and reliability. In complementary fusion, each sensor captures different aspect of the same phenomenon and the acquired data is compositely analyzed for high level information. And when it is not possible to get information from a signal source independently, cooperative fusion is used. In cooperative fusion, multiple signals are analyzed simultaneously to obtain the information. It is the most frequently used sensor fusion model.

In the same manner, the data abstraction or fusion for processing can be achieved on three different levels such as data-level fusion, feature-level fusion, and decision-level fusion. If the same physiological phenomenon is measured using multiple homogeneous sensors, the data-level fusion can be used because the sensor data can be directly fused. On the other hand, if data is generated from different heterogeneous sources it cannot be combined at data-level, and feature-level or decision-level fusion techniques must be adopted. Table 2 shows different fusion levels and particular models that can be adopted with that level in conjunction with parameters, applications and techniques.

After the fusion process, data must be further processed to extract the required information. The processing can be done using three different approaches given as centralized, distributed, and hybrid. The centralized approach processes the data in a fusion center, whereas in distributed approach each sensor performs independent processing of its own data and transfers the result to the fusion node for further processing. In hybrid data fusion, collection and pre-processing are performed with a distributed approach while a central node is responsible for performing decision-level computations.

Table 2. Fusion parameters, applications and techniques at the different fusion levels

Fusion Level	Model	Parameter	Use	Technique
Data-level	competitive	number of sources, sampling rate, sensing synchronization, sensing periodicity, data buffering, aggregation strategy, sensor node platform	spectral data mining, data adaptation, estimation of parameters, robustness and calibration, source recovery	digital signal processing, coordinate transforms, Kalman filtering, weighted averaging, independent component analysis
Feature-level	competitive, complementary, cooperative	feature domain, feature extraction method, feature normalization, overlapping, processing model	classification	pattern recognition, clustering, neural networks
Decision-level	competitive, complementary, cooperative	decision fusion method, source diversity, classification periodicity, processing model	decisional action	expert systems, artificial intelligence

(Gravina et al., 2017)

Wearable BAN Design

The wearable healthcare monitoring solutions are much beneficial as compared to the traditional healthcare systems in terms of operational cost, scalability and restricted access to remote monitoring. Along with numerous advantages, the wearable sensor has some drawbacks like it is very uncomfortable to continuously wear multiple sensors for physiological data collection. If we use simple devices like bracelets or smart watches the data collected is not of that accuracy. Besides all these the user may have negative psychological effects of continuously wearing monitoring devices. The user might feel that he/she has some health problems which further causes stress and negative emotions. More seriously, the negative psychological effects may result in mental illness, especially when the patient feels lonely or depressed (Chen et al., 2017). Hence the BAN should be designed in such an innovative way that it will provide more comfortable, sustainable, and energy efficient structure to acquire the physiological data.

To acquire complicated medical-level data, multifaceted devices with high accuracy are needed. As the complexity of these devices increase the system complexity, inconvenience also increases. So in order to be truly convenient for any wearable sensor network, it must be very comfortable and should not affect or disturb the normal life of that person. Here, the authors have mentioned some of the innovative wearable's that can really make the wearable network imperceptible to the user and hence can improve the user experience to a great extent if incorporated into the BAN.

1. **Smart Clothing:** With continuous improvement in wearable technology smart clothing proposes multiple connected devices to offer more meaningful information. These wearables are better than tradition monitoring systems in terms of accuracy, usability, comfort, washability, and real time monitoring. Smart clothing will improve the quality of experience (QoE) and quality of service (QoS) in the next generation because while wearing these wearables the user will not experience any different feeling than that of a jacket or pullover (Chen et al., 2017; Chen et al., 2016).
2. **Body Fluid Biomarkers and Sensors:** Body fluid sensors are one of the most established tools in traditional diagnostics. Blood and urine are the most frequently used body fluids for getting the different physiological parameters. Other body fluids that are readily available and do not require any invasive sampling are tears (Chu et al., 2011), sweat (Schazmann et al., 2010) and saliva (Papacosta & Nassis, 2011). These body fluids contain nearly 1500 types of proteins and some of them are present in sufficiently high concentration and can be used for medical monitoring purpose (Tricoli, Nasiri, & De, 2017).
3. **Implantable and Edible Biosensors:** In implantable and edible biosensors all components of the sensor, including the circuitry and transmitters must be of the biocompatible or biodegradable material that does not cause inflammation or any adverse reaction into the host (Steinmetz & Jones, 2016). Also, to function over a long period, these biosensors need to have renewable and safe energy sources. These type of devices go beneath the skin via bloodstream or ingestion into the digestive tract to acquire the physiological biosignals. In this respect, MIT scientists have recently tested a device to monitor the heart rate and respiratory rate using sound waves in the gastrointestinal tract (Traverso et al., 2015).
4. **Intelligent Tattoos, Patches and Bio-Stamps:** These biosensors are attached to the epidermis of the human body and are capable to sense the physiognomies on or under the skin physically, electrochemically or chemically. Electrochemical sensors, screen printing technologies and flexible electrodes can provide high comfort to the patient without compromising any of the functionalities. The idea of intelligent patches, tattoos, innovative fabrication techniques and electrodes has fledged in recent years but is still mostly limited to laboratories (Zhu, Liu, Shuang, Nair, & Li, 2017; Coyle et al., 2015). Figure 2 shows some of these innovative wearable, implantable or edible physiological sensors.

Figure 2. Innovative wearable, implantable or edible physiological sensors

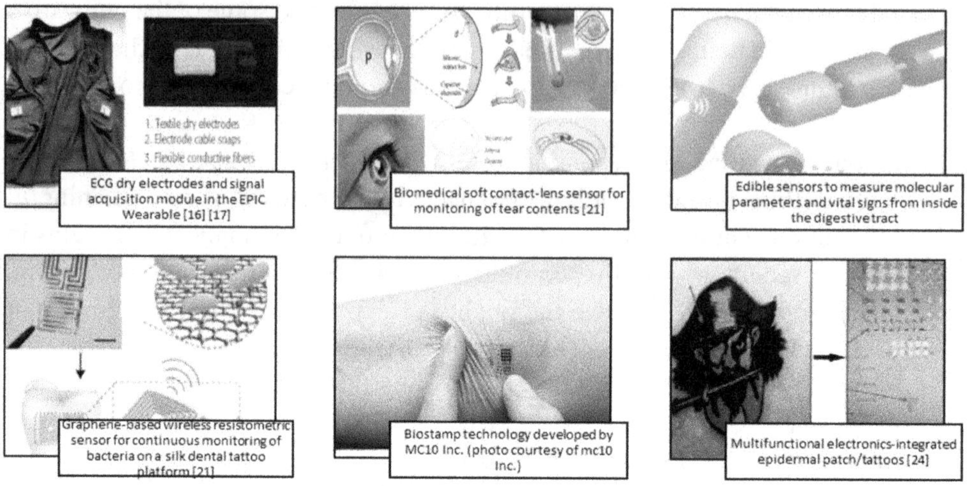

Contextual Information

The precision of any remote monitoring system depends on how well the acquired physiological data is correlated with the patient's current context. The context awareness for a system is defined as the state of knowledge of external and internal entities that cause the change in the user's condition, thus necessitating a different interpretation of the data in hand (Talaei-Khoei, Ray, Parameshwaran, & Lewis, 2012). In the case of wearable healthcare, contextual information can be obtained from the vital signs, low level activities (Viswanathan, Chen, & Pompili, 2012), environmental variables, occupancy, and object usage in the home environment. Figure 3 shows different parameters that can be used to draw contexts from the acquired data (Yuan, 2014).

In addition to these, the data collected by kinematics sensors (accelerometer and gyroscope), GPS (location), gesture recognition units, fall detection units can improve the accuracy of the system to a great extent. The collected contextual data must be processed in close collaboration with the physiological data to generate correct contextual information. The contextual information generated from this analysis can be further used for automated physiological diagnosis of the patient. For example, the heart rate variability of a cardiac patient can be correlated with contextual information such as a state of exertion, rest/on-move using physical activity recognition to get the perceptions of the patient's health condition. The system will need intensive machine learning based algorithms and real time distributed sensing to draw such contexts from the obtained data.

Figure 3. Information used for generating or identifying the contexts

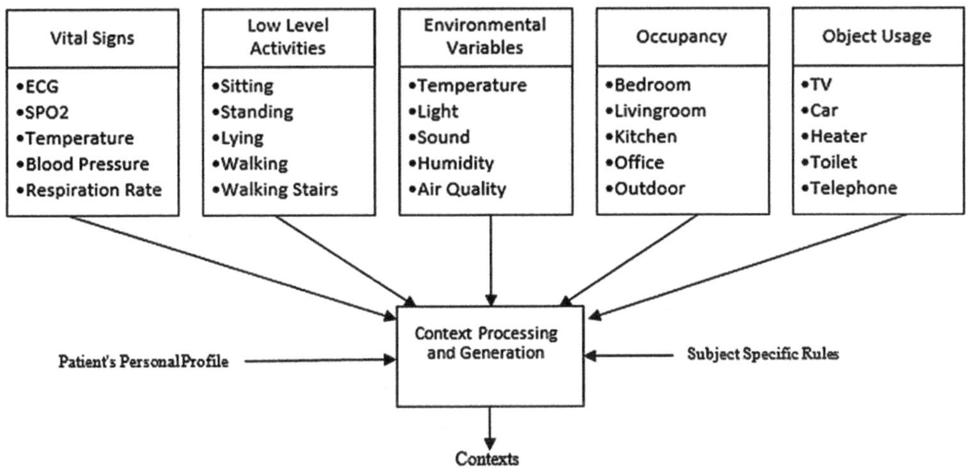

The context aware systems provide relevant services and information to the patient where relevancy of the information is totally dependent on the user's current action. The context awareness, of the system can be active or passive in nature. In active context awareness the system adapts in accordance with the changing contexts whereas in passive context awareness the system becomes aware of the changes but does not adapt accordingly. In clinical decision making systems active awareness is considered better for achieving the anticipated healthcare goals. For the contexts generation from contextual data a hierarchical structure can be used i.e. we can first identify the low level activities and then these low level activities are further used to deduce the high level activities. The ambient sensing data like environmental variables, occupancy and object usage can further improve the accuracy of activity prediction and contexts (Cavallari et al., 2014).

Figure 4. High level context generation rules

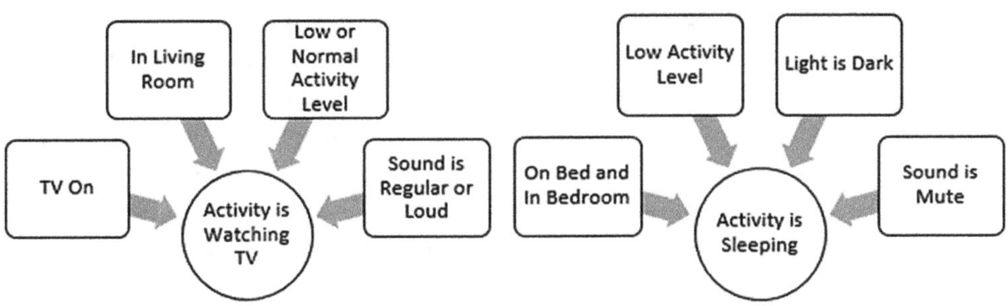

For example, we can consider sitting or walking as low level contexts since these are recognized through accelerometer and gyroscope sensor data. These contexts are then further processed to get high level activity interpretation like sleeping or exercising in collaboration with other related contexts. Figure 4 shows some high level context generating rules in WHMS. These interpretation rules should differ in accordance to the individual person or changing contexts. The authors will discuss these interpretation rules and reasoning framework in later Sections.

In contextual information, we can also include the emotional state of a patient because it is a major driving force intended for medical conditions in many chronic diseases. The performance of emotional interface data is directly influenced by the quality of collected data. To achieve high accuracy in emotional analysis we need more and more data. However, it is very difficult to meet the requirements of emotional data with limited resources of wearable devices. To solve the bottleneck created by limited resources and diversified data we can use hybrid big emotion data analysis (Chen et al., 2015). This technique is mainly based on physiology, video and text data for sentiment or emotion analysis. The physiological data includes voice, pupil, posture, respiration, body temperature, heart rate, blood pressure and body characterization. On the contrary, video based analysis mainly focuses on multi-information fusion and visual features, mostly involving the video and image cognition and segmentation. In text based analysis we analyze and reason the subjective text with emotional words from social networks and messaging application. The emotional analysis can offer a prodigious edge in terms of accuracy enhancement for the WHMS.

MOBILE BASE UNIT (MBU)

It is the second subsystem of WHMS and forms 2nd logical layer of the system. Handheld devices like smartphones, tablets, PDAs are most suitable choice for mobile based unit. These devices have the processing power like a computer to process the data, storage to store the data and network to pass the data to the BESys. Smartphones are the devices that are already owned by nearly 34% of the world's population. In a developing country like India where maximum population resides in villages mobile networks are accessible to nearly 94% of the population.

The primary functionalities offered by MBU includes biosignal interpretation, primary biosignal processing, biosignal transfer, and user system interaction. The MBU processes the biosignals on the primary level to determine any irregularities. If it finds any anomalies in the data it immediately asks for the user response and issues a notification for the clinical server to alert them about the abnormality. The primary biosignal processing is entirely centered on learning models and knowledge base provided to the MBU by BESys. For complete processing of biosignals the data should be further transferred to the BESys. While transferring the data from MBU to BESys the prime concerns are data security and data interpretation.

A minor change in the biosignal data can lead to a big misinterpretation of patient's health condition. So, the security and biosignal delivery is also very important for MBU. To provide security to the biosignal data we can use end to end encryption. In the prevailing patient monitoring systems dedicated hardware units for biosignal compression (Bortolotti et al., 2016), power saving (Wang, Lin, Jin, & Xu, 2016), and encryption were included (Kim, Lee, & Yoo, 2013). This unit apparently improves the speed, security and power efficiency of the systems but it also increases the cost and number of wearable units in the system. Mobile or handheld devices used for the MBU can provide a very effective solution to these hitches by implementing the algorithms on these devices. It will introduce a time lag in data forwarding but it can potentially solve the raised issues.

The data sent from MBU to the BESys should be structured according to the global healthcare standards such as IHE DEC PCD-01 Technical Framework, HL7 V 2.6 Messaging, ISO/IEEE std 11073 semantics (Lee & Do, 2018). The ISO/IEEE 11073 standard messages have the smallest data size which is particularly suitable for devices having very small computing power. On the contrary PCD-01 and HL7 standards will be useful for the environments that are connected to the clinical information systems and require patients' information. In particular cases, where reuse of information is frequent HL7 is quite advantageous over PCD-01 framework. The frameworks provide assistance for data interpretation on different platform and data sharing among different hospitals and clinical systems. The data, set to follow the following standard will aid features like easy connectivity, platform independence, interoperability, and efficient exchange of medical data.

MBU also provides a Graphical User Interface (GUI) for user interaction. It is very important for gathering the data via simple questionnaires apart from the data gathered by biosensors. GUI helps the patient by timely providing feedback, passing clinician messages, and reminding them about medication via notifications. It also helps in preventing false alarm generation by user interactions. The graphical interface provided on the MBU can also be used to gather contextual information by questionnaires. The data generated by this user system interaction can be used for text based sentiment analysis. It can also provide some important insights about the user's current activity and emotional state.

The devices (smartphones, tablets, PDAs) used for MBU have themselves become an outstanding alternative for wearable sensing due to the diversity of sensors they support. Sensors like accelerometers and gyroscopes along with the processing power make them a robust tool for performing activity recognition (Reyes-Ortiz et al., 2016; Anguita et al., 2013). The activity recognition module mainly includes a machine learning module and a probabilistic support vector machine that takes feature vectors as input for activity prediction. If the module is implemented autonomously on the smartphone it saves a lot of processing on the BESys and if it is employed in collaboration with BAN sensors it significantly improves the accuracy of activity prediction.

At the end, the data acquired by the MBU is forwarded to the BESys for further processing. The biosensors together produce data at the rate of nearly 154 kbps. It is a very difficult task to continuously transfer such a big amount of data over mobile networks. To handle this problem we can compress the data as already discussed or we can adopt a mechanism wherein the data will be sent continuously only when MBU finds any discrepancies in the biosignal otherwise the data will be sampled and transferred to the BESys at predefined regular intervals (Jiang et al., 2016). In this manner, we can easily transfer the generated data on 4G mobile network.

BACK-END SERVER (BESys)

The back-end server can be considered as the most important and critical part of the WHMS. It will receive physiological and contextual data from MBU for further processing. BESys lastly processes the data for knowledge abstraction and decision support. It passes the analysis and threshold to the clinician and MBU. The algorithm used for processing the data on BESys will be varying according to the user or disease monitoring needs. The main components of BESys will include clinical knowledge library, data mining unit, knowledge discovery unit, decision support unit, threshold determination unit, algorithmic learning unit, clinical fact base, data storage and mining unit, cloud and backup storage unit, data requisition unit, clinical server application, data lose recovery unit, and emergency control unit.

To provide evidence based decision support BESys need efficient data processing methods to process large volume of data into relevant information. Big data analytics has the potential and capabilities to provide back bone for predictive healthcare monitoring system. Big data analytics basically refers to the techniques used to examine and accomplish intelligence from the large datasets. Therefore big data analytics can be viewed as a part of knowledge abstraction from the data. To extract the knowledge from data we need selection of data analytic methods (Sivarajah, Kamal, Irani, & Weerakkody, 2017). Figure 5 shows a typical data analytics process to resolve and regulate the WHMS actions. A brief description of these action determining approaches is given as follows.

Figure 5. Healthcare data analytics process with selected methods

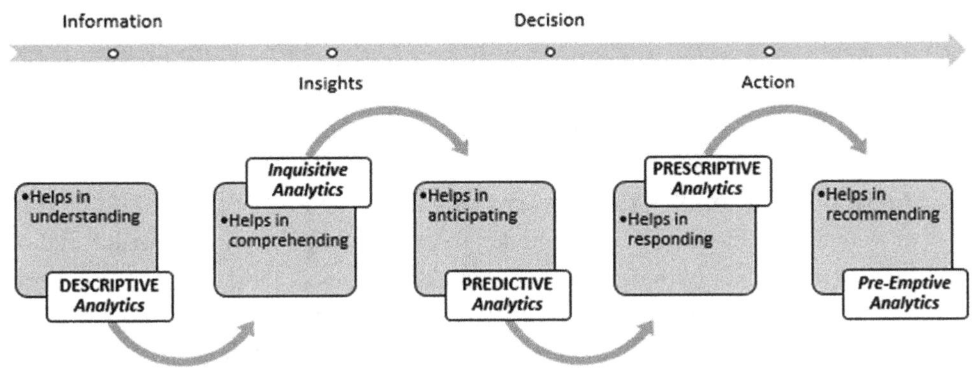

- Descriptive analytics inspects data and information to define the current state of a situation in a way that developments, patterns and exceptions become evident, in the form of producing standard reports, ad hoc reports, and alerts (Joseph & Johnson, 2013). The descriptive analytics basically helps in understanding "What happened".
- Inquisitive analytics is about probing data to certify/reject business propositions, for example, analytical drill down into data, statistical analysis and factor analysis (Bihani & Patil, 2014). It helps in comprehending "Why has something happened or is happening."
- Predictive analytics is concerned with forecasting and statistical modeling to determine the future possibilities (Waller & Fawcett, 2013). It fundamentally helps in anticipating "What is likely to happen".
- Prescriptive analytics is about optimization and randomized testing to assess how to enhance the services while decreasing the expenses. The prescriptive analytics help in responding to "So What?" and "Now What?"
- Pre-emptive analytics is about having the capacity to take precautionary actions on events that may undesirably influence the system's performance, for example, identifying the possible perils and recommending mitigating strategies far ahead in time (Smith et al., 2012). It helps in recommending "What needs to be done now".

These analytical techniques provide improved decision-making and system performance by making everything more translucent and measureable, while further uncovering inconsistencies as well as potential concerns and opportunities. The use of data analytic techniques infuses certain capabilities and intelligence into the system. Following Section covers these capabilities of WHMS while the subsequent subsections encompass different mechanisms used in BESys to realize these capabilities.

Capabilities Introduced by Means of Big Data Analytics Into WHMS (Wang, Kung, & Byrd, 2018)

1. **Analytical Capability for Patterns of Care:** The analytics capabilities of a system are referred as the competency to process huge amount of structured or unstructured data by means of different techniques (Chen, Chiang, & Storey, 2012; Simon, 2013). In WHMS the analytical capabilities can be used to identify the patterns of care and determine connections between huge monitoring records. The analytical capability will empower the system to process gigantic amount of data in near real time and capture patient's visual as well as medical records. It can also identify the previously unnoticed patterns in the patient data and hence deliver a broader view for evidence based medical system.
2. **Unstructured Data Analytical Capability:** The big data analytic system acquires the data from physiological sensors and context aware data in the form of low level activities, environmental variables, occupancy, and object usage. The acquired data is stored in a distributed file or database system. It is further processed to add indispensable information to the data warehouse (Belle et al., 2015; Zhang et al., 2017). Figure 6 shows the process of creating a data warehouse for WHMS. In data warehousing process, the acquired data is first preprocessed and then filtered using various filtering techniques such as map reduce. The warehousing process makes WHMS capable to process the semi structured or unstructured data like biomedical signals, clinical images, transcripts and reports. This ability plays a very important role in the success of big data analytics in healthcare. It improves the system efficiency in terms of cost control by identifying the unnecessary extra investigative tests and treatments.
3. **Decision Support Capability:** It determines the capability of a system to recommend or make decision about a particular medical condition and generate a report for the same. This decision making ability produces information and knowledge, statistical analysis, and summaries about health conditions of the patient and shares particular optimal statistics with the patient, physician and caretakers in the dashboard provided on the clinical server and MBU. The information is also instrumental in providing evidence based medicine, detecting emergency health conditions, and providing personalized patient care. The system continuously evaluates comprehensive perceptions and results with proper contextual information to improve the strategies for long term decision making (Yin & Jha, 2017; Bourouis, Feham, Hossain, & Zhang, 2014).

4. **Predictive Capability:** It is the capability of a system to produce and assess the real time data for accurate health condition prediction. The capability also refers to prognostication of future health conditions and contemplation of new acumen based on sophisticated statistical tools and datasets (Shmueli, & Koppius, 2011; Wessler, 2013). To incorporate predictive capabilities the system will heavily rely on machine learning, neural networks, deep convolution networks, and regression analysis algorithms. The platform enhances the system's capability in terms of context aware recommendations and predictions about future events that may take place. The capability is extensively used to reduce the degree of uncertainty and to provide supporting preventive care (Bardhan, Oh, Zheng, & Kirksey, 2014). Besides these, the framework also assists in the identification of best clinical practices and future healthcare trends. The framework provides a proactive platform for cost reduction based on in-depth analysis of patient's lifestyle, habits, and disease monitoring (Kayyali, Knott, & Van, 2013).
5. **Traceability:** The traceability of a system is the capability to track output data from system components and service units. The data such as physiological biosignals, clinical data, activities, patient behavior, sentiment analytics and context data are normally collected in near real time from different identities. The big data analytic algorithms help us to capture these data concurrently from diverse sources. Traceability not only decreases the conflicts but also reduces the complications in associating the data to healthcare process optimization (Groves et al., 2013). Primary goal of this capability is to provide WHMS

Figure 6. The process of creating the data warehouse for health care

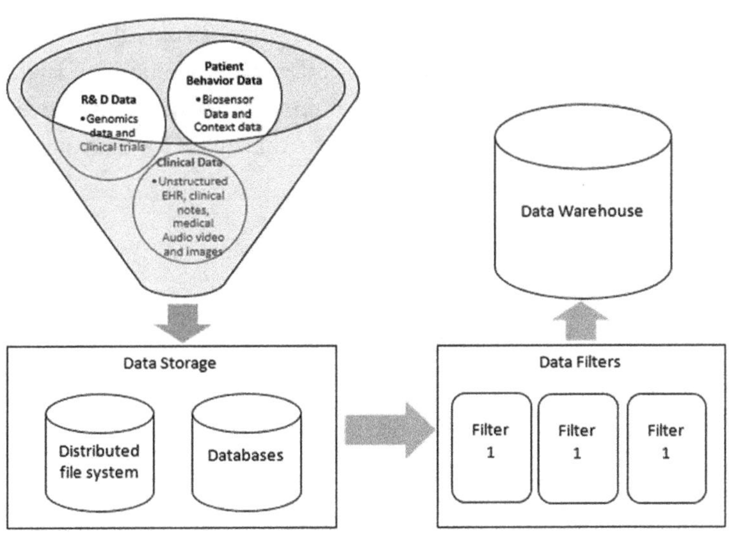

with more consistency, perceptibility and effortlessly reachable data. It can augment the monitoring system to get an edge by tracing promising solutions from various datasets in accordance with the patient needs.

These big data analytic capabilities will help us in getting required proficiency in the BESys. In succeeding subsections we will further comprehend different algorithms and techniques that will help us to get the required data analytic capabilities into the WHMS.

The Intelligent Reasoning Framework

The core functionalities offered by the reasoning framework include generation of continuous contexts from contextual information, anomaly detection, abnormality prediction, and generation of notification in the emergency situation. The intelligent reasoning framework engine can be configured using different knowledge bases or custom made rules (Yuan & Herbert, 2014; Horst & Sinitsyn, 2011). But these rules must be substantiated to ensure consistency and correctness of the reasoning framework (Riesbeck & Schank, 2013). A hybrid reasoning framework for WHMS has been shown in Figure 7.

A hybrid reasoning framework is the most suitable choice of reasoning framework for WHMS. The intelligent hybrid reasoning framework uses case based reasoning mechanisms (Van, Woo, & Choi, 2009) with fuzzy based knowledge base (Ali et al., 2017) to overcome the limitations of a single reasoning model. The fuzzy based reasoning framework proves to be very useful specifically in the case of medical and pharmaceutical systems. In these particular domain the reasoning rules not only consists of explicit knowledge but it also embraces the experience of domain experts. On the other hand case based reasoning framework utilizes the knowledge from prior solved cases to improve the efficacy of inference mechanism. Figure 8 shows some sample context associated rules to draw inferences from high level activities. The inference drawn from these rules can be further used for anomaly detection.

Figure 7. Intelligent Hybrid Reasoning Framework

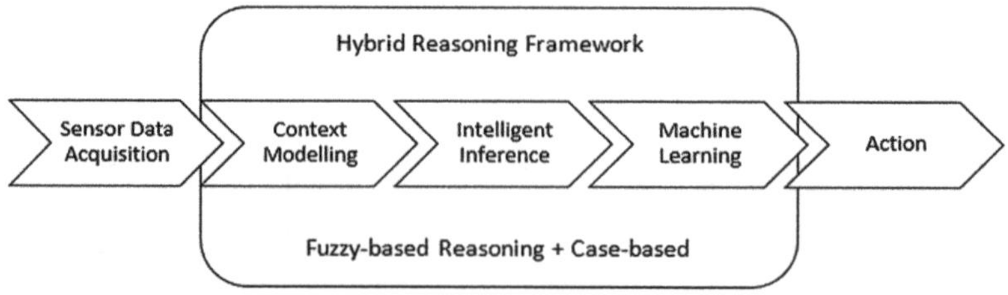

Figure 8. Medical context associated rules for anomaly detection

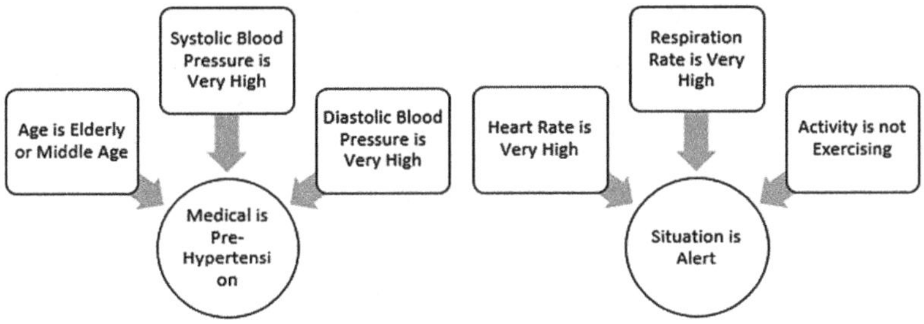

In hybrid reasoning, the physiological data acquired by the biosensors are provided to the machine learning unit through an intelligent interface. The different physiological parameters acquired through biosensors are processed in close collaboration with the contexts to reach certain actions. Context awareness in the WHMS provides an inherent intelligence to the reasoning framework to enhance the healthcare services. The reasoning engine processes the data in near real time and immediately generates the notification for abnormalities found in health conditions. To make reasoning engine more transparent, sophisticated, and accountable source of reasoning the output is recorded to provide description of a decision to the patient, clinician or caretakers.

The reasoning framework also provides context rule based activity recognition by collectively processing the smartphones inertial sensor data (Su, Tong, & Ji, 2014; Reyes-Ortiz et al., 2016) with wearable sensor data (Ordóñez & Roggen, 2016). The framework first creates segments of acquired sensor data. Subsequently, various features are extracted from the segmented data. These features are further used to create various classification models using machine learning algorithms. The patient activities will be classified in real time using a combination of two fusion models. The first technique based on thresholds will be used for simple activity recognition. In contrast to the first technique, second technique is based on machine learning, and will be used for the recognition of complex activities (Krishnan & Cook, 2014; Ronao & Cho, 2016). The machine will be trained by multiple datasets using an unsupervised learning scheme so that it can adapt in accordance with the particular user.

The Data Mining and Machine Learning Framework

In recent years, patient monitoring systems have shown a tremendous growth in the areas of automated healthcare delivery. Various systems based on data mining and machine learning algorithms have been proposed and implemented (Lucas &

Lucas, 2016; Manogaran & Lopez, 2017). The focus of these monitoring systems has shifted towards the big data driven decision making. The models for these healthcare monitoring systems are moving towards the proactive care and anomaly prediction from reactive care and anomaly detection respectively. This transformation has been taking place with the help of deeper data mining techniques that produces deeper insights of knowledge from the collected data.

The system primarily considers three main dimensions while processing the data for mining and learning. The first dimension contemplates the preprocessing of acquired data along with the contexts (occupancy, environment in which the monitoring is taking place, and object uses) and clinical data (patient's social and demographic information, medical history and various type of medical data including diagnoses, medications, lab tests, procedures, unstructured data (i.e. doctor's notes), image data (that is x-rays, MRI) and much more (Shaji, Ramesh, & Menon, 2016). The second dimension directly relates to the information extraction from data, provided by the first dimension. It mainly considers the type of subject and analysis preferences. Eventually, the three main data mining tasks i.e. anomaly detection, prediction and decision making have been performed by the third dimension. Figure 9 shows the data mining approach used for WHMS along with the mentioned dimensions (Banaee, Ahmed, & Loutfi, 2013).

Anomaly detection is the first task associated with this unit, in which we try to identify the infrequent patterns that do not conform to the expected data behavior. These abnormal behaviors help the system and clinician to take the accurate decision in short time. We can use classification based techniques like support vector machine (Lee, Kung, & Verma, 2012), Markov model (Zhu, 2011) and wavelet analysis (Gialelis et al., 2011) for anomaly detection. These techniques detect abnormalities by classifying the dataset into normal classes and outliers.

The second module assists the system to discover the events which have not yet occurred but expected to occur in the near future. The approach is very important since it helps in the prevention of critical conditions by taking proactive measures. This unit of the WHMS becomes very important from the perspective of forthcoming

Figure 9. Data mining approach for wearable healthcare monitoring system

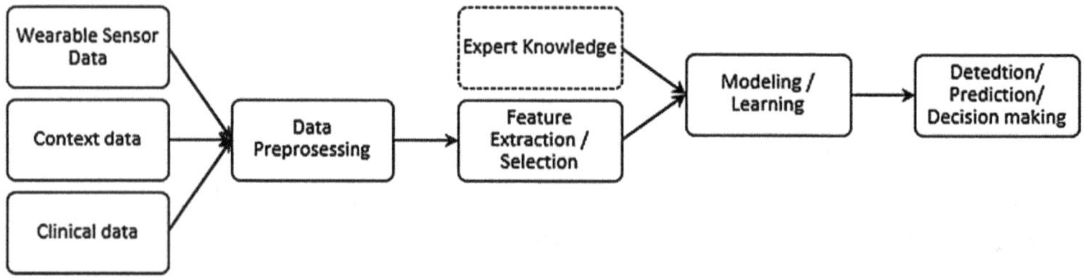

Figure 10. Back-end server decision support system

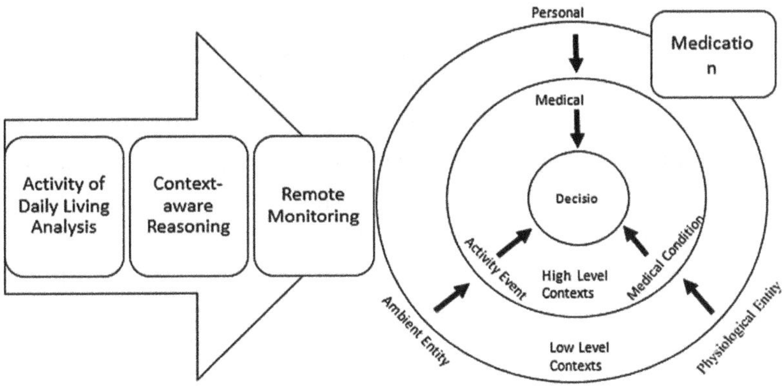

systems. The researchers are expecting a shift towards the proactive monitoring from reactive monitoring. The difficulty in implementation of the predictive unit is maximum since predicting the future is still a very critical task. The unit can be implemented using unsupervised learning models (Yoo et al., 2012) and predictive decision making algorithms (Bellazzi & Zupan, 2008; Yeh, Wu, & Tsao, 2011).

Decision making diagnosis is third and most important unit of the system. The decisions made by this unit are mostly based on knowledge retrieved from vital signs and clinical EMRs. The system cannot make a decision about any events or complications by only considering biosignal abnormality patterns. So in order to make a meaningful decision for the system, the unit needs more robust and global information. In the particular setup information and events produced by first two units becomes very important for this unit. These (abnormal conditions, outliers, alarms, and future prediction) are the events for which it is expected to take the decision. In Figure 10 the authors have shown a decision support unit for WHMS.

The unit takes monitoring, context, analysis, and clinical data to provide a decision based on certain rules. It can also suggest some medication in consultation with the clinician or physician. The deep learning based algorithms like deep neural network or deep convolution networks are the best suited choices for decision support systems (Ravi et al., 2017; Summers et al., 2017; Miotto et al., 2017). The data mining and machine learning unit collectively need to process a large amount heterogeneous data generated from various diverse sources. Mining such data still pose many challenges like high dimensionality, data scarcity, irregularity, bias, missing data and noise (Lee et al., 2017).

Cloud Based Data Analytics

The outburst of sensor technology has opened whole new opportunities for wearable sensing. We have seen some of these sensor technologies in above Sections. The WHMS continuously acquire healthcare data that includes physiological parameters, contextual data and sentiment data from various sensors. This continuous stream of data collected from multiple patients, in collaboration with clinical statistics, produces an enormous amount of data that requires near real time data processing. Through data analytic techniques such as machine learning, computational mathematics, and deep neural networks we can process this large volume of heterogeneous data in a competent manner to explore the data for patterns (Lo'ai et al., 2016). The lack of data is never a problem for such type of systems but the lack of information is. To process such a huge amount of data and to get the deeper insights from the data massive processing power is required. The traditional methodologies such as distributed systems and DBMS are not suitable to handle such a big amount of data in terms of availability and scalability (Manogaran & Lopez, 2018).

We can satisfy our requirements using the cloud computing platform because the solution offered by cloud has greater efficiency, scalable data analysis and reduced cost. We can deploy multiple instances of BESys on groups of cloud servers to get processing, storage and networking resources. The resources provided by the cloud platform can be easily scaled up or scaled down according to our system needs. Figure 11 shows a general structure of cloud based data analytics platform that processes the data provided by the clinical back-end server.

The multiple instances of machine learning nodes deployed on the cloud server process the uploaded data analogously. The learning models generated by these nodes are then evaluated and best model is selected for further processing. The WHMS can make use of unsupervised classification model to classify and tag the new input data. The learning model is enhanced continuously in unsupervised mode as progressively more data is uploaded on to the server. These adapted models are then further used by the MBU to process the limited amount of data. The cloud based data analytics platform not only improves the data processing capabilities of the system but also improves its security, scalability and availability.

Figure 11. Structure of cloud based data analytics platform

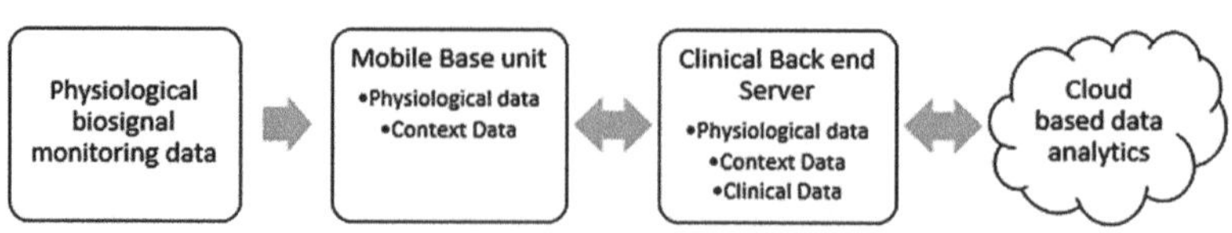

We have described various subsystems of BESys individually to provide a better understanding of their working. However, these subsystem works in very close collaboration with one another and we cannot draw a clear line that separates these subsystems of BESys.

CONCLUSION AND FUTURE SCOPE

In this chapter, the authors have presented a novel architectural approach for the design of wearable healthcare monitoring systems. The main objective of this architectural design was to realize a fast, reliable, secure, accurate and economical system. To achieve these objectives the authors have designated some preeminent architectural alternatives available for the system based on the various constraints. From the architectural perspective, the authors have presented the WHMS in three layers or subsystems. The components, functionalities, requirements, and realization mechanisms along with their merits and demerits have been presented for each layer. The resolution of design issues like data fusion, data delivery, data processing, security, accuracy, and efficiency were the main emphasis points of this architecture design. While choosing any alternative for WHMS our main concentration was on providing an answer to the question raised in the Introduction Section. Through these answers directly or indirectly the authors have tried to achieve accuracy enhancement, cost reduction and pervasiveness for WHMS. Most of the alternatives chosen for WHMS do not directly relate to any specific disease and hence improve the generosity of the system. The provided architectural alternative will surely improve the efficiency and accuracy of WHMS. But, in order to achieve end user readiness these systems still need a lot of improvement in selected regions. The regions that need further improvement mainly include wearability related issues of BAN, user privacy and back-end server accuracy.

REFERENCES

Alemdar, H. (2015). *Human activity recognition with wireless sensor networks using machine learning* (Doctoral dissertation). Bogaziçi University.

Ali, F., Islam, S. R., Kwak, D., Khan, P., Ullah, N., Yoo, S. J., & Kwak, K. S. (2017). Type-2 fuzzy ontology–aided recommendation systems for IoT–based healthcare. *Computer Communications*.

Anguita, D., Ghio, A., Oneto, L., Parra, X., & Reyes-Ortiz, J. L. (2013, April). A Public Domain Dataset for Human Activity Recognition using Smartphones. ESANN.

Banaee, H., Ahmed, M. U., & Loutfi, A. (2013). Data mining for wearable sensors in health monitoring systems: A review of recent trends and challenges. *Sensors (Basel), 13*(12), 17472–17500. doi:10.3390131217472 PMID:24351646

Bardhan, I., Oh, J. H., Zheng, Z., & Kirksey, K. (2014). Predictive analytics for readmission of patients with congestive heart failure. *Information Systems Research, 26*(1), 19–39. doi:10.1287/isre.2014.0553

Bellazzi, R., & Zupan, B. (2008). Predictive data mining in clinical medicine: Current issues and guidelines. *International Journal of Medical Informatics, 77*(2), 81–97. doi:10.1016/j.ijmedinf.2006.11.006 PMID:17188928

Belle, A., Thiagarajan, R., Soroushmehr, S. M., Navidi, F., Beard, D. A., & Najarian, K. (2015). Big data analytics in healthcare. *BioMed Research International.* PMID:26229957

Bihani, P., & Patil, S. T. (2014). A comparative study of data analysis techniques. *International Journal of Emerging Trends & Technology in Computer Science, 3*(2), 95-101.

Bortolotti, D., Mangia, M., Bartolini, A., Rovatti, R., Setti, G., & Benini, L. (2016). Energy-aware bio-signal compressed sensing reconstruction on the WBSN-gateway. *IEEE Transactions on Emerging Topics in Computing*, 1. doi:10.1109/TETC.2016.2564361

Bosse, E., Roy, J., & Grenier, D. (1996, May). *Data fusion concepts applied to a suite of dissimilar sensors.* In *Electrical and Computer Engineering, 1996. Canadian Conference on* (Vol. 2, pp. 692-695). IEEE. 10.1109/CCECE.1996.548247

Bourouis, A., Feham, M., Hossain, M. A., & Zhang, L. (2014). An intelligent mobile based decision support system for retinal disease diagnosis. *Decision Support Systems, 59*, 341–350. doi:10.1016/j.dss.2014.01.005

Cavallari, R., Martelli, F., Rosini, R., Buratti, C., & Verdone, R. (2014). A survey on wireless body area networks: Technologies and design challenges. *IEEE Communications Surveys and Tutorials, 16*(3), 1635–1657. doi:10.1109/SURV.2014.012214.00007

Chen, H., Chiang, R. H., & Storey, V. C. (2012). Business intelligence and analytics: From big data to big impact. *Management Information Systems Quarterly*, 1165–1188.

Chen, M., Ma, Y., Li, Y., Wu, D., Zhang, Y., & Youn, C. H. (2017). Wearable 2.0: Enabling human-cloud integration in next generation healthcare systems. *IEEE Communications Magazine, 55*(1), 54–61. doi:10.1109/MCOM.2017.1600410CM

Chen, M., Ma, Y., Song, J., Lai, C. F., & Hu, B. (2016). Smart clothing: Connecting human with clouds and big data for sustainable health monitoring. *Mobile Networks and Applications*, *21*(5), 825–845. doi:10.100711036-016-0745-1

Chen, M., Zhang, Y., Li, Y., Hassan, M. M., & Alamri, A. (2015). AIWAC: Affective interaction through wearable computing and cloud technology. *IEEE Wireless Communications*, *22*(1), 20–27. doi:10.1109/MWC.2015.7054715

Chu, M., Shirai, T., Takahashi, D., Arakawa, T., Kudo, H., Sano, K., & Mochizuki, M. (2011). Biomedical soft contact-lens sensor for in situ ocular biomonitoring of tear contents. *Biomedical Microdevices*, *13*(4), 603–611. doi:10.100710544-011-9530-x PMID:21475940

Coyle, S., Curto, V. F., Benito-Lopez, F., Florea, L., & Diamond, D. (2015). Wearable bio and chemical sensors. In Wearable Sensors (pp. 65-83). Academic Press.

Elmenreich, W. (2002). *An introduction to sensor fusion*. Vienna University of Technology.

Espina, J., Falck, T., Panousopoulou, A., Schmitt, L., Mülhens, O., & Yang, G. Z. (2014). Network topologies, communication protocols, and standards. In *Body sensor networks* (pp. 189–236). London: Springer. doi:10.1007/978-1-4471-6374-9_5

Gialelis, J., Chondros, P., Karadimas, D., Dima, S., & Serpanos, D. (2011, October). *Identifying Chronic disease complications utilizing state of the art data fusion methodologies and signal processing algorithms*. In *International Conference on Wireless Mobile Communication and Healthcare* (pp. 256-263). Springer.

Gravina, R., Alinia, P., Ghasemzadeh, H., & Fortino, G. (2017). Multi-sensor fusion in *body sensor networks: State-of-the-art and research challenges. Information Fusion*, *35*, 68–80. doi:10.1016/j.inffus.2016.09.005

Groves, P., Kayyali, B., Knott, D., & Van Kuiken, S. (2013). The 'big data' revolution in healthcare. *The McKinsey Quarterly*, *2*, 3.

Horst, H. J., & Sinitsyn, A. (2011). An approach to structuring reasoning for interpretation of sensor data in home-based health and well-being monitoring applications. *2011 5th International Conference on Pervasive Computing Technologies for Healthcare (PervasiveHealth) and Workshops*, 47-54. 10.4108/icst.pervasivehealth.2011.246099

ISO/IEEE 11073-20601:2016. (2016). *Health informatics - Personal health device communication - Part 20601: Application profile - Optimized exchange protocol*, IT applications in health care technology, 2016-06, 2.

Jiang, P., Winkley, J., Zhao, C., Munnoch, R., Min, G., & Yang, L. T. (2016). An intelligent information forwarder for healthcare big data systems with distributed wearable sensors. *IEEE Systems Journal, 10*(3), 1147–1159. doi:10.1109/JSYST.2014.2308324

Joseph, R. C., & Johnson, N. A. (2013). Big data and transformational government. *IT Professional, 15*(6), 43–48. doi:10.1109/MITP.2013.61

Kayyali, B., Knott, D., & Van Kuiken, S. (2013). *The big-data revolution in US health care: Accelerating value and innovation.* McKinsey & Company.

Kim, J., Lee, B. J., & Yoo, S. K. (2013, July). Design of real-time encryption module for secure data protection of wearable healthcare devices. In *Engineering in Medicine and Biology Society (EMBC), 2013 35th Annual International Conference of the IEEE* (pp. 2283-2286). IEEE.

Krishnan, N. C., & Cook, D. J. (2014). Activity recognition on streaming sensor data. *Pervasive and Mobile Computing, 10*, 138–154. doi:10.1016/j.pmcj.2012.07.003 PMID:24729780

Latré, B., Braem, B., Moerman, I., Blondia, C., & Demeester, P. (2011). A survey on wireless body area networks. *Wireless Networks, 17*(1), 1–18. doi:10.100711276-010-0252-4

Lee, C., Luo, Z., Ngiam, K. Y., Zhang, M., Zheng, K., Chen, G., & Yip, W. L. J. (2017). Big healthcare data analytics: Challenges and applications. In *Handbook of Large-Scale Distributed Computing in Smart Healthcare* (pp. 11–41). Cham: Springer. doi:10.1007/978-3-319-58280-1_2

Lee, K. H., Kung, S. Y., & Verma, N. (2012). Low-energy formulations of support vector machine kernel functions for biomedical sensor applications. *Journal of Signal Processing Systems for Signal, Image, and Video Technology, 69*(3), 339–349. doi:10.100711265-012-0672-8

Lee, S., & Do, H. (2018). Comparison and Analysis of ISO/IEEE 11073, IHE PCD-01, and HL7 FHIR Messages for Personal Health Devices. *Healthcare Informatics Research, 24*(1), 46–52. doi:10.4258/hir.2018.24.1.46 PMID:29503752

Lo'ai, A. T., Mehmood, R., Benkhlifa, E., & Song, H. (2016). Mobile cloud computing model and big data analysis for healthcare applications. *IEEE Access: Practical Innovations, Open Solutions, 4*, 6171–6180. doi:10.1109/ACCESS.2016.2613278

Lucas, P. J., & Lucas, P. (2016). *Bayesian analysis, pattern analysis, and data mining in health care health care.* Academic Press.

Manogaran, G., & Lopez, D. (2017). A survey of big data architectures and machine learning algorithms in healthcare. *International Journal of Biomedical Engineering and Technology*, *25*(2-4), 182–211. doi:10.1504/IJBET.2017.087722

Manogaran, G., & Lopez, D. (2018). Health data analytics using scalable logistic regression with stochastic gradient descent. *International Journal of Advanced Intelligence Paradigms*, *10*(1-2), 118–132. doi:10.1504/IJAIP.2018.089494

Miotto, R., Wang, F., Wang, S., Jiang, X., & Dudley, J. T. (2017). Deep learning for healthcare: Review, opportunities and challenges. *Briefings in Bioinformatics*. doi:10.1093/bib/bbx044 PMID:28481991

Murphy, R. R. (1996). Biological and cognitive foundations of intelligent sensor fusion. *IEEE Transactions on Systems, Man, and Cybernetics. Part A, Systems and Humans*, *26*(1), 42–51. doi:10.1109/3468.477859

Negra, R., Jemili, I., & Belghith, A. (2016). Wireless body area networks: Applications and technologies. *Procedia Computer Science*, *83*, 1274–1281. doi:10.1016/j.procs.2016.04.266

Ordóñez, F. J., & Roggen, D. (2016). Deep convolutional and lstm recurrent neural networks for multimodal wearable activity recognition. *Sensors (Basel)*, *16*(1), 115. doi:10.339016010115 PMID:26797612

Paliwal, G., & Bunglowala, A. (2017). Software Product Lines for Mobile Patient Monitoring Systems Using FoDA a Grammar. *Biochem Ind J.*, *11*(2), 112.

Paliwal, G., & Kiwelekar, A. W. (2013, March). A comparison of mobile patient monitoring systems. In *International Conference on Health Information Science* (pp. 198-209). Springer. 10.1007/978-3-642-37899-7_17

Paliwal, G., & Kiwelekar, A. W. (2015). A Product Line Architecture for Mobile Patient Monitoring System. In *Mobile Health* (pp. 489–511). Cham: Springer. doi:10.1007/978-3-319-12817-7_22

Papacosta, E., & Nassis, G. P. (2011). Saliva as a tool for monitoring steroid, peptide and immune markers in sport and exercise science. *Journal of Science and Medicine in Sport*, *14*(5), 424–434. doi:10.1016/j.jsams.2011.03.004 PMID:21474377

Pawar, P., Jones, V., Van Beijnum, B. J. F., & Hermens, H. (2012). A framework for the comparison of mobile patient monitoring systems. *Journal of Biomedical Informatics*, *45*(3), 544–556. doi:10.1016/j.jbi.2012.02.007 PMID:22406009

Ravì, D., Wong, C., Deligianni, F., Berthelot, M., Andreu-Perez, J., Lo, B., & Yang, G. Z. (2017). Deep learning for health informatics. *IEEE Journal of Biomedical and Health Informatics*, *21*(1), 4–21. doi:10.1109/JBHI.2016.2636665 PMID:28055930

Reyes-Ortiz, J. L., Oneto, L., Samà, A., Parra, X., & Anguita, D. (2016). Transition-aware human activity recognition using smartphones. *Neurocomputing*, *171*, 754–767. doi:10.1016/j.neucom.2015.07.085

Riesbeck, C. K., & Schank, R. C. (2013). *Inside case-based reasoning*. Psychology Press.

Ronao, C. A., & Cho, S. B. (2016). Human activity recognition with smartphone sensors using deep learning neural networks. *Expert Systems with Applications*, *59*, 235–244. doi:10.1016/j.eswa.2016.04.032

Schazmann, B., Morris, D., Slater, C., Beirne, S., Fay, C., Reuveny, R., & Diamond, D. (2010). A wearable electrochemical sensor for the real-time measurement of sweat sodium concentration. *Analytical Methods*, *2*(4), 342–348. doi:10.1039/b9ay00184k

Shaji, S., Ramesh, M. V., & Menon, V. N. (2016). Real-time processing and analysis for activity classification to enhance wearable wireless ecg. In *Proceedings of the Second International Conference on Computer and Communication Technologies* (pp. 21-35). Springer. 10.1007/978-81-322-2523-2_3

Shmueli, G., & Koppius, O. R. (2011). Predictive analytics in information systems research. *Management Information Systems Quarterly*, *35*(3), 553–572. doi:10.2307/23042796

Simon, P. (2013). *Too big to ignore: the business case for big data* (Vol. 72). John Wiley & Sons.

Sivarajah, U., Kamal, M. M., Irani, Z., & Weerakkody, V. (2017). Critical analysis of Big Data challenges and analytical methods. *Journal of Business Research*, *70*, 263–286. doi:10.1016/j.jbusres.2016.08.001

Smith, M., Szongott, C., Henne, B., & Von Voigt, G. (2012, June). *Big data privacy issues in public social media.* In *Digital Ecosystems Technologies (DEST),* 2012 6th IEEE International Conference on (pp. 1-6). IEEE. 10.1109/DEST.2012.6227909

Steinmetz, L. M., & Jones, A. (2016). *Sensing a revolution.* Academic Press.

Su, X., Tong, H., & Ji, P. (2014). Activity recognition with smartphone sensors. *Tsinghua Science and Technology*, *19*(3), 235–249. doi:10.1109/TST.2014.6838194

Summers, M. J., Madl, T., Vercelli, A. E., Aumayr, G., Bleier, D. M., & Ciferri, L. (2017). Deep Machine Learning Application to the Detection of Preclinical Neurodegenerative Diseases of Aging. *DigitCult-Scientific Journal on Digital Cultures*, *2*(2), 9–24.

Talaei-Khoei, A., Ray, P., Parameshwaran, N., & Lewis, L. (2012). A framework for awareness maintenance. *Journal of Network and Computer Applications*, *35*(1), 199–210. doi:10.1016/j.jnca.2011.06.011

Thomopoulos, S. C. (1990). Sensor integration and data fusion. *Journal of Field Robotics*, *7*(3), 337–372.

Traverso, G., Ciccarelli, G., Schwartz, S., Hughes, T., Boettcher, T., Barman, R., & Swiston, A. (2015). Physiologic status monitoring via the gastrointestinal tract. *PLoS One*, *10*(11), e0141666. doi:10.1371/journal.pone.0141666 PMID:26580216

Tricoli, A., Nasiri, N., & De, S. (2017). Wearable and miniaturized sensor technologies for personalized and preventive medicine. *Advanced Functional Materials*, *27*(15), 1605271. doi:10.1002/adfm.201605271

Van Nguyen, T., Woo, Y. C., & Choi, D. (2009, April). Ccbr: Chaining case based reasoning in context-aware smart home. In *Intelligent Information and Database Systems, 2009. ACIIDS 2009. First Asian Conference on* (pp. 453-458). IEEE. 10.1109/ACIIDS.2009.20

Viswanathan, H., Chen, B., & Pompili, D. (2012). Research challenges in computation, communication, and context awareness for ubiquitous healthcare. *IEEE Communications Magazine*, *50*(5), 92–99. doi:10.1109/MCOM.2012.6194388

Waller, M. A., & Fawcett, S. E. (2013). Data science, predictive analytics, and big data: A revolution that will transform supply chain design and management. *Journal of Business Logistics*, *34*(2), 77–84. doi:10.1111/jbl.12010

Wang, A., Lin, F., Jin, Z., & Xu, W. (2016). Ultra-low power dynamic knob in adaptive compressed sensing towards biosignal dynamics. *IEEE Transactions on Biomedical Circuits and Systems*, *10*(3), 579–592. doi:10.1109/TBCAS.2015.2497304 PMID:26800548

Wang, Y., Kung, L., & Byrd, T. A. (2018). Big data analytics: Understanding its capabilities and potential benefits for healthcare organizations. *Technological Forecasting and Social Change*, *126*, 3–13. doi:10.1016/j.techfore.2015.12.019

Wessler, M. (2013). *Big data analytics for dummies*. John Wiley & Sons.

Yang, G. Z., Andreu-Perez, J., Hu, X., & Thiemjarus, S. (2014). Multi-sensor fusion. In *Body sensor networks* (pp. 301–354). Springer London. doi:10.1007/978-1-4471-6374-9_8

Yeh, J. Y., Wu, T. H., & Tsao, C. W. (2011). Using data mining techniques to predict hospitalization of hemodialysis patients. *Decision Support Systems*, *50*(2), 439–448. doi:10.1016/j.dss.2010.11.001

Yin, H., & Jha, N. K. (2017). A Health Decision Support System for Disease Diagnosis Based on Wearable Medical Sensors and Machine Learning Ensembles. *IEEE Transactions on Multi-Scale Computing Systems*, *3*(4), 228–241. doi:10.1109/TMSCS.2017.2710194

Yoo, I., Alafaireet, P., Marinov, M., Pena-Hernandez, K., Gopidi, R., Chang, J. F., & Hua, L. (2012). Data mining in healthcare and biomedicine: A survey of the literature. *Journal of Medical Systems*, *36*(4), 2431–2448. doi:10.100710916-011-9710-5 PMID:21537851

Yuan, B. (2014). *Context-aware real-time assistant architecture for pervasive healthcare*. Academic Press.

Yuan, B., & Herbert, J. (2014). Context-aware hybrid reasoning framework for pervasive healthcare. *Personal and Ubiquitous Computing*, *18*(4), 865–881. doi:10.100700779-013-0696-5

Zhang, Y., Qiu, M., Tsai, C. W., Hassan, M. M., & Alamri, A. (2017). Health-CPS: Healthcare cyber-physical system assisted by cloud and big data. *IEEE Systems Journal*, *11*(1), 88–95. doi:10.1109/JSYST.2015.2460747

Zhu, X., Liu, W., Shuang, S., Nair, M., & Li, C. Z. (2017). Intelligent tattoos, patches, and other wearable biosensors. In Medical Biosensors for Point of Care (POC) Applications (pp. 133-150). Academic Press. doi:10.1016/B978-0-08-100072-4.00006-X

Zhu, Y. (2011). Automatic detection of anomalies in blood glucose using a machine learning approach. *Journal of Communications and Networks (Seoul)*, *13*(2), 125–131. doi:10.1109/JCN.2011.6157411

Chapter 8
Fuzzy-Based Predictive Analytics for Early Detection of Diabetes

Vijayalakshmi Kakulapati
Sreenidhi Institute of Science and Technology, India

Devara Vasumathi
Jawaharlal Nehru Technological University, India

Mahender Reddy S
Sreenidhi Institute of Science and Technology, India

B. S. S. Deepthi
Mamatha Medical College, India

ABSTRACT

Today, diabetes is the most costly and burdensome chronic disease. The severity of diabetes is reducing with anticipation, premature recognition, and the early supervision impediments in people. These symptoms are the optimization of the diagnosis phase of the disease through the process of evaluating symptomatic characteristics and daily habits of patients. Big data analytical tools play a useful task in executing significant real-time investigation on the huge volumes of data and are also used to foresee the crisis situations earlier than it occurs. This chapter accomplished an efficient assessment of the applications of machine learning algorithms and tools in the diabetes investigation relating to genetic background and environment. With improving accuracy for early detection and prevention of diabetes, this chapter implemented a fuzzy linear and logistic regression model with fuzzy clustering for predicting early detection of diabetes.

DOI: 10.4018/978-1-5225-7131-5.ch008

INTRODUCTION

In recent year's, the population of diabetic patients in the world has been increased more than 382 million. Surveys and researches have predicted that the prevalence of diabetes will increase by 55% in the next decade. The observation of diabetic (Federation, I. df diabetes atlas 2013, Kaul et al.,2013) impact in claim to be one death every 6 to 10 seconds. Diabetes is a multifaceted devastating illness that can result in severe impediments such as high glucose levels in body blood, which leads to opposing insulin (Beloufa et al.,2013; Thirugnanam et al.,2012; Varma et al.,2014).

The main causes of this complex disease diabetes mellitus are a permutation of genetic aspects, ecology and way of life. Many researchers analyzed the large amount of data associated with the diabetic disease (Zhu et al., 2015). By using traditional methods dealing with huge corpora has frequently caused by measures to take the decision about improbability factors complexity (Nguyen et al., 2015; Sanz et al., 2014). To reduce this type of complications in estimating the diabetic patient prospective with intelligent techniques that requires in pertaining the investigation with the data to retrieve efficiency and effectiveness (Varma et al., 2014). To achieving effectiveness, applying Fuzzy Logic of linear and logistic regression analysis on huge data and also performed pattern analysis with predictive performance analysis

To determine and predict the occurrences of diabetic conditions, which utilized the present and old data with statistical or analytical models that includes a diversity of methods in predictive analysis (Mishra et al.,2012). Health care systems are applying big data analytics, techniques like Analytical prediction, decision making analysis. In this chapter utilize the prognostic analysis algorithm in Hadoop to forecast the category of diabetes, associated impediments and treatment to be analyzed. The methodology proposed in this chapter provides an efficient way to predict early detection of diabetic.

Researchers implement many numbers of associated works about the use of intelligent methods in the medical sector for detection and prevention of diabetes (Muthukaruppan et al.,2012, Sikchi et al., 2012, Kumar et al.,2013, Sikchi et al.,2013). Physicians make use of computational techniques to aid in the analysis and provide medicinal analysis suggestions as is filled of vagueness. For dealing with vagueness, efficient techniques are incorporating by Fuzzy Logic and neural network (Opeyemi et al.,2012).

Different classification techniques (komi et al.,2017) used different symptoms of diabetes such as levels of glucose, BP, Thickness of skin, insulin, BMI, pedigree function and age. In their research pregnancy parameters are not include to predict diabetes. An alternative method for the classical regression analysis is Fuzzy regression, in which some elements are representing by fuzzy numbers. The vagueness of this regression be converted into ambiguity not indiscriminately, which is known as the possibility (Zimmerman et al.,1991). Fuzzy regression is used in numerous areas such as predicting and diagnosis of disease (Tsaur et al.,2001; Tseng et al.,2002). The function of computational intelligence (Lukmanto et al., 2015), by a utilization of fuzzy hierarchical model which has the ability to carry out early detection against DM. A set of membership functions and rules of fuzzy rather than by the rules of two-valued logic (Raiahi-madvar et al., 2009) is conducted inference in the fuzzy expert system.

By definition of Fuzzy Logic is a form of several appropriated logic conceived (Zadeh, 1965) truth values of variables lies between 0 and 1. Fuzzy Logic based on the theme of degree, inaccurate, linguistic and observation. This logic meanly deals with natural languages and knowledge representation with formalization of reasoning modes. This mainly contains four principal features of logic, set theoretic, relational and epistemic (Zadeh, 2004).

The predictable regression model is describing by intelligent, specific and variations between experimental and approximate values of the dependent inconsistent are the consequence of inaccuracy of examination. There are two models are discussed in this chapter, the linear regression model and the logistic regression model. For fuzzy non-linear models utilizes fitting particular parametric algorithm (Buckley et al.,2000) which explores functions to facilitate best fit the information together with linear, polynomial, exponential, and logarithmic functions. Fuzzy non linear regression (Buckley et al.,1999; Celmins et al.,1991) considers information through the diversity of crisp contributions-fuzzy productivity and fuzzy contributions-fuzzy productivity. Still, it's very difficult for increasing the technique of fuzzy nonlinear regression so as to pertain to factual information.

The core intention of this work is to predict early detection of the diabetic condition established on the symptoms and provide prevention of this disease. Here, we analyzed the fuzzy model was developed to predict the diabetic accuracy. The accuracy is obtaining by predicted values are evaluated with investigational values. This prediction analysis offers a proficient treatment and health care to diabetes with enhanced results.

RELATED WORK

Researchers have investigated many several techniques for predicting diabetes utilizing different prediction models. The omitted values and disorder values in the collected data of diabetic are substituted by arrangement of classification; neural network genetic regression models (Bhat et al.,2009). This pre-processed data is using for the prediction of diabetic by applying the neural network model. Data mining regression techniques are applying on diabetes data to predictive analysis of treatment of diabetic which identified patterns by utilizing SVM methods providing better treatment process for diabetes for different age group (Abdullah et al.,2012). In this method prescribed medicine treatment applying for diabetic patients gives better results for old patients than young patients.

The treatment of the back propagation neural network and Fuzzy Logic and to recognized in the presence of exudates in the image of fundus (Habash et al.,2013). Fuzzy C-Means clustering algorithm (Lee et al.,2011) is use to identify DM (diabetes mellitus) retinopathy characteristics like blood vessel structure, micro aneurysms and stage. Fuzzy expert systems are illustrating the understandable modelling in improbability and extend by developed five-layer fuzzy ontology in diabetic data. Hybrid Fuzzy Logic (Aribarg et al.,2012; Ganji et al.,2011; Beloufa et al.,2013) and the artificial bee colony algorithm employ classification of the ant colony is to retrieve fuzzy rules which is called as FCS-ANTMINER. The modified artificial bee colony algorithm used to carry out the diagnosis process of diabetes. The main goal of this modified algorithm uses evolutionary algorithm for creating the best possible fuzzy classification for helping in general practitioner assessment.

For predicting early detection of diabetes by applying the machine learning algorithm through the Gini index-Gaussian Fuzzy decision trees (Varma et al.,2014) which categorize the divide point and construct a nodule of the Gini index binary tree. Collecting long-suffering physiological information as contribution and convert into vector input during the procedure of converting information with regulated values among 0 and 1 by applying various classification methods (WHO, 2018) to identify T2DM(Type 2 Diabetes Mellitus). These vector values are taking as training data for classification that can identify patient potential against diabetes mellitus.

The intention of the proposed technique is to compact with the complication of healthcare data as the preservative representation is dealing with high dimensional data. As a variety of attempts to add fuzzy-based applications to prevent that has the facility to carry out early recognition of diabetics.

DETECTION AND PREVENTION OF DIABETES MELLITUS

Detection of Diabetes Mellitus

When a patient complains of polyuria, polydipsia, polyphagia, weight loss associated with impaired vision should be suspected of having diabetes and the following tests are to be performed for early detection and treatment of the case.

Testing Urine

Testing of the Urine is for glucose, in pasting after 2 hours a meal is generally employed in medical exercise in identifying diabetes. This test is generally complete, but sometimes milder forms of disease cannot be detecting in this test, i.e. this test lacks sensitivity, so the results of this test is confirming by the oral glucose test or blood sugar testing.

Blood Sugar Testing

Blood sugar is tested in fasting, post prandial and random blood samples.

Other Methods of Detection of Diabetes Include:

1. Checking blood sugar in fasting
2. Enduring glucose
3. Triglycerides
4. High Blood sugar contains in the family history
5. Abdomen extent
6. Height
7. Abdomen-to-hip ratio

It is a persistent; the lifetime state that influences the patient body's aptitude to exploit the energy to be specific glucose originates in foodstuff. If a patient effected by diabetic observed as a single entity, which is seen as a diverse set of diseases such as chronic hyperglycaemia, resulting from various aetiologies, ecological and hereditary performing together. The main origin of this is the malfunctioning creation of the hormone insulin, a hormone that controls glucose, fat and amino acid metabolism, it can also be due to the defective absorption of glucose in cells though insulin is produced in normal amounts. Chronic hyperglycaemia, no matter what cause directs to a number of problems.

Table 1. Types of diabetic and their sugar levels.

Target Levels by Type	Upon Waking	Before Meals (Pre Prandial)	At Least 90 Minutes After Meals (Post Prandial)
Non-diabetic*		4.0 to 5.9 mmol/L	under 7.8 mmol/L
Type 2 diabetes		4 to 7 mmol/L	under 8.5 mmol/L
Type 1 diabetes	5 to 7 mmol/L	4 to 7 mmol/L	5 to 9 mmol/L
Children w/ type 1 diabetes	4 to 7 mmol/L	4 to 7 mmol/L	5 to 9 mmol/L

Maximum persons experiencing from the ailment is not recognized or the suggestion from the doctor is known as an iceberg disease. The result of adverse life alteration and metropolitan food habits are the major cause of diabetic disease. The frequency of occurrence of diabetic in metropolitan is double when compared to rural areas. Most of the general public is still inadequate consciousness regarding the actual cause of diabetic disease.

Generally diabetes is categorized into 3 classes:

1. DM (Diabetes mellitus)
    a. Type 1 is identified by insulin dependent DM
    b. Type 1 is identified by non-insulin dependent DM
    c. scarcity communicated DM
    d. minor to Pancreatic, hormonal, drug persuaded, hereditary and other irregularities
2. Prejudiced glucose acceptance
3. Hyperglycaemia during pregnancy(Gestational diabetes mellitus)

For control diabetes by consuming tablets or taking the form of injection is absolutely not the method to organize glucose levels. The major aim of supervision of diabetes is to prevent end-organ problems. The diabetes patient frequently visits the physicians to check their glucose levels and hemoglobin. Patient experiences scarcity in eye sight, blazing or piercing pain in their foot from neuropathy, or indications of end-stage renal disease or uremia and then early detection of diabetes symptoms of different situations. For this, the treatment and diagnosis of retinopathy, neuropathy, and nephropathy suggestion from the health care professionals provides primary diabetic care.

Diabetes symptoms are categorized into damage in small blood vessels is known as microvascular and damage in larger blood vessels is known as macro vascular.

Probable Symptoms are:

- Heart disease.
- Damage in Nerves is also known as Neuropathy
- Damage of Kidney is also known as Nephropathy.
- Damage in Eye is also known as Retinopathy
- Damage or burning in Foot
- Change in Skin conditions.
- destruction in Hearing
- Alzheimer's disease.

The Significance of Eye Care

Diabetic disease leads to blindness. To avoid blindness, the patient is educating about the prerequisite of accustomed enlarged-eye assessments. An enlarged eye assessment and a complete retinal test by an ophthalmologist should be done on a regular basis. If patients can put on emphasis that diabetes can be postponed and many times keep away from visual disability if damage to eyes is noticed at its initial phases. The larger blood vessels are damaged are also known as macrovascular. Microvascular impediments contain eye damage leads to sightless, kidney damage leads to failure in renal and nerves damage leads to impotence and severe infections leading to amputation. In macrovascular impediments contain heart attacks, strokes, and scarcity in blood circulation to foot.

- **Origin:** Eye sight problems occurred in diabetic patients due to small blood vessels damage to the back layer of the eyeball, the retina, conspicuous to the steady failure of optical, constant visual deficiency.
- **Symptoms:** The patients have misty revelation at the same time as additional visual symptoms.
- **Detection:** The patient gone for regular eye testing
- **Curing:** The diabetic patient should maintain good metabolic controls postponement the inception and development of eye disease. The patient gone for the regular eye checkup also provides premature exposure and diagnosis can avoid blindness.

Nephropathy (Etiology)

Diabetic patients are also affected by kidney disease, due microvascular abnormalities in the kidneys which leads to kidney failure, and ultimately death. This problem is the main reason for dialysis and transplantation of the kidney.

- **Symptoms:** The diabetic patients have no symptoms in the beginning, however, as ailment advancements the patient may feel tired, anemic, sense is not clear, and even enlarge unsafe electrolyte inequality
- **Diagnosis:** Premature analysis can be through a urine and blood test for protein as well as kidney functioning.
- **Curing:** The patients diagnosed at the beginning of the disease, numerous evaluates can impede the development of kidney failures which contain controlling of high blood glucose, interference with the prescription in the premature point of kidney spoil, and control of nutritional protein.

Nerve Disease (Neuropathy)

This can cause in diabetic including hyperglycemia damage and the flow of blood in nerves are decreased due to small blood vessels damaging which can This nerve damage can result to loss of sense, limbs damage, and impotence in men. This is the most common symptom in diabetic patients.

- **Symptoms:** The complications are lack of sensation, pain in extremities and impotence. Lack of sensation at feet can lead to enduring not be acquainted with cuts and on the increase of infectious foot which can lead to amputation not recognize in the early stage.
- **Analysis:** Premature analysis is through early detection of complications by patients and physicians as well as by suspicious assessment at regular periods.
- **Curing:** Premature detection of diabetic leads to controlling the blood, avoid these obstacles.

Foot disease in the diabetic patient caused due to alterations in blood vessels and nerves, regularly leads to ulceration and consequent limb elimination. This is also major complications of diabetes with insufficient footwear which results from both vascular and neurological ailment procedures. Good care and identification of damage in foot can avoid amputations.

Cardiovascular Disease

- **Etiology:** Hyperglycemia harms veins through a procedure called "atherosclerosis", or stopping up of conduits. This narrowing of courses can prompt a diminished blood stream to heart muscle which leads to a heart attack, or to brain stroke, or to the furthest points (WHO, 2018) leads to hurt and diminished curing of contaminations.
- **Indications:** Begin from chest pain to foot pain, to perplexity and paralysis.
- **Analysis:** These symptoms are detected in the early stage setback development, detection of further possibility issues, for instance, smoking, high BP, high cholesterol in serum cholesterol and heftiness is significantly more critical.
- **Curing:** The above possible issues are controlling along with glucose in blood can avoid heart related impediments.

Renal replacement therapy is the main motive for involving in diabetes, the major reason of sightlessness in effective age groups and the frequent reason of non-traumatic elimination. However, most by far of these overwhelming occasions could be averted, deferred, or their effect limited. The usefulness of diabetes concern and the insistent supervision of hazard issues into high-quality medical concerns.

Complications of Diabetes

If microvascular and microvascular illness present in humans having complications in common which inception of impediments diminishes healthy life (Koopman Schap, 2003). Over 7000 diabetic unwearied with Type 2 is the result in 8 European observations (Williams, 2002). In their study 72% suffer with one impediment and 24% suffering with equally microvascular and microvascular impediments. Within 6 months gap, 13% patients were joining in the infirmary, with an indicate length of remain of twenty-three days. The yearly normal cost per patient is evaluated as Euro 2834. 55% of this aggregate was endorsed to expenses of hospitalization, with just 7% inferable from expenses of insulin and oral glucose-bringing down specialists (Jonsson, 2002).

Prevention

To predict and prevent diabetes is as:

1. Individual life fashion intrusions
2. Controlling of Blood pressure
3. Glycemic index
4. Regular eye check-up
5. Individual can care their foot care with the high hazard of diabetic sores.

Prevention Tips

For preventing diabetes in the early stage the following are few tips for general public.

Vegetables and Fruit are rich in fiber, minerals and vitamins and also less fat and calorie contents. This kind of diet is known as prudent diet.

- Eat plenty of fruits and vegetables
- Mix diverse vegetables or fruits to acquire the utmost vitamins and minerals.
- Fruits and vegetables can be fresh, frozen, canned or dried
- Taking fruit juice intake is the limit up to 150 ml for every day, which contains more carbohydrates and fibre previously gone down which preserves patient blood sugars to mount more rapidly.
- Generally fruits contain natural sugars, which can increase blood sugar levels. It is suggested to diabetes control their intake quantity of fruit juice per day.

Suggestions for using fruits and vegetables**:** For prevention of diabetes humans can take care of their health by using the following tips in their dietary.

- In daily breakfast add some fruit slices to oats.
- Every afternoon has some chopped vegetables
- In each meal add at least two vegetables, for example, onions, tomatoes and spinach to pasta.

Stuffy Carbohydrates

The significant resource of food to produce energy in diabetes is carbohydrates broken into glucose, which is utilized to stimulate human body cells.

- Keep an eye to contain some carbohydrates in the diet.
- Choose multigrain/seeded bread to increase energy
- Limit the intake of food proportion. If the proportion is exceeding, it will increase blood glucose levels.

Suggestions for using carbohydrates: In daily breakfast take seeded bread or wholegrain cereals

- In lunch choose a potato which roast in the oven or the sugary potato for the added fibre.
- Eat chapatti or Nan.
- Eat brown rice instead of normal rice.

The Product of Dairy Alternatives

These products are rich in calcium, vitamins and minerals.

- Use less fat and sugar contents as intake to condense fat, calorie and sugar and prefer on behalf of products of dairy with less sweet for instance, soy milk.

Suggestions for using dairy products:

- Take skimmed milk instead of full-fat milk.
- Low-fat fruits are a healthy breakfast.
- Baked potatoes with cottage cheese instead of fat contain cheese.
- Be inclined to consume smaller amounts of food for healthy life.

Non-vegetable like meat, fish, egg and vegetable like beans, pulses, nuts and other proteins

These foods are rich in protein and a source of iron.

- Choose these foods are in daily life.
- For healthy heart consume fatty fish per week in limited proportion.
- Processed meat can consume in small quantity.
- For vegetarian people, these proteins can be available with beans, pulses and lentils which will condense fat and enhance fibre intake.

Suggestions for using these foods:

- Consume eggs in the form of boiled, scrambled, poached, in an omelet.
- In dinner choose non-vegetables like grilled meat, fish or meat alternatives and serve with vegetables
- Whenever hungry choose some nuts and seeds.
- Consume extra beans and pulses to dietary or replace meats

Liquids

These are keeping hydrated.

- Drink more than six glasses of liquid for every day which consist of non-sugar drinks or alternative for liquid for calorie-free is water.

Suggestions for using liquids:

- Prefer mostly 400 mg caffeine a day don't bear healthiness issues. For pregnant don't choose more than 200 mg caffeine a day.
- Calculate calories in each meal count
- A bottle of water always carry
- Avoid full sugar contain juices and take non sugar contain juices or better take water.
- Before taking diet choose glass of water to avoid more portion of food

Salted

- Intake food must be a low quantity which reduces BP, heart stroke and diabetic.
- Avoid processed food and ready meals which contains more salt contents.

- Consume fresh food which will avoid taking more salt.

Suggestions for consuming salt:

- On the dining table, remove salt
- Use pepper, seeds of cumin, mirchi peels.
- Take homemade sauces and food.
- Reduce processed meats similar to bacon and salami those contains more salt.
- Utilize salt cubes for soups, gravy.

Foods High in Fat and Sugar

Now a day people are getting more fat food more than normal diet such as more sugar foods and cholesterol food, juices can add to gain in their weight, food contains more sugar can acquire rise in blood glucose.

Suggestions for using foods contain fat and sugar

- Avoid make use of fat contains oils in cooking
- Avoid butter with olive oil.
- Use a spray oil
- Choose low fat variety food while buying food check their labels

Foods Causing Blood Glucose Levels to Raise

Carbohydrate foods cause glucose levels to mount.

- Bread, rice, pasta, potatoes and cereals.
- Milk, fruit and sweets in purified forms, dairy products and fruit juice having more carbohydrates.

Natural sugars form in starchy carbohydrates and foods which gives a well balanced diet. But be careful while eating not to a take large proportion of these foods.

Glycemic Index

People consuming food is quickly digested and absorbed or not can be known by the glycemic index (GI) and increase in glucose levels can be detected. Low GI gives energy slowly and helps diminish quick instability in blood glucose levels. Fruit and vegetable lentils, pulses, beans and wholegrain starchy varieties contain healthy low GI. Chocolate is a better example for unhealthy low GI. Low GI foods will cause high blood glucose. To avoid this, people should focus on their eating principle and proportion of food control.

Food Portion Amount

Continue with checking the portion of eating food is help to steady or weight loss which will manage glucose levels.

- Eat in small plates
- Choose proportionate food.
- Consume food has low-calorie such as salads and vegetables
- Consume food slowly.
- Don't watch television or playing on a computer while eating.
- Reduce temptations

The Benefits of Weight Loss

Overweight can improve glucose levels in the human body. Weight loss can help decrease in glucose and fat levels which sequentially helps to diminish the stroke threat and diabetes.

Loss of weight in terms of the percentage as 5-10% of the human body is adequate to achieve major healthiness.

EXPERIMENT EVALUATION

The approach of Predictive Analysis can facilitate practitioners precisely anticipate and take action to the enduring requirements. The predictive analysis also offers the facility to cost effective and medical assessments. In this, for implementation purpose utilizes the map-reduce algorithm in the Hadoop environment to foresee and categorize the category of diabetes, obstacles correlated through it and the diagnosis category is predicted. An open source platform Hadoop is processing data distributed platform. This system can provide the two different functions of organizing information and analytical tool (Raghupathi et al.,2014). This system processing the huge quantity of medical data by distributed partitioned data to dissimilar clusters, each cluster resolves diverse divisions of the larger difficulty and then incorporates for the final outcome. In Hadoop system, there are two main components which are processing the job: one is Map/Reduce and another one is HDFS. The first component is programming the model to progression collected data by splitting into tiny chunks of jobs. It utilizes disseminated algorithms, on a collection of systems in a group, to process broad data. Map/Reduce contains two types of functions: The first one is the Map () function and another one is the Reduce () function. The job of Map () locates on the master node and splits the participation data or job into minor sub jobs, then it allocates to slave nodes to facilitate process minor jobs and send the outcome to the master node. All the sub jobs are executed in parallel on multiple systems. The job of the second one is the Reduce () function accumulates the outcome of all the sub jobs and merges them to generate a collective final outcome and then it returns as the outcome to the query. HDFS duplicates the information block that exists on the other systems in the data center and supervises distribution of data to different locations of the system.

Fuzzy Logic (FL) is also known as several-rated logic, which allows intermediate values as real numbers between 0 and 1. Fl is also called as an accurate logic of indefinite reasoning in which the membership functions and simplified limitations are precise (Zadeh, 2009).

The proposed fuzzy based system which that provides diagnosis carry out and investigational out comes demonstrated that the fuzzy system is moderately enhanced than inefficient urologist and around 94% as a well as efficient urologist did. The proposed fuzzy system designed to accomplish as follows

1. By employing Fuzzy Logic able to detection of diabetics and its risks
2. Provides precautions for the risk of the diabetic
3. Fuzzy variables in every input and output
4. Member function is related to every fuzzy Variable
5. The strength of rules is determined based on the membership function.

Fuzzy regression models are defined by revealing the vagueness of designed methods (Kacprzyk et al.,1992; Poleshchuk et al.,2012; Shapiro, 2006). Output values are estimating by the indeterminate nature of the fuzzy regression model and the coefficients of fuzzy regression in the structure of vague numbers. The fuzzy linear regression model (Buckley et al.,2008; Heshmaty et al.,2009; Tanaka et al.,1982) is specified by the improvement of the imprecise degeneration representation is the vague model's improvement by means of the formalization of vagueness to a certain extent, statistical periods via fuzzy intervals.

Fuzzy Linear Regression Model

This model is utilized to estimate the useful association amid the needy and self-determining inconsistent in a fuzzy situation. There are several types of fuzzy regression are developed and diverse methods are investigated to approximation fuzzy factors. Generally, fuzzy regression models are two types of analysis: those are the Possibilistic approach and the fuzzy least square model. In the method of model detection, the accumulation procedure reduces the imprecision of overall function throughout the minimization of computation of fuzzy regression coefficient vagueness

$$\text{Min J} = \min \sum_{i=1}^{n} \left(C_i\right) \text{where } h_j \leq H, j=1,2,....m$$

An extension of K-mean clustering algorithm is also known as fuzzy C-means, which determines the centroids of clusters; the contribution data set is allocated to cluster with least distance from centroid. Though, sometimes new input data can be reduced for other than one which was avoided by C-means algorithm (Sakshi Gujral, 2017) as it utilizes fuzzy separation that reports for the membership function. Therefore, consequences generating are more precise.

- **Benefits:**
    - MF (membership function) assists in giving enhanced consequences for the classification.
    - Results are more real-time due to the unsupervised learning technique
- **Drawbacks:**
    - More consume time.
    - Suspect to wrong assessments at early stages.
- **Dataset:** For Implementation result, collect data from the dataworld and this data set contains variables like age, blood pressure, body mass index, pedigree function and blood cholesterol. The data set contains 3000 records; out of these utilized for analysis purpose 100 records.
- **Preprocessing:** The collected data set pre-processed each record to remove irrelevant information such as stop word removal. After pre-processing, the diabetic records are as follows.

BMI is a measure of body fat i.e,

$$\text{BMI} = \text{weight (kg)} \div \text{height}^2 \text{ (m}^2\text{)}$$

The correlation among them calculated for 20 sample records is 0.1765446

Table 2. Probabilities of BMI and pedigree function

Blood Pressure	Skin Thickness	Insulin	BMI	Diabetes Pedigree	Age	Outcome	Probability
72	35	0	33.6	0.627	50	1	0.5863
66	29	0	26.6	0.351	31	0	0.3811
64	0	0	23.3	0.672	32	1	0.5863
66	23	94	28.1	0.167	21	0	0.3811
40	35	168	43.1	2.288	33	1	0.5863
74	0	0	25.6	0.201	30	0	0.3811
50	32	88	31	0.248	26	1	0.5863
0	0	0	35.3	0.134	29	0	0.3811
70	45	543	30.5	0.158	53	1	0.5863
96	0	0	0	0.232	54	1	0.5863
92	0	0	37.6	0.191	30	0	0.3811
74	0	0	38	0.537	34	1	0.5863
80	0	0	27.1	1.441	57	0	0.3811
60	23	846	30.1	0.398	59	1	0.5863
72	19	175	25.8	0.587	51	1	0.5863

Table 3. Predictable interval limits for the pedigree function and the outcome using linear regression

S. No	fit	lwr	upr
1	0.5863333	-0.5838399	1.756507
2	0.3811429	-0.8207481	1.583034
3	0.5863333	-0.5838399	1.756507
4	0.3811429	-0.8207481	1.583034
5	0.5863333	-0.5838399	1.756507
6	0.3811429	-0.8207481	1.583034
7	0.5863333	-0.5838399	1.756507
8	0.3811429	-0.8207481	1.583034
9	0.5863333	-0.5838399	1.756507
10	0.5863333	-0.5838399	1.756507
11	0.3811429	-0.8207481	1.583034
12	0.5863333	-0.5838399	1.756507
13	0.3811429	-0.8207481	1.583034
14	0.5863333	-0.5838399	1.756507
15	0.5863333	-0.5838399	1.756507

Figure 1. Density graphs for pedigree function and the outcome

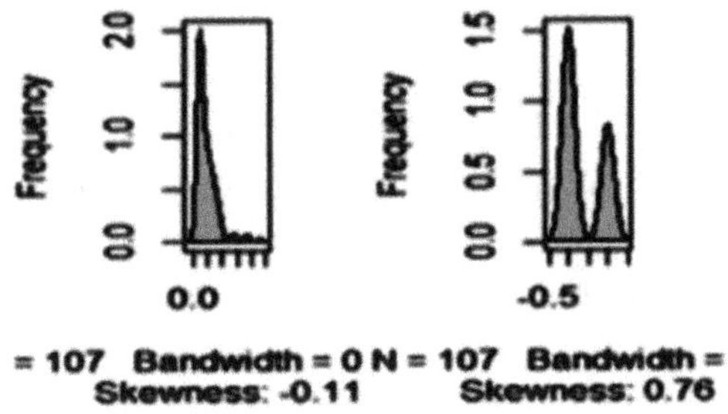

Table 4. A summary of linear model

Min	1Q	Median	3Q	Max
-0.4099	-0.2	-0.1019	0.1056	1.7251

Table 5.

	Estimate Std	Error	t Value	Pr (>|t|)
(Intercept)	0.42590	0.04442	9.588	0.000000000000000516
Outcome	0.13700	0.07454	1.838	0.0689

Residual standard error: 0.369 on 105 degrees of freedom
Multiple R-squared: 0.03117, Adjusted R-squared: 0.02194
F-statistic: 3.378 on 1 and 105 DF, p-value: 0.0689

Figure 2. The pedigree function varies in between 0 or 1

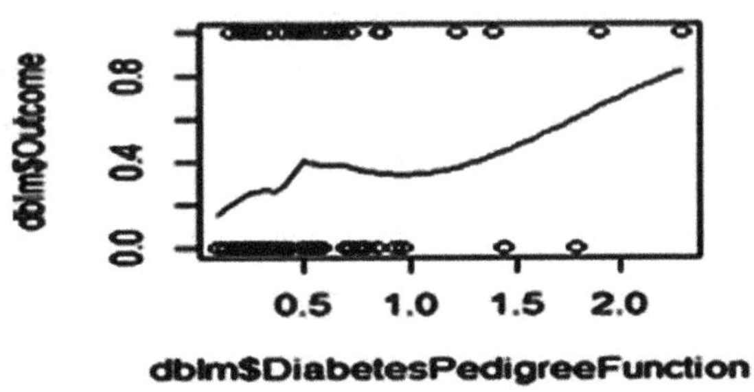

Fuzzy Logistic Regression

The data set which contains $Xi = (xi1, xi2, ..., xin)\ i = 1, 2, . . . n$, where Xi is the vector of observations like BMI, pedigree function, blood pressure and blood cholesterol for the i-th case. μi, the consequent observation, is a number in (0,1) and indicates the option of i-th case have the appropriate property, i.e. μi = Poss(Yi=1).

The total number of input data to the outcome in the dataset 0's are 69 and 1's are 38.

IV_df (the degree of freedom value) value for the dataset input records:

$$\text{Sensitivity}=\frac{\#\text{Actual1's and predicted as1's}}{\#\text{of Actual1's}}=0.34$$

$$\text{Specificity}=\frac{\#\text{Actual0's and predicted as0's}}{\#\text{of Actual0's}}=0.836$$

Table 6. The degree of freedom value for input records

Vars	IV
Age	1.4392
Glucose	1.2966
BMI	0.0000
Diabetes Pedigree Function	0.0000
Blood Pressure	0.0000
Skin Thickness	0.0000
Insulin	0.0000

Table 7. Standard values for the input data

Input Data	Estimate	Std.Error	Z value	Pr(>|z|)
(Intercept)	-7.03546	2.19078	-3.211	0.00132**
Age	0.08246	0.03799	2.171	0.02994*
Glucose	0.01653	0.01187	1.393	0.16362
BMI	0.06053	0.03927	1.541	0.12320
Diabetes Pedigree Function	0.39475	0.86882	0.454	0.64957

where Sensitivity is the percentage of 1's correctly predicted by the model, and specificity is the percentage of 0's correctly predicted.

Crisp clustering vector:

```
(1) 3 2 3 2 3 1 2 1 3 3 1 3 3 3 3 1 1 1 1 1 3 1 3 1 3 3 3 2 3 3
1 3 2 1 3 2 3 1 2 1 3 3 1 3 3 3 3 2 2 1 2 2
(53) 2 3 3 2 3 1 3 2 1 3 2 3 1 2 1 1 2 3 2 3 3 3 2 1 2 2 1 2 1
1 2 2 3 1 1 2 3 2 2 3 2 3 3 3 2 2 2 1 3 3 3 2
(105) 2 1 1
```

Table 8. Classification of diabetic patients

S.No.	Type	Age	BS.Fast	BS.pp	Plasma.R	Plasma.F	HbA1c	Class
1	Type1	50	6.8	8.8	11.2	7.2	62	1
2	Normal	31	5.2	6.8	10.9	4.2	33	0
3	Type1	32	6.8	8.8	11.2	7.2	62	1
4	Normal	21	5.7	5.8	10.7	4.8	49	0
5	Type1	33	6.8	8.8	11.2	7.2	62	1
6	Normal	30	5.2	7.4	8.7	5.6	41	0
7	Type2	26	5.8	4.2	11.4	8.4	53	1
8	Normal	29	5.2	7.4	8.7	5.6	41	0
9	Type2	53	6.9	8.4	11.2	7.2	62	1
10	Type2	54	6.3	4.2	12.2	7.8	57	1

Table 9. Diabetics symptoms

S.No.	Glucose	Blood Pressure	Skin Thickness	BMI	Pedigree Function	Age
1	148	72	35	33.6	0.627	50
2	85	66	29	26.6	0.351	31
3	89	66	23	28.1	0.167	21
4	197	70	45	30.5	0.158	53
5	110	92	0	37.6	0.191	30
6	189	60	23	30.1	0.398	59
7	166	72	19	25.8	0.587	51
8	125	70	26	31.1	0.205	41
9	147	76	0	39.4	0.257	43
10	97	66	15	23.2	0.487	22

Table 10. Female diabetic patient's symptoms

Pregnancies	Glucose	Blood Pressure	Skin Thickness	Insulin	BMI	Pedigree Function	Age	Outcome
6	148	72	35	0	33.6	0.627	50	1
1	85	66	29	0	26.6	0.351	31	0
8	183	64	0	0	23.3	0.672	32	1
1	89	66	23	94	28.1	0.167	21	0
0	137	40	35	168	43.1	2.288	33	1
5	116	74	0	0	25.6	0.201	30	0
3	78	50	32	88	31	0.248	26	1
10	115	0	0	0	35.3	0.134	29	0
2	197	70	45	543	30.5	0.158	53	1
8	125	96	0	0	0	0.232	54	1

Table 11. Assign different probabilities in different clusters.

S.No	Cluster 1	Cluster 2	Cluster 3
1	0.13747722	0.44171891	0.10918240
2	0.84606353	0.26284424	0.31761429
3	0.21499722	0.69145018	0.15333761
4	0.46472340	0.38690507	0.24603484
5	0.21304949	0.71453144	0.15205670
6	0.92960424	0.43399216	0.31224912

Number of data objects:107
Number of clusters: 3

Table 12. Initial cluster prototypes

	Glucose	Blood Pressure	Skin Thickness	BMI	Pedigree Function	Age
Cluster 1	85	65	0	39.6	0.930	27
Cluster 2	71	48	18	20.4	0.323	22
Cluster 3	115		0	35.3	0.134	29

Prognostic Pattern Matching

Every time the data was implemented in Hadoop environment, directly the map reduces the task is executed. In this, the procedure estimated and the investigated threshold assessment value achieved.

Table 13. Final cluster prototypes

	Glucose	Blood Pressure	Skin Thickness	BMI	Pedigree Function	Age
Cluster 1	115.6435	71.42539	20.65017	31.16322	0.4630614	3.11240
Cluster 2	105.1784	68.33592	21.71815	30.18715	0.4348529	30.31015
Cluster 3	122.3727	72.72936	19.69803	31.58360	0.4756178	34.51896

Table 14. Distance between the final cluster prototypes

Cluster 1	Cluster 2	Cluster 3
129.00978	50.04377	338.69144

Table 15. Difference between the initial and final cluster prototypes

	Glucose	Blood Pressure	Skin Thickness	BMI	Pedigree Function	Age
Cluster 1	30.643506	6.425393	20.650166	-8.436779	-0.4669386	6.112398
Cluster 2	34.178408	20.335919	3.718146	9.787148	0.1118529	8.310154
Cluster 3	7.372666	72.729359	19.698026	-3.716399	0.3416178	5.518955

Root Mean Squared Deviations (RMSD): 54.9309
Mean Absolute Deviation (MAD): 517.1077

Table 16. Membership degrees matrix (top and bottom 5 rows)

	Cluster 1	Cluster 2	Cluster 3
1	0.4640805	0.3085429	0.5239170
2	0.5570335	0.6929775	0.4437818
3	0.2083424	0.1408080	0.2286273
4	0.5974639	0.7502265	0.4778776
5	0.4268892	0.3326092	0.4297700
...			
103	0.4995598	0.3784440	0.5096888
104	0.5048914	0.6193198	0.4029992
105	0.4687733	0.5220600	0.3886028
106	0.7019584	0.5976787	0.6864056
107	0.2773600	0.2356186	0.2548805

Table 17. Descriptive statistics for the membership degrees by clusters

	Size	Min	Q1	Mean	Median	Q3	Max
Cluster 1	30	0.08669724	0.2993262	0.4977418	0.5231006	0.6952497	0.9285412
Cluster 2	33	0.20039546	0.5220600	0.6612678	0.6929775	0.8138359	0.9573988
Cluster 3	44	0.159976 85	0.3585530	0.4914684	0.5021205	0.6152516	0.9428153

Table 18. Dunn's Fuzziness Coefficients

Dunn_coeff	normalized
0.8273677	0.7410516

Table 19. Within cluster sum of squares by cluster

1	2	3
71773.34	16111.08	48589.20

(between_SS / total_SS = 4.48%)

Figure 3. Fuzzy plot for the diabetes dataset

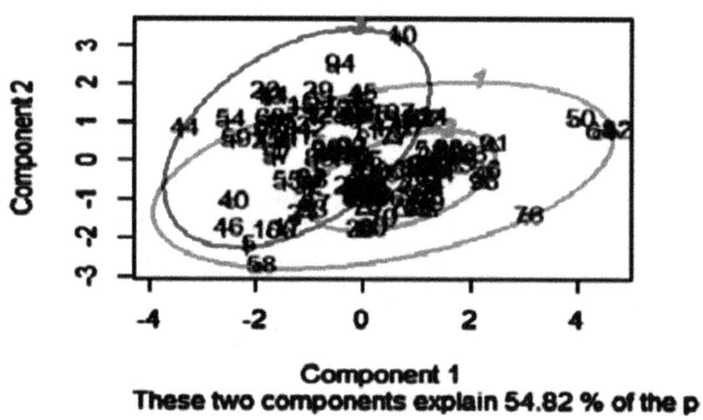

Dealing Out Investigated Reports

The huge diabetic data set is analyzed; the absolute end results are disseminated. Through online communication to share the data of patients among healthcare

Figure 4. K means cluster plot for the diabetes dataset

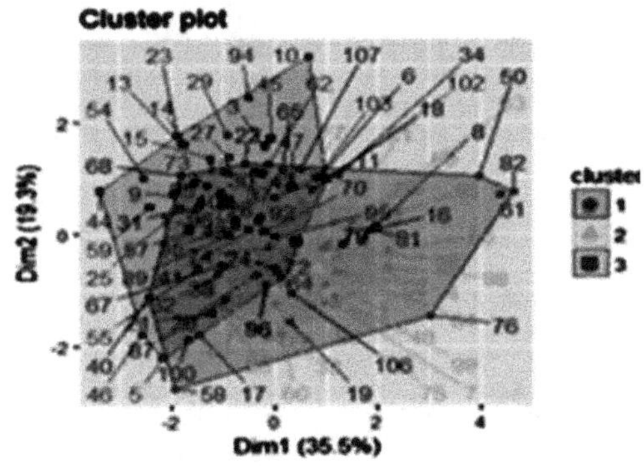

Figure 5. General cluster plot for all the fields of the dataset

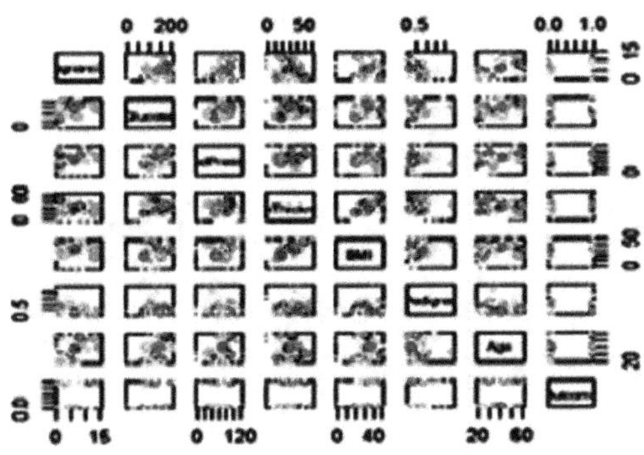

Figure 6. K means the general cluster plot for glucose blood pressure thickness BMi pedigree and age

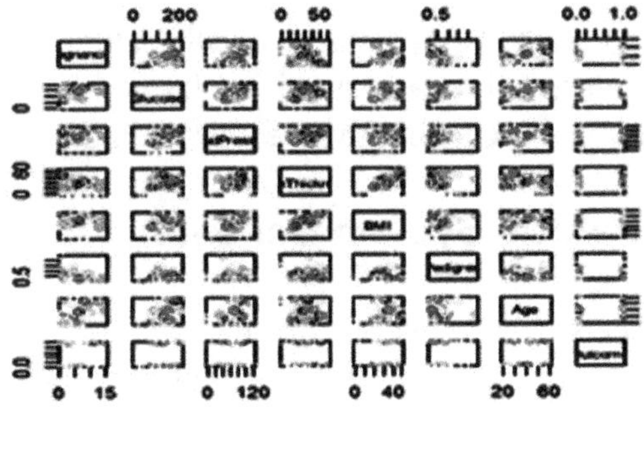

Figure 7. Cluster plot general using membership function

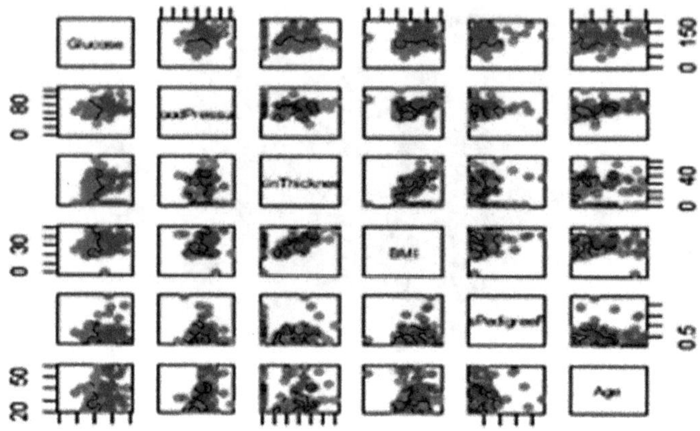

Figure 8. Fuzzy cluster plot using membership function

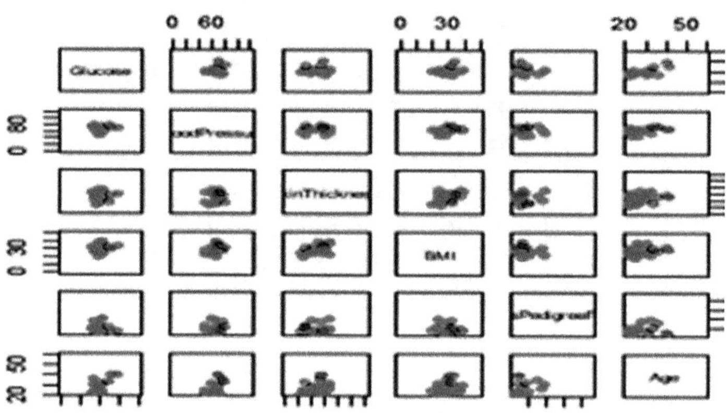

providers, which leads to acquire, appropriate healing in different locations.

Training data and testing data are classified based on the decimal values i.e integral values for training and decimal values for testing.

The Predictive Analysis System Benefits

The complexity of diabetes leads several correlate diseases for instance, the failure of heart, brain strokes, blindness and failure of kidneys etc. By predicting the hazard assessment by the intensity of diabetes physical condition, showing the results within the table can be analyzed by the physician. Early detection of diabetes can facilitate for better and immediate diagnosis more easily and efficiently. The major aim of

Table 20. Categorization of diagnosis persons

<table>
<tr><th rowspan="3">Terminology</th><th colspan="2">Categorization 1</th><th colspan="2">Categorization 2</th></tr>
<tr><th colspan="2">Pedigree<0.2(healthy)
Pedigree(0.2-0.6)(normal)
Pedigree(0.6-1.0)(to be diagnosed)
Pedigree(>1)(serious)</th><th colspan="2">Pedigree<0.25(healthy)
Pedigree(0.25-0.75)(normal)
Pedigree(0.75-1.25)(to be diagnosed)
Pedigree(>1.25)(serious)</th></tr>
<tr><th>Residual Standard Error</th><th>F-Statistic</th><th>Residual Standard Error</th><th>F-Statistic</th></tr>
<tr><td>healthy</td><td>0.02515</td><td>1.537</td><td>0.03995</td><td>1.068</td></tr>
<tr><td>normal</td><td>0.1197</td><td>0.1289</td><td>0.03995</td><td>1.068</td></tr>
<tr><td>To be diagnosed</td><td>0.1048</td><td>0.7983</td><td>0.1284</td><td>1.17</td></tr>
<tr><td>Serious</td><td>0.4374</td><td>0.05305</td><td>0.3928</td><td>0.4706</td></tr>
</table>

this system leads to the enhanced method on each diabetes patient. Hence, decrease and accumulate future generation from diabetic disease.

CONCLUSION

The Big Data generated by different online systems execute in Hadoop shows enhanced outcomes approximating the ease of use and affordability of healthcare services. Diabetic plays a major health hazard in world wide. Diabetic patient health data is analyzed which will provide better understanding of the diabetic complication to take place. In this work utilize predictive analysis of diabetic treatment by applying Fuzzy Logic linear and logistic regression on BMI using big data analytics which yields improved data and analytics with the maximum outcomes in the healthcare domain.

In this chapter predicting and diagnosis of diabetes by using fuzzy regression models with c mean clustering techniques by analyzing their family background. These are used for early detection for diabetes and provide better suggestion for preventing the diabetic. The method makes use of the fuzzy regression technique and can be applied to a convenient analysis of categorical data for predictive analysis.

By converting numerous medical records of diabetics to analyzed the make use of the result, which helps the diabetic patient be aware of the complications to be happen. The prognostic analysis technique of diabetic healing may provide improved data and analytics defer the enormous consequences in the medical field. The Fuzzy Logic System for diabetic diagnosis with membership functions, input variables, and output variables. For this method can check whether someone has any diabetic hazard or not. The main goal of this research centered for the diabetes patients in world wide. Better diagnosis can be suggested when it is early detected in patients. Here, the chapter concludes with performance metrics of premature recognition of diabetes and prevention.

FUTURE ENHANCEMENT

In the future work for improving accuracy for prediction and, the diagnosis of diabetes would be worked out further using types of diabetes and behavior analysis of the diabetic patient. Uses of clustering methods for predict the better diagnosis and treatment of diabetes.

REFERENCES

Aljumah, Ahamad, & Siddiqui. (2012). Application of data mining: Diabetes health care in young and old patients. *Journal of King Saud University – Computer and Information Sciences, 25*, 127–136.

Aribarg, T., Supratid, S., & Lursinsap, C. (2012). Optimizing the modified fuzzy ant-miner for efficient medical diagnosis. *Applied Intelligence*, *37*(3), 357–376. doi:10.100710489-011-0332-x

Beloufa, F., & Chikh, M. (2013). Design of fuzzy classifier for diabetes disease using modified artificial bee colony algorithm. *Computer Methods and Programs in Biomedicine*, *112*(1), 92–103. doi:10.1016/j.cmpb.2013.07.009 PMID:23932385

Bhat, Rao, & Shenoy. (2009). An Efficient Prediction Model for Diabetic Database Using Soft Computing Techniques. In *Architecture*. Springer-Verlag.

Buckley, Feuring, & Hayashi. (n.d.). Multivariate non-linear fuzzy regression: an evolutionary algorithm approach. *International Journal of Uncertainty*.

Buckley, J. J., & Feuring, T. (2000). Linear and non-linear fuzzy regression: Evolutionary algorithm solutions. *Fuzzy Sets and Systems*, *112*(3), 381–394. doi:10.1016/S0165-0114(98)00154-7

Buckley, J. J., & Jowers, L. J. (2008). *Fuzzy Linear Regression I. Studies in Fuzziness and Soft Computing* (Vol. 22). Springer.

Celmins. (1991). A practical approach to nonlinear fuzzy regression. *SIAM Journal on Scientific and Statistical Computing, 12*, 521–546.

Ganji, M. F., & Abadeh, M. S. (2011). A fuzzy classification system based on ant colony optimization for diabetes disease diagnosis. *Expert Systems with Applications*, *38*(12), 14650–14659. doi:10.1016/j.eswa.2011.05.018

Gujral. (2017). Early Diabetes Detection using Machine Learning: A Review. *International Journal for Innovative Research in Science & Technology, 3*(10).

Habashy, S. M. (2013). Identification of diabetic retinopathy stages using fuzzy C-means classifier. *International Journal of Computers and Applications*, *77*(9).

Jonsson, B. (2002). Revealing the cost of Type II diabetes in Europe. *Diabetologia*, *45*(S1), S5–S12. doi:10.100700125-002-0858-x

Kacprzyk, M. F. (Ed.). (1992). *Fuzzy Regression Analysis. Studies in Fuzziness and Soft Computing*. Physica-Verlag HD.

Kaul, K., Tarr, J. M., Ahmad, S. I., Kohner, E. M., & Chibber, R. (2013). Introduction to diabetes mellitus. In *Diabetes* (pp. 1–11). Springer.

Komi, M., Li, J., Zhai, Y., & Zhang, X. (2017, June). Application of data mining methods in diabetes prediction. In *Image, Vision and Computing (ICIVC), 2017 2nd International Conference on* (pp. 1006-1010). IEEE. 10.1109/ICIVC.2017.7984706

Koopman Schap, M. (2003). Coping with Type II diabetes: The patient's perspective. *Diabetologia*, *45*, 302–303.

Kumar, A. S. (2013). Diagnosis of diabetic using Advanced Fuzzy resolution Mechanism. *International Journal of Science and Applied Information Technology*, *2*(2), 22–30.

Lee, C. S., & Wang, M. H. (2011). A fuzzy expert system for diabetes decision support application. *Systems, Man, and Cybernetics, Part B: Cybernetics. IEEE Transactions on*, *41*(1), 139–153.

Lukmanto, R. B., & Irwansyah, E. (2015). The Early Detection of Diabetes Mellitus (DM) Using Fuzzy Hierarchical Model. *Procedia Computer Science*, *59*, 312–319. doi:10.1016/j.procs.2015.07.571

Mishra & Silakari. (2012). Predictive Analytics: A Survey, Trends, Applications, Oppurtunities & Challenges. *International Journal of Computer Science and Information Technologies, 3*(3), 4434-4438.

Muthukaruppan, S., & Er, M. J. (2012). A hybrid particle swarm optimization based fuzzy expert system for the diagnosis of coronary artery disease. *Expert Systems with Applications*, *39*(14), 11657–11665. doi:10.1016/j.eswa.2012.04.036

Nguyen, T., Khosravi, A., Creighton, D., & Nahavandi, S. (2015). Classification of healthcare data using genetic Fuzzy Logic system and wavelets. *Expert Systems with Applications*, *42*(4), 2184–2197. doi:10.1016/j.eswa.2014.10.027

Opeyemi, O., & Justice, E. O. (2012). Development of Neuro-fuzzy System for Early Prediction of Heart Attack. *International Journal of Information Technology and Computer Science*, *4*(9), 22–28. doi:10.5815/ijitcs.2012.09.03

Poleshchuk, E. (2012). *A fuzzy linear regression model for interval type-2 fuzzy sets. NAFIPS 2012*. Fuzzy Information Processing Society.

Raghupathi, W., & Raghupathi, V. (2014). Big data analytics in healthcare: Promise and potential. *Health Information Science and Systems*, *2*(1), 3. doi:10.1186/2047-2501-2-3 PMID:25825667

Riahi-Madvar, H., Ayyoubzadeh, S. A., Khadangi, E., & Ebadzadeh, M. M. (2009). An expert system for predicting longitudinal dispersion coefficient in natural streams by using ANFIS. *Expert Systems with Applications*, *36*(4), 8589–8596. doi:10.1016/j.eswa.2008.10.043

Sanz, J. A., Galar, M., Jurio, A., Brugos, A., Pagola, M., & Bustince, H. (2014). Medical diagnosis of cardiovascular diseases using an intervalvalued fuzzy rule-based classification system. *Applied Soft Computing*, *20*, 103–111. doi:10.1016/j.asoc.2013.11.009

Shapiro, A.F. (2006). *Fuzzy regression models*. Retrieved on 10.4.2013 from file:///C:/Users/mcaesar/Downloads/arch06v40n1-ii%20(1).pdf

Sikchi, S. S., Sikchi, S., & Ali, M. S. (2012). Design of fuzzy expert system for diagnosis of cardiac diseases. *International Journal of Medical Science and Public Health*, *2*(1), 56–61. doi:10.5455/ijmsph.2013.2.56-61

Sikchi, S. S., Sikchi, S., & Ali, M. S. (2013). Fuzzy Expert Systems (FES) for Medical Diagnosis. *International Journal of Computer Applications, 63*(11), 7-17.

Tanaka & Asai. (1982). Linear regression analysis with fuzzy model. IEEE Transactions and Systems, Man and Cybernetics, 12(6), 159-171.

Thirugnanam, M., Kumar, P., Srivatsan, S. V., & Nerlesh, C. (2012). Improving the prediction rate of diabetes diagnosis using fuzzy, neural network, case based (fnc) approach. *Procedia Engineering*, *38*, 1709–1718. doi:10.1016/j.proeng.2012.06.208

Tsaur, R. C., Wang, H. F., & Yang, J.-C. O. (2002). Fuzzy regression for seasonal time series analysis. *International Journal of Information Technology & Decision Making*, *1*, 165–175. doi:10.1142/S0219622002000117

Tseng, F. M., & Tzeng, G. H. (2002). A fuzzy seasonal ARIMA model for forecasting. *Fuzzy Sets and Systems, 126*(3), 367–376. doi:10.1016/S0165-0114(01)00047-1

Varma, K. V., Rao, A. A., Lakshmi, T. S. M., & Rao, P. N. (2014). A computational intelligence approach for a better diagnosis of diabetic patients. *Computers & Electrical Engineering, 40*(5), 1758–1765. doi:10.1016/j.compeleceng.2013.07.003

Varma, K. V., Rao, A. A., Lakshmi, T. S. M., & Rao, P. N. (2014). A computational intelligence approach for a better diagnosis of diabetic patients. *Computers & Electrical Engineering, 40*(5), 1758–1765. doi:10.1016/j.compeleceng.2013.07.003

Wang, L. X. (1999). Article. *Fuzziness and Knowledge-Based Systems, 7*, 83–98. doi:10.1142/S0218488599000076

Williams, R., Van Gaal, L., & Lucioni, C. (2002). Assessing the impact of complications on the costs of Type II diabetes. *Diabetologia, 45*(S1), S13–S17. doi:10.100700125-002-0859-9

World Health Organization (WHO). (2018). About Diabetes. Retrieved from http://www.who.int/diabetes/action_online/basics/en/index3.html

Zadeh, L. A. (1965). Fuzzy sets. *Information and Control, 8*(3), 338–353. doi:10.1016/S0019-9958(65)90241-X

Zadeh, L. A. (2004). *Fuzzy Logic Systems: Origin, Concepts, and Trends*. Retrieved November 29, 2015, from http://wi-consortium.org/wicweb/pdf/Zadeh.pdf

Zadeh, L. A. (2009). Toward extended Fuzzy Logic—A first step. *Fuzzy Sets and Systems, 160*(21), 3175–3181. doi:10.1016/j.fss.2009.04.009

Zhu, J., Xie, Q., & Zheng, K. (2015). An improved early detection method of type-2 diabetes mellitus using multiple classifier system. *Information Sciences, 292*, 1–14. doi:10.1016/j.ins.2014.08.056

Zimmerman, H. J. (1991). *Fuzzy Set Theory and its Applications*. Boston: Kluwer Academic. doi:10.1007/978-94-015-7949-0

Chapter 9
A Fourier-Bessel Expansion-Based Method for Automated Detection of Atrial Fibrillation From Electrocardiogram Signals

Ashish Sharma
National Institute of Technology Goa, India

Shivnarayan Patidar
National Institute of Technology Goa, India

ABSTRACT

This chapter presents a new methodology for detection and identification of cardiovascular diseases from a single-lead electrocardiogram (ECG) signal of short duration. More specifically, this method deals with the detection of the most common cardiac arrhythmia called atrial fibrillation (AF) in noisy and non-clinical environment. The method begins with appropriate pre-processing of ECG signals in order to get the RR-interval and heart rate (HR) signals from them. A set of indirect features are computed from the original and the transformed versions of RR-interval and HR signals along with a set of direct features that are obtained from ECG signals themselves. In all, 47 features are computed and subsequently they are fed to an ensemble system of bagged decision trees for classifying the ECG recordings into four different classes. The proposed method has been evaluated with 2017 PhysioNet/CinC challenge hidden test dataset (phase II subset) and the final F1 score of 0.81 is obtained.

DOI: 10.4018/978-1-5225-7131-5.ch009

INTRODUCTION

The atrial fibrillation (AF) is one of the most common and sustained abnormal heart rhythm encountered in clinical practices (Potte & Le Lorier, 2015). It is one of the growing epidemics worldwide causing considerable mortality and morbidity due to risk of stroke, hospitalization, cardiac failure, coronary artery disease, death, etc. (Nabar & Pathan, 2016). As per one recent study, about 0.5 percentage of the global population covering 33.5 million individuals are diagnosed with AF (Chugh et al., 2014). Nevertheless, AF occurs in 1-2% of the general population. And it is estimated that nearly 2.3 million patients in the United States are suffering from AF and this figure may rise to 16 million by 2050 2050 (Issa et al., 2012; Rieta et al., 2013).

Basically, AF is a type of cardiac pathology which is characterized by a rapid and random contraction or quivering of the atria. In electrophysiological context, asynchronous and high rate of bio-potential are discharged in the atrial cells that causes to quivering of atria. Consequently, the normal and regular impulses produced by the sinus node are suppressed by the rapid electrical discharges produced in the atria and adjacent parts of the pulmonary veins. The resulting irregular contractions of the atria deteriorate the pumping action of heart. This, in turn, leads to a hypercoagulative state and increased risk of stroke (Fuster et al., 2001; Sohara et al., 1997). On the basis of duration of occurrence, AF can manifest in the following three different forms: paroxysmal, persistent and permanent AF (January et al., 2014). Normally, the episode of AF lasts only for a very short duration in case of paroxysmal form. The symptoms include the sudden increase in the heart rate such that the effect goes off on its own after a while (de Vos et al., 2010). In case of persistent AF, duration of episode lasts for more than seven days and may repeat often. In permanent AF, the episode stays forever.

It is noteworthy that, in case of paroxysmal AF, episodes are of very shorter duration which makes it difficult for diagnosis in short sessions (Savelieva & Camm, 2000). Hence, the detection of AF becomes a major cardiovascular challenge. For that reason, suspected AF patients are often prescribed a Holter monitor, event recorder or a point of care diagnostic tool for recording their electrocardiography (ECG) at the instant when they experience symptoms. However, the Holter monitoring is diagnostically 33 to 35% effective than event recorders, while automatically triggered recorders detect more arrhythmias (72 to 80%) than patient-triggered devices (17 to 75%). This shows huge potential for the Holter monitoring and automated event-driven recorders for AF detection. And, so far, a lot of progress has been made in AF detectors based on both atrial activity and ventricular response analysis-based methods. In addition, around 30 percent of the patients do not show basic or clear symptoms and therefore AF remains undetected. Even though the cases are symptomatic, it is not always easy to differentiate between AF and other cardiac abnormality. Despite the above mentioned challenges and consequences, early detection of AF alone can contribute to reduced risk of heart failure and stroke (Camm et al., 2012; Colloca, 2013).

Traditionally, the ECG, echocardiography and other routine test are preferable tools used by the physician for the diagnosis of cardiovascular diseases (Patidar et al., 2015). Whenever the symptoms of AF or other cardiac abnormality are suspected, performing the ECG is the first routine investigation of choice. The manual ECG based diagnosis can provide efficient AF detection. The manual interpretations of ECG for the diagnosis AF involve analyses of the irregular heart rate and the absence of p-wave (Patidar et al., 2015). However, the interpretations of the ECG recordings need enough expertise. Even, in case of the popular imaging modalities which are currently used such as echocardiography, the modalities itself and the involved diagnostic procedures are quite expensive and therefore their availability is limited to health care centers in urban areas. Hence, the specific skills required together with the high cost of the equipment in the present scenario is leading to increased vulnerability in many of the high risk patients, with cardiovascular diseases, as it goes undetected and thus endangering their lives (Silber et al., 1982 ; San Rom´ an et al., 1998).

The above mentioned technical and practical challenges in detecting AF and other cardiovascular disease create a need for a smart prescreening system. Such prescreening system should be automatic, cost effective, easy to use and be capable enough to distinguish the AF and other cardiovascular disease. The recent advancement in field of signal processing, high performance computing and data mining techniques have open the way for the development of such a smart prescreening system. Even, it encourages using such technology in smart hand-held or wearable devices.

This chapter describes a novel design of algorithm for subsequent development of such a smart prescreening system. This work emphasizes the use of single-lead ECG systems over multiple-lead ones to avoid the recording, execution and space complexities (Clifford et al., 2017).

BACKGROUND

In literature, different algorithms have been suggested for automatic detection of AF using the ECG signals. Most of these algorithms are based on atrial activity analysis and ventricular response analysis. The atrial activity analysis based algorithms are built on the concept of p-wave analysis. These algorithms consider the fact that in the presence of AF, the normal characteristic features of p-waves are lost due to the unsynchronized electrical firing in the atria and the time-varying fibrillatory-f waves over-ride the p- wave (Ladavich et al., 2015; Du et al., 2014). Figure 1 shows the fibrillatory-f waves in an ECG record of a typical AF.

Regarding the previous state-of-the-art concerning atrial activity analysis, one study suggests the average number of f-waves in a TQ interval can be used as a characteristic parameter for the detection of AF (Du et al., 2014). An echo state neural network based approach involving estimation of the time-varying nonlinear transfer function from two-lead signals, one with atrial activity and the other without it have been proposed (Petrenas., 2012). The Gaussian mixture model based methodology has been proposed where the model is trained by features extracted from p-wave for its identification (Ladavich et al., 2015). This method shows similar performance as compared to RR interval based strategies. In the recent past, several works on wavelet transform have shown the potential for screening the AF (Ródenas et al., 2015; García et al., 2016). To summarize the facts, most of atrial activity based methods are capable enough to detect the short episodes of AF in paroxysmal AF cases. On the other hand these methods have found to perform poorly in presence of noise as these p-waves are prone to contamination with noise and artifacts (Park et al., 2009; Sarkar et al., 2008). Hence, detection of AF using atrial activity analysis necessitates the use of better quality of ECG signals with high resolution and lower noise contamination (Colloca; 2013).

The ventricular response analysis for AF detection is more reliable as compare to the atrial activity based analysis. In fact, the accurate detection of TQ waves from the ECG signals is a challenging task in atrial activity based analysis as its performance is significantly get effected in noisy cases. Basically, the ventricular

Figure 1. Example of an AF signal showing fibrillatory-f waves within the p wave intervals

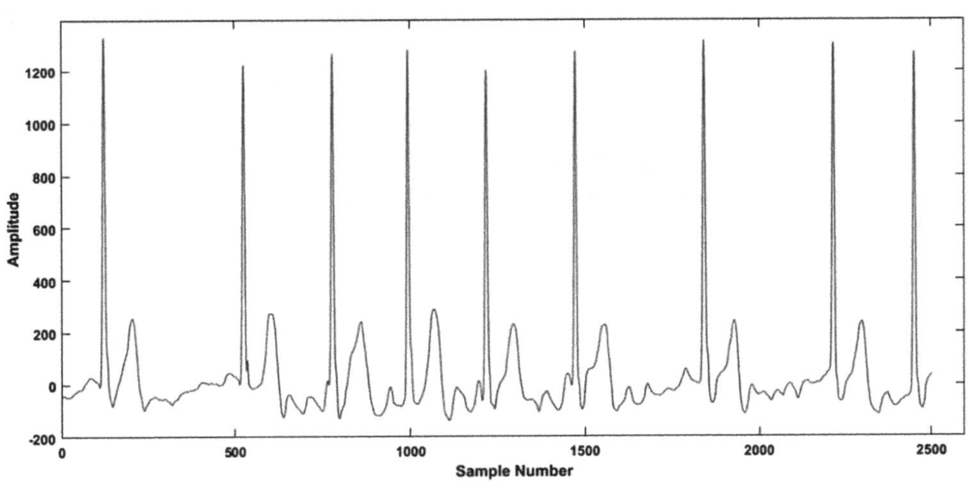

Figure 2. Example of an AF signal showing variation in RR intervals

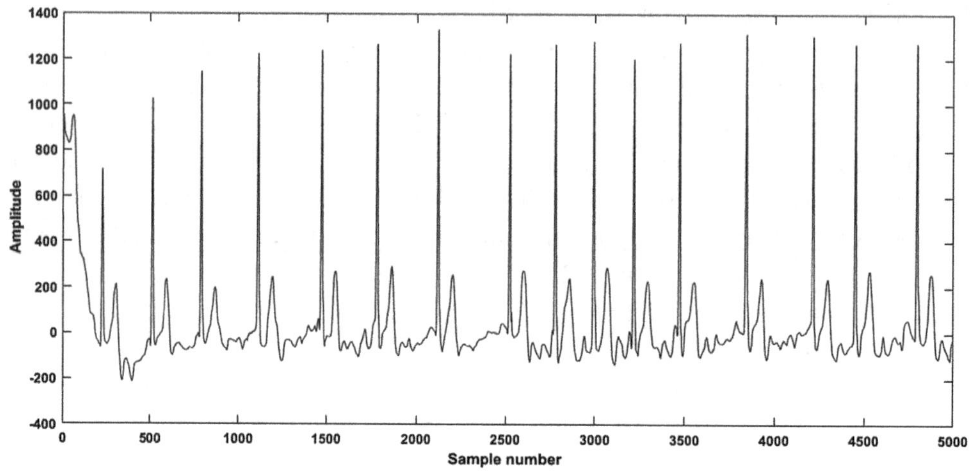

response analysis relies on the variations of the RR intervals. In presence of the AF episodes, the irregular and uncorrelated ventricular response is triggered that in turn generates the irregular RR-interval patterns. Figure 2 shows the variation in RR intervals of a representative ECG recording of AF.

Many ventricular response analysis based strategies for detection of AF are available in the literature. One of the study involves the application of sample entropy, detrend fluctuation analysis and the local dynamics of RR intervals which intends to discriminate among normal sinus rhythm, AF and sinus rhythm with ectopy (Carrara et al., 2015). The AF and non-AF classes of ECG signals are classified based up on the Poincare plot of RR intervals that plots the variability of inter-beat intervals and their corresponding features (Park et al., 2009). The Lorenz plot and the plot of successive differences of the inter-beat of RR-intervals and their spread are also explored to detect AF beats (Sarkar et al., 2008). The standard density histograms of the RR-intervals and successive differences of RR-intervals are proposed for detecting the AF beats (Taten & Glass, 2001). The histogram of the first difference of RR-intervals is explored for AF detection (Huang et al., 2011). The sample entropy and its optimized version are used as feature for detecting the AF beats (Alcaraz et al., 2010; Lake et al., 2011). The normalized fuzzy entropy, symbolic dynamics and Shannon entropy based time-domain methodologies are also described for the detection of AF (Zhou et al., 2014).

MAIN FOCUS OF THE CHAPTER

Regarding automatic detection of AF, there are many challenges that need to be carefully addressed. Firstly, in real-time environment, the involved medical-decision making needs to have proper modelling strategies in terms of number of classes considered. In this regard, a variety of solutions are available in the literature ranging from ordinary two classes to more general four class classification approach.

Most of the previous studied methods intend to address the detection of AF with the two class classification involving AF and normal cases. It is noteworthy that predicting the other cardiac abnormality cases as normal in such studies is more sever and related prescreening system cannot be adopted in practice. Even the outcomes are unpredictable in presence of noise. In fact, there are very limited studies available in literature, which demonstrates the classification among three different classes involving normal, AF and other cardiac abnormality. This type of classification scheme reduces the chances of predicating an abnormal case as normal in presence of any other cardiac abnormality.

In reality, the noises and artifacts in ECG recordings corrupt the required information and always remains a challenge for the detection algorithm because it reduces the overall accuracy of the system. This motivates the use of four class classification approach with noisy recording constituting the fourth class other than the above described classes. This addition of fourth class helps the operator to re-record the signals for meaningful diagnosis. In a nutshell, the detection of AF detection can be addressed well with four class classification approach (Clifford et al.; 2017).

Secondly, the classifier training and prediction performance can be better generalized by including more and diversified training samples with a separate test data. However, most of the available methods are proven better only for carefully chosen and noise free data. Even the data used was also limited for training and testing the algorithms. Lack of separate test data was also seen to be the one of the severe issue with these developed methods.

Thirdly, single lead configuration and shorter recordings is one of the highly desirable characteristics for a prescreening system. These characteristics make the system easy to implement and user friendly in hand-held or wearable devices. Nevertheless, these features make such systems more compatible with Internet of Things.

Lastly, nonlinear and non-stationary nature of the ECG signal makes it more difficult to frame simple scheme for multi-class analysis (Ródenas et al., 2015; García et al., 2016). As a result, it necessitates application of variety of transforms and operations for quantifying and revealing most of the embedded clinical information during classification for better diagnostic decision making.

SOLUTIONS AND RECOMMENDATIONS

The signal flow graph of the proposed methodology for diagnosis of AF using single-lead ECG signals of shorter durations is presented in Figure 3. The method includes the following main subsections: pre-processing, applied transform and operator, diagnostic predictors and classification using an optimally designed ensemble system of bagged decision trees. The proposed method begins by deriving RR-intervals and heart rate (HR) signals from the pre-processed ECG signals. A set of direct and indirect predictors are then extracted. The direct predictors are computed from pre-processed ECG signals themselves. A part of indirect predictors are computed from (a) RR and HR signals and (b) FB expansion along with its spectrum applied on RR and HR signals. The rationale of using FB expansion is that the clinical information is found to be more evident in the FB coefficients (FBC) and their spectrum than that of RR and HR signals themselves. In the same line of thought, TEO is applied on (i) pre-processed ECG, (ii) RR and HR signals, and (iii) FBC and their spectrum of RR and HR signals to obtain the other part of predictors. In all, 47 predictors are computed and subsequently they are fed to an ensemble system of bagged decision trees for classifying the ECG recordings into the following four different classes: normal, AF, others and noisy. The details of each of these subsections and dataset used are described as follows.

Dataset

Single-lead ECG signals of shorter durations are used in this work to develop an algorithm for detection of AF. Originally, all the ECG recordings were collected using the AliveCor device and used for the PhysioNet/ CinC Challenge 2017. The ECG signals were recorded with a sampling rate of 300 Hz and have been subsequently band-pass filtered within the AliveCor device. The database contains overall 12,186 single-lead ECG recordings of which 8528 recordings with their labels are openly available for training the models involved in the algorithms, although, a closed database of 3658 recordings were used for testing purpose. This test set is not availed publicly and it remained private for the purpose of scoring during the challenge and for some time afterwards. Four categories of ECG recordings were present in the databases: AF, normal sinus rhythm, other rhythms and noisy recordings. Figure 6 (a-b) and Figure 7 (a-b) illustrates the representative ECG signals respectively for the said four classes (Clifford et al.; 2017).

Figure 3. The proposed framework for automatic diagnosis of AF using ECG signals

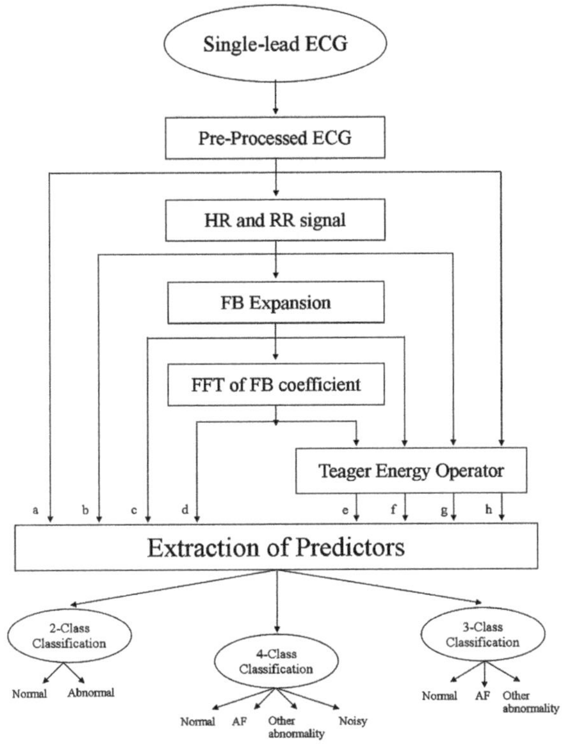

Pre-Processing

The RR intervals can be obtained from raw ECG signals by adequate pre-processing. In this work, one state-of-the-art is used to pre-process and detect the R peaks in ECG signals (Clifford et al.; 2017). In general, the stages of pre-processing involve removal of low-frequency baseline wander, unwanted high-frequency noises and 50 Hz power line interference. A band-pass filter with lower and higher cut-off frequencies of 0.3 and 50 Hz is used to reduce the baseline wander and unwanted high frequency noises. The notch filter is used to eliminate the power line interference. The RR peaks intervals (t_{RR}) between successive QRS complexes is used to obtain the RR-interval signals in seconds. The HR signals in beats per minute is derived from RR-interval signals by using the following expression:

$$HR = \frac{60}{t_{RR}}\left(bpm\right) \tag{1}$$

After pre-processing the obtained RR and HR signals, they are used for further stages of automatic AF detection.

Applied Transform and Operation

In context to signal processing, transform and operators are commonly used for mapping the raw data from one domain to another more informative domain. A brief introduction of the transform and operator used in this work are described as follows:

Fourier-Bessel Expansion

Fourier-Bessel series expansion: A signal $x(t)$ can be represented in terms of Fourier-Bessel series expansion with zero-order Bessel function $J_0(t)$ or first order Bessel function $J_1(t)$ The signal $x(t)$ in the interval $0 < t < P$ has been expressed using $J_0(t)$ as follows (Schroeder, 1994).

$$x(t) = \sum_{k=1}^{M} b_k J_0(\lambda_k t / P) \tag{2}$$

where, $\{\lambda_k; k = 1,2,3 \ldots\ldots M\}$ are the roots of $J_0(t) = 0$, in ascending order way. The Fourier- Bessel coefficients set $\{ b_k \}$ are expressed as follows:

$$b_k = 2\int_0^P tx(t) J_0(\lambda_k t / P) dt / [P J_1(\lambda_k)]^2 \tag{3}$$

The Bessel functions of the first and second kinds are the solution to Bessel equation and presented in the form of integer order for the range of -1 to +1. The Bessel function of first kind for the order of 0, 1 and 2 are *J(0)*, *J(1)* and *J(2)* respectively shown in figure 4. Normally, the order *M* is selected as the length of the signal so that the entire frequencies in the signal under study can be spanned. In this work, the order *M* is set as length of the signal. The advantage of Bessel basis functions in the Fourier series as compare to the sinusoidal basis functions in the Fourier series representation are aperiodic and decay nature within the range P. Hence, the Fourier-Bessel series expansion method is suitable for analysis of non-stationary signals like electroencephalogram (EEG), ECG, phonocardiogram (PCG) etc.

Figure 4. The Bessel function of first kind for different order v = 0, 1 and 2

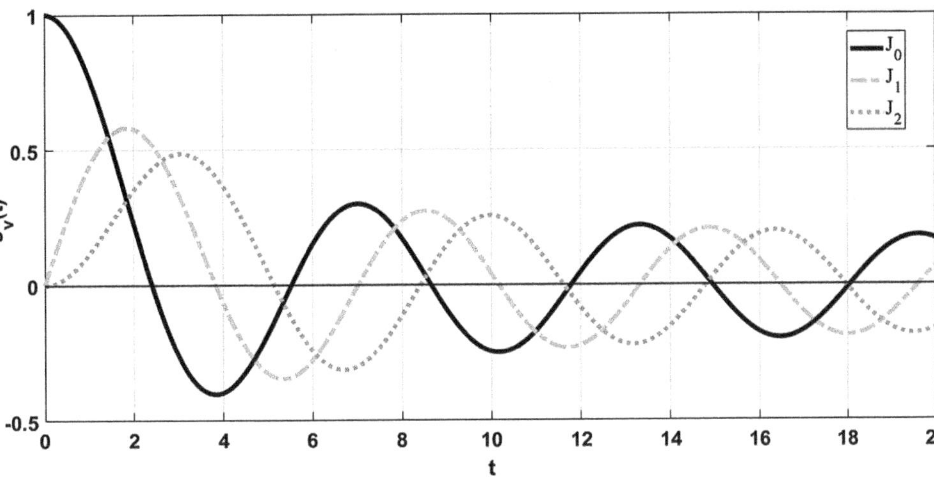

Teager Energy Operator

The Teager energy operator is a non-linear operator which is commonly used for estimating the instantaneous frequency and instantaneous amplitude within non-stationary signals. In this work, the Teager energy tracking operator is used for enhancing the feature level details in the ECG and other signals under studies because they have non-linear characteristics embedded in them. In fact, cardiovascular system is a quite complex system, therefore we assume that non-linear dynamics of the ECG signals would reveal the cardiac abnormality if TEO is applied appropriately. The TEO for a discrete signal $x[n]$ can be computed by as follows (Kaiser, 1990; Kaiser, 1993):

$$\psi[x[n]] = x^2[n] - x[n-1]x[n+1] \tag{4}$$

Diagnostic Predictors

In order to detect AF, a set of useful predictors are strategically derived from ECG signals and the signals obtained after applying the transform and operator as discussed in the above subsection. Here, we briefly introduce the predictors used in this work.

Shannon Entropy

Shannon entropy (*ShEn*) is one of statistical descriptor of the uncertainty within the signal (Shannon, 1948). It describes the shape of the distribution of the templates or patterns within the signals. Indeed, the value of ShEn is large if the distribution of patterns is flat and the series is said to have maximum amount of information. On the contrary, the value of *ShEn* is small if there are subsets of patterns that are more likely or missing or infrequent.

The normalized form of ShEn is given as follows:

$$ShEn = -\frac{\sum_n p_n \log(p_n)}{\log(m)} \tag{5}$$

where n is the range of signal amplitude, p_n is the probability of the signal having amplitude A_n. For N samples in the signal, the amplitude range of signal is linearly divided into n m bins such that the ratio m/N remains constant. Here, we have set the ratio m/N at 0.01.

Sample Entropy

The sample entropy (*SampleEn*) is a non-linear statistical measure which is used to investigate the complexity of the physiological time-series for diagnostic usage (Richman & Moorman, 2000). To be precise, $SampleEn(m, r, N)$ is the negative natural logarithm of the conditional probability that two patterns similar for m samples remain similar at the next sample. In calculating the probability, however, sample entropy does not cover the self-similar patterns. It can be defined as follows:

$$SampleEn(m, r, N) = -\ln\frac{A}{B} \tag{6}$$

The ratio A/B is precisely the conditional probability that two patterns within a tolerance r for m samples remain within tolerance r of each other at the next sample. Where, A and B are the number of forward matches of length $m+1$ and m respectively with i^{th} pattern or subseries. Generally, lower values of sample entropy indicate higher self-similarity in the time-series or less noisy time-series. Sample entropy is mostly independent of the signal lengths and gives relatively consistent results under various circumstances. Usually, r is set *0.2* times the standard deviation.

Spectral Entropy

Spectral entropy (*SpEn*) has its root in Shannon's entropy. It measures the complexity in the power spectrum of signals (Fell et al., 1996; Shannon, 1948).

The *SpEn* is defined as

$$SpEn = -\frac{\sum_{j=f_L}^{f_H} P_j}{\log\left(N_f\right)} \tag{7}$$

where P_j represents the power levels of the signal at j^{th} frequency in the band $\left[f_L\ f_H\right]$ and N_f is the number of frequencies within this band. In this work, we have covered all the frequencies present in the signal. Heuristically, the entropy measures the uncertainty of the event at frequency f and therefore provides a measure of signal complexity. Signals showing broad and flat power spectrum would have higher entropy as against the one which is narrowed and peaked.

Robust Empirical Permutation Entropy

The robust empirical permutation entropy (*RePE*) is the extended version of permutation entropy (*PE*), It is robust with respect to the observational noise in the time series. The empirical permutation entropy was originally introduced in (Bandt & Pompe, 2002) as a natural complexity measure of time series. The main idea involves measurement of complexity based on comparison of the amplitudes of neighboring samples in the time series. For a fix length of selected samples, on comparison among their neighboring values, patterns are formed. These patterns are computed continuously for each shift with a defined lag. The probability distribution of each pattern adds the information of time series complexity.

For a given time series $x\left(t\right); t = 1, \ldots, N,$ whose length is N, there are two parameters that need to be determined for the computation of *PE*, the order d and time lag τ. The total number of possible patterns for a given value of order d is all the possible permutation $d!$. The *PE* is defined as:

$$PE = -\sum_m P_m \log\left(P_m\right), \tag{8}$$

where,

$$P_m = \frac{t_m}{N - d + 1} \tag{9}$$

P_m is the probability of occurrence of the mth pattern and t_m represents the number of occurrences of the mth pattern in the time series.

However, in *RePE*, a threshold is added while comparing the neighboring samples of the time series of order d and lag τ (Keller et al.,2014).

For positive $\zeta \in R$, a given time series $x(t)$, whose length is N, order d and time lag τ, the ordinal pattern vector $x_t, x_{t-\tau}, x_{t-2\tau}, \ldots x_{t-d\tau}$, are $\zeta -$robust if

$$\#\left\{(i,j) : 0 < i < j < \left|x_{t-i\tau} - x_{t-j\tau}\right|\right\} < (d+1)d8 \tag{10}$$

The RePE for the ζ - robust is defined as:

$$RePE = -\sum_m P_m \log\left(P_m\right) \tag{11}$$

where P_k is defined as:

$$P_k = \frac{\#\left(m^{th}\, robust\, ordinal\, pattern\right)}{\#\left(total\, robust\, ordinal\, pattern\right)} \tag{12}$$

Statistical Predictors Based on Derived Signals at Different Stage

A set of statistical predictors such as Mean (*M*), Median (*Md*), Mode (*Mo*), variance (σ^2), standard deviation (σ), kurtosis (*Ku*) and skewness (*Sk*) is computed for the signal derived at different level of transformation. The signal generated at different stage is HR, RR interval, FBC of HR, TEO of FBC of HR, TEO of RR, Kurtosis of ECG, Median of ECG. All the details of the selected predictors corresponding to various transform signals are depicted in Table 3.

Morphological Predictors

The morphologies of the ECG signal play a significant role while detecting the cardiac abnormalities. They cover physiological information in connection with the functionality of the heart. Basically, the electrocardiographic morphology analysis involves the interpretation of the shape of the ECG signals. It includes the amplitude, width and the prominence of the different waves present in the ECG. It also includes their relative measures between the different waves in a segment. Therefore, in order to enhance the classification performance of the considered classes of rhythms, a few morphological parameters are also used in this work as predictors which are described as follows: Width of R and S peaks and their ratio, prominence of R peaks, Difference of R and S peaks, Difference of width of R and S peaks and the difference of the location of R and S peaks. Figure 5 shows different measures. The simplified peak detection algorithm is used for the computation of the different peak, location, prominence and their width. The statistical predictors such as Mean (M), Median (Md), Mode (Mo), variance (σ^2), standard deviation (σ), kurtosis (Ku) and skewness (Sk) are then computed for these morphological measures. Table 3 lists all the relevant morphological predictors used in this study.

Figure 5. A segment of Electrocardiogram signal shows morphology of ECG and its critical measures.

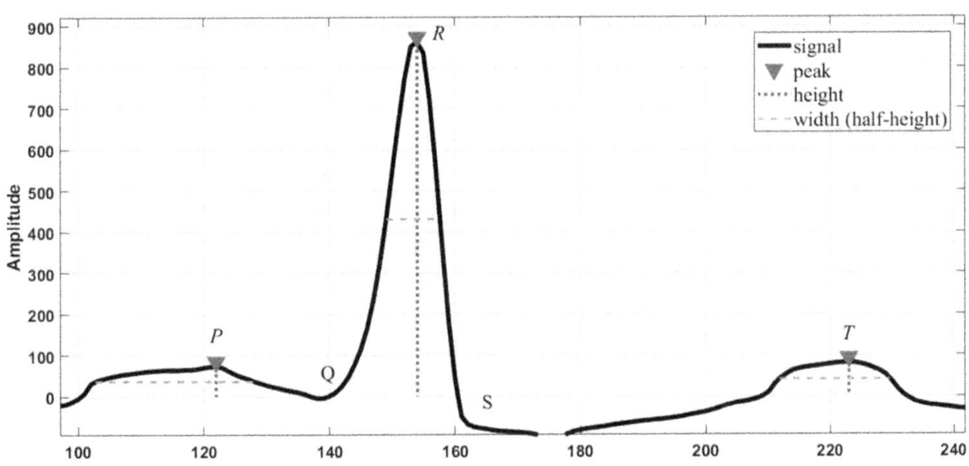

Classification Using an Ensemble System of Bagged Decision Trees

Ensemble classification (Polikar,2006) strategically generates a set of classifiers and combines them to get better performance than every one of them to address a particular machine learning problem. Basically, ensemble learning aims to enhance the predictive performance of a model. This approach uses an intuitive fact that we as human being often seeks several opinions from multiple experts and combine their views based on their worth in order to frame an important decision. Along the same lines, an ensemble method uses multiple classifiers to make better decision by combining the decisions of several weak learners into one high-end ensemble predictor. In an ensemble system of bagged decision tree, decision trees are used as the classification models and their decisions are combined by bootstrap aggregation (Breiman, 1996). For bagging with training set of size N, the decision trees are developed on the bootstrap replicas of the training dataset which are formed by randomly choosing M observations out of N with replacement, where N is the training set size. The predictions of the individual classifiers are then combined using majority vote to cast the final decision. Thus, for any given observation, the class casted by majority of classifiers forms the ensemble decision. Screening M out of N observations with replacement omits on an average 37% of the observations as out-of-bag for each decision tree. These out-of-bag observations are used to measure the predictive power of the classifier and assess the significance of each individual predictors involved in the decision-making process. The true ensemble error is the average out-of-bag error as measured by comparing the out-of-bag predicted responses with the observed responses for the entire training set. The out-of-bag estimated predictors of significance can be obtained by performing random permutations of out-of-bag data across one variable at a time and estimating corresponding increase in the out-of-bag error. The higher increase indicates more significance of the predictor in classification. Thus, the salient feature of bagging is that it reliably estimates the predictive power and significance of predictors during the training process without needing the test data.

Classification Performance Measures

The classification performance of the ensemble system of bagged decision trees has been evaluated using the generated confusion matrix. Based on the obtained confusion matrix, the accuracy (*Acc*) as well as F_1 measure are computed as metrics for performance measure. The counting rules to obtain the F_1 scores (equations (13) to (17)) from the confusion matrix of each considered class are defined in Table 1.

$$F_{1n} = \frac{2 * N_n}{\sum N + \sum n} \tag{13}$$

$$F_{1a} = \frac{2 * A_a}{\sum A + \sum a} \tag{14}$$

$$F_{1o} = \frac{2 * O_o}{\sum O + \sum o} \tag{15}$$

$$F_{1p} = \frac{2 * P_p}{\sum P + \sum p} \tag{16}$$

$$F_1 = \frac{F_{1n} + F_{1a} + F_{1o} + F_{1p}}{4} \tag{17}$$

Table 1. Confusion matrix for four class performance evaluation

		Predicted Calcification				
		Normal	AF	Other	Noisy	Total
Reference Classification	Normal	N_n	N_a	N_o	N_p	$\sum N$
	AF	A_n	A_a	A_o	A_p	$\sum A$
	Other	O_n	O_a	O_o	O_p	$\sum O$
	Noisy	P_n	P_a	P_o	P_p	$\sum P$
	Total	$\sum n$	$\sum a$	$\sum o$	$\sum p$	

The F_1 measure is used to compute the accuracy of predication among the different classes. It is an average of the accuracies of four F_1 scores of the different classes.

Results

The proposed work for automated diagnosis of AF is implemented in Matlab 2017. And the work has been evaluated using one established publicly available 2017 PhysioNet/CinC Challenge dataset. The pre-processing is done to obtain the RR and HR signals as described previously. The predictors are derived from FB expansion and TEO which in turn are applied strategically on ECG signals. A set of carefully chosen direct and indirect predictors as listed in Table 2 and Table 3 are extracted. Figure 3 shows the predictor extraction workflow. The direct predictors are computed from pre-processed ECG signals themselves as depicted in the Figure 3 with arrow marked by (a). A part of the indirect predictors are computed from (i) HR signals and (ii) FB expansion along with its spectrum as marked by (b), (c) and (d) respectively . In order to obtain the other part of predictors, we have applied TEO on the above set of signals obtained at different levels of proposed framework as marked by (e)-(h).

Several considerations are forced while choosing the number of predictors to extract: More predictors use more memory and computational time. Fewer predictors can produce a poor classifier. Figures 6 and 7 illustrate the ECG signals and their valuable transformed versions for considered four classes. It is prima facie evident from these figures that FB expansions and their spectra are qualitatively more informative as compared to ECG, RR and HR signals. And the embedded minute changes in these transformed signals can be quantified by meticulously choosing the appropriate predictors. Similarly, Figure 8 and Figure 9 show the changes in the signals of the Figure 6 and Figure 7 after applying TEO. Again, these transformed versions of the

Table 2. List of predictors used for classification

Sr. No.	Predictors	Input Signals		
		ECG	HR/RR	FBC-HR/ FBC-RR
1	Sample Entropy	34, 35	10/11	/12
2	Spectral entropy	21	19	
3	RePE	5	/6,7	8,9
4	Shannon entropy	22		1
5	Shannon entropy of TEO		/2,3,4	
6	Energy of TEO		13	

Figure 6. Example of signals and their valuable transformed versions for (a) normal and (b) AF. Where, (c, d) correspond to HR signals, (e, f) plot of FB coefficients vs. order of HR signals and (g, h) FFT of (e, f) respectively.

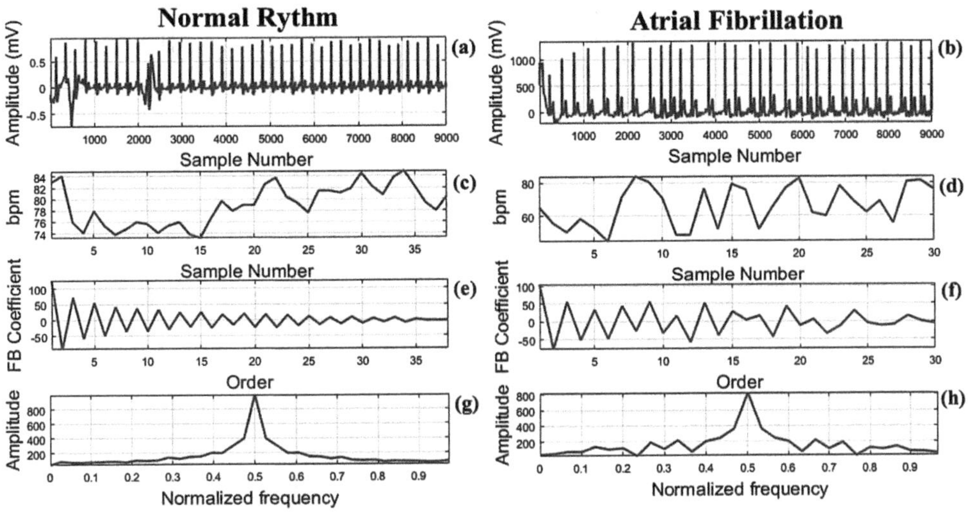

Figure 7. Example of signals and their valuable transformed versions for (a) other rhythms and (b) noisy ECG signals. Where, (c, d) correspond to HR signals, (e, f) plot of FB coefficients vs. order of HR signals and (g, h) FFT of (e, f) respectively

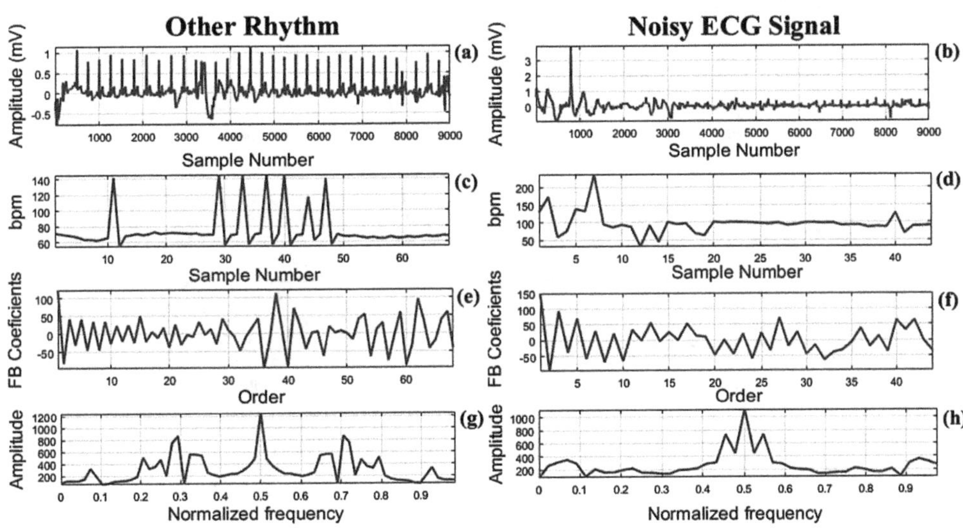

Figure 8. TEO based transformed signals of Figure 6 for (a) normal and (b) AF, (c, d) HR signals, (e, f) FB coefficients of HR signals and (g, h) FFT of FB coefficients.

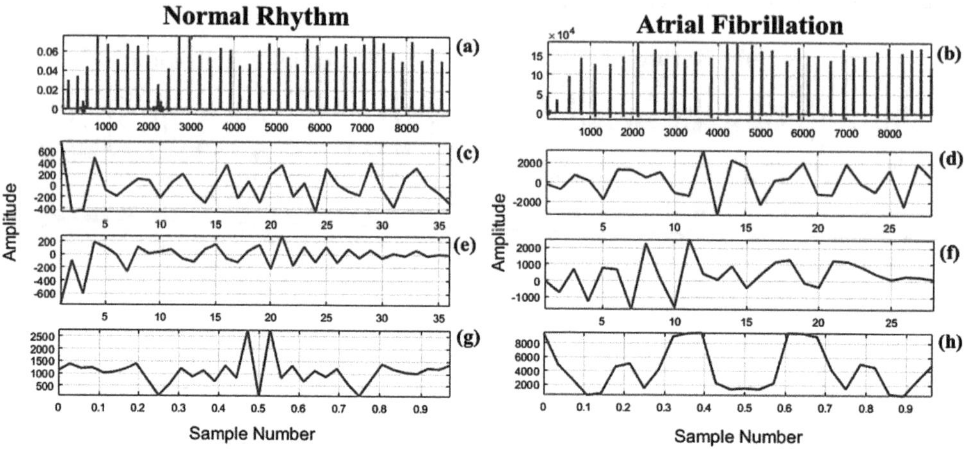

Figure 9. TEO based transformed signals of Figure 7 for: (a) other rhythms and (b) noisy ECG signals, (c, d) HR signals, (e, f) FB coefficients of HR signals and (g, h) FFT of FB coefficients

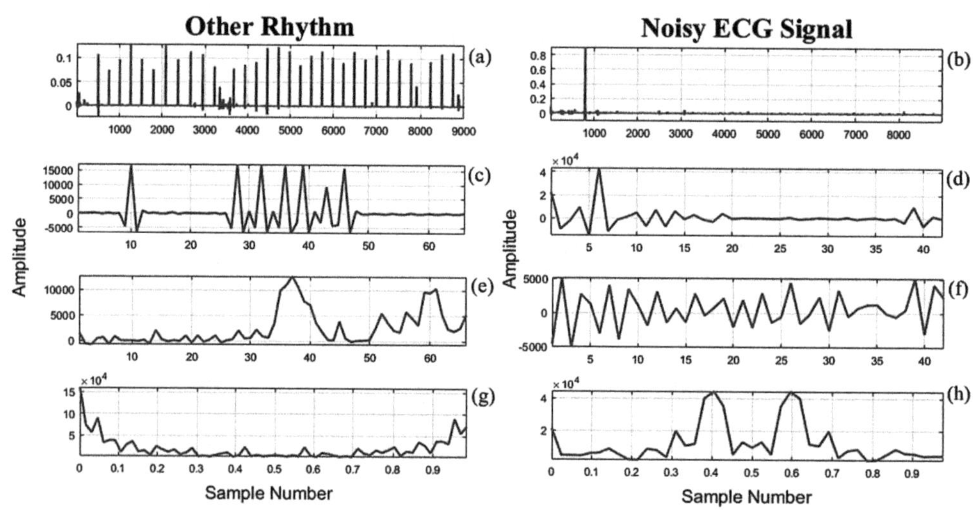

signals also carry significant information that can be used for characterization of the different classes of ECG signals. In order to quantify the qualitative information in Figure 6 to Figure 9, a set of predictors are empirically selected. We have found 47 clinically significant predictors as listed in Table 2 and Table 3 that ultimately yielded robust 10-cross validation based results during training.

Table 3. List of predictors used for classification

Sr. No.	Input Parameters	Predictors						
		μ	Md	Mo	σ	σ2	Ku	Sk
1	HR/RR Signals	27	28 /23	29 /24	30		/25	/26
2	FBC of HR			20				
3	TEO of HR				18		14	
4	TEO of ECG						15	
5	TEO of FBC of HR				17			16
6	Kurtosis of ECG		31					32
7	Median of ECG		33					
8	Widths of R peaks			37	39	41		
9	Widths of S peaks			38		42		
10	Prominences of R peaks				40			
11	Ratios of widths of R & S peaks	36						
12	Diff. of R & S peaks	43	45					
13	Diff. of widths of R & S peaks	44						
14	Diff. of locations of R & S peaks						46	

An ensemble of bagged decision trees is used for classifying the ECG recordings into the following four different classes: normal, AF, others and noisy. Using the auto search engine in Matlab, we have generated the optimal ensemble classifier model based on the bootstrap aggregation which is popularly known as bagging. We have tested our ensemble classifier model for its dependence on training data and its suitability and capability for instances which are out of the training dataset. In line with this, we have found similar results for training and hidden test data which emphases that the trained model covers the picture of the involved pathology in a more realistic way.

A graph to illustrate the importance of each predictors used in decision making for the ensemble classifier is shown in Figure 10. It indicates the relative relevance of a set of 47 predictors. The out-of-bag classification error as a function of the number of decision trees, as illustrated in Figure 11, is used to construct the ensemble. The optimal ensemble classifier was constructed by using 490 weak learners that are decision trees with minimum leaf size of 3 and with training instances of 8528. The salient feature of bagged ensemble is that it reliably estimates the classification accuracy and predictor's importance during the training process without needing the test data.

Figure 10. The predictor's importance in diagnosis of AF using ECG signals

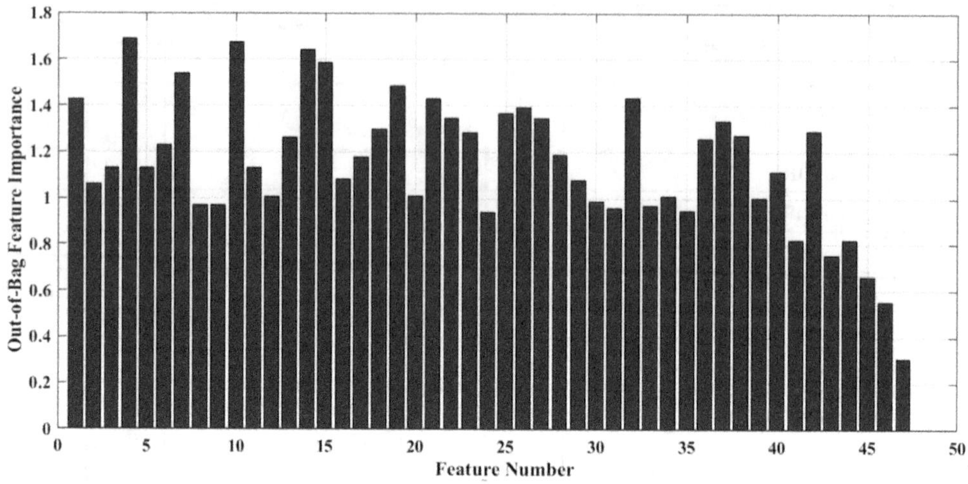

Figure 11. Plot of out-of-bag classification error for increasing number of weak learners

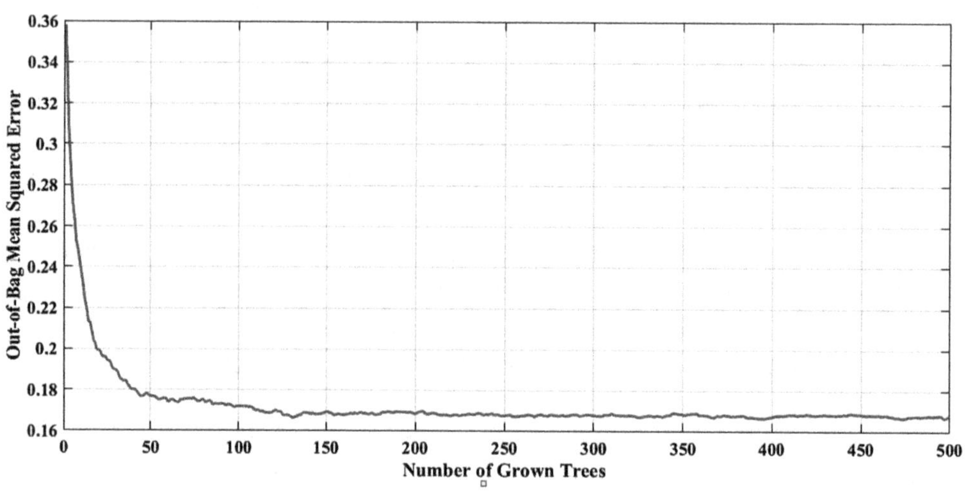

We have evaluated our approach for its applicability in three different scenarios:

1. The first scenario suggests the use of a four class model for involved classification in the medical device. Such devices are relevant when unskilled medical staff operates the device in the clinics and hospitals and even at home. When integrated with hand-held gadgets, diagnostic system based on such model

can even be used by a lay man in non-clinical setup. In addition, such medical devices are quite useful for mass screening of AF patients accurately.

2. In the second scenario, we assume that the medical device would be used by an expert in the field who is capable enough to discard the noisy records before it passes into the further stages of automated analysis. This implies that the integration of three-class model, for involved classification, in the medical device is sufficient. This in turn would ensure more reliable results. The rationale is that three-class model is more accurate over four-class model for the same predictors if developed appropriately.
3. Finally, the first aid type or primarily level diagnostic tool to detect any cardiovascular diseases (CVDs) is also preferred in day-to-day clinical practice. And such systems are quite useful for mass screening of patients suffering from CVDs. Thus it justifies the applicability of a two class model for involved classification in the medical device.

The outcomes for all the above mentioned scenarios are discussed in the following subsections respectively. These outcomes assume the uniform settings for predictors and classifier as stated and found before.

Detection of AF and Other Cardiac Abnormalities in Noisy Scenario: A Four-Class Problem

The experimental outcomes of detection of AF considering possibility of other cardiac abnormalities and noisy scenario are depicted in Table 4 that provides the derived statistics on the training performance of the considered four class model. The average F_1 scores of classes with normal rhythm, AF, other rhythm and noisy are achieved as follows: 90%, 80%, 73%, 54% with overall average F_1 score of 74% for the training data using 10-cross validation. The average accuracy of 84% is obtained.

Table 5 provides the predictive performance statistics on hidden test data. The test F_1 scores of classes with normal rhythm, AF and other rhythms are achieved as follows: 91%, 80%, 72%, with overall average F_1 score of 81% for the test data ignoring the scores of noisy class.

Detection of AF and Other Cardiac Abnormalities: A Three-Class Problem

Here, we discuss the correct classification among the main classes which normally remains after rejecting the unwanted noisy records in advance. The experimental outcomes of this study are depicted in Table 6 that provides the derived statistics on the training performance of the considered three-class model. The average F_1

Table 4. Training statistics of four-class predictive performance

Type of Data	No. of Instances	F1n	F1a	F1o	F1p	F1n + F1a + F1p	F1overall	Acc
Training	8528	90	80	73	54	81	74	84

Table 5. Testing statistics of four-class predictive performance

Type of Data	No. of Instances	F_{1n}	F_{1a}	F_{1o}	F_{1p}	$F_{1n} + F_{1a} + F_{1p}$	$F_{1overall}$	Acc
Testing	3658	91	80	72	NA	81	NA	NA

scores of normal, AF, other classes are achieved as follows: 91%, 82%, 74% with overall average F_1 score of 82% for the training data using 10-cross validation. The average accuracy of 85% is obtained.

Detection of CVDS: A Two-Class Problem

The experimental outcomes of detection of CVDs are presented in Table 7 that provides the training performance parameters of the considered two-class model. The obtained average F_1 scores of normal and abnormal classes are 92% and 83% respectively. The overall average F_1 score is achieved as 87% for the training data using 10-cross validation. The average accuracy of 87% is obtained.

Table 6. Training statistics of three-class predictive performance

Sr. No.	No. of Instances	F_{1n}	F_{1a}	F_{1o}	$F_{1overall}$	*Acc*
Training	8249	91	82	74	82	85

Table 7. Training statistics of two-class predictive performance

Sr. No.	No. of Instances	$F_{1normal}$	$F_{1abnormal}$	$F_{1overall}$	*Acc*
Training	8249	92	83	87	87

On comparison with the state-of-the-art for four-class problem, the proposed algorithm appeared in the top algorithms that scored within 2% of the maximum achieved F_1 score of 83. Table 8 shows the compared methods with respect to their performances. This study reveals that the predictors derived using FB expansion and TEO are quite promising for better characterization of different ECG signals to detect and identify AF and other CVDs.

FUTURE RESEARCH DIRECTIONS

The methodology described in this chapter has shown a bench mark performance on evaluating with the hidden data set. This demonstrates that an automated screening system is feasible for incorporating in smart hand-held or wearable deceives at a very low cost for the prescreening purpose. However, regardless of proven performance capacity of the methodology, it needs many further improvements in terms of strategies involving information characterization. These changes in the strategies may increase the number of features in turn increasing the accuracy of the other cardiac abnormalities and noisy classes. A large dataset can also be recorded and used at the level of training, validation and testing of the method for enhancement the prediction performance of the overall system.

Table 8. Comparison of the proposed method with the other top scorers of the challenge.

Entrant	Test	Validation	Train	k-Fold Cross Validation
Teijeiro et al.	0.83	0.91	0.89	8
Datta et al.	0.83	0.99	0.97	5
Zabihi et al.	0.82	0.96	0.95	10
Hong et al.	0.82	0.99	0.97	NA
Baydoun et al.	0.82	0.85	0.96	NA
Bin et al.	0.82	0.87	0.87	100
Zihlmann et al.	0.82	0.91	0.88	5
Xiong et al.	0.81	0.90	0.87	5
Proposed method	0.81	0.97	0.96	10

In fact, the other cardiac abnormalities class can represent a variety of arrhythmias with different morphological characteristics. Hence, this class can be further divided into more number of the subclasses with respect to a particular disorder.

Furthermore, we note the some more key limitations of this work described as follows. The F_1 metric based performance measure may not be the most appropriate for developing such screening system. A better metric can be proposed for better evaluation of classification performances and comparing different algorithms or changes within the algorithms. The training data could be improved further to cover more diversity in the data. Even a group of different algorithms with diversity in terms of involved signal processing and machine learning techniques can be developed and voting among them can further boost the overall performance of the medical-decision making.

In addition, the proposed framework can be extended to other healthcare diagnostic applications for detecting diabetes, eye diseases, and neural diseases etc.

CONCLUSION

An automatic prescreening system for early and accurate diagnosis of AF can save many human lives. In this chapter, the effectiveness of the Fourier Bessel expansion of RR and HR signals with respect to its role in characterization of arrhythmias has been explored. A four class classification schemes for a single-lead ECG signals of short durations has been adopted. The method has shown substantial performance on a large and diverse dataset with noisy records. Furthermore, the algorithm demonstrates the same performance during training and on a separate out-of-the sample test dataset. This work has the clinical potential to be realized into an automatic real-time detection and identification tool for AF and other cardiac abnormalities. The resulting device based on this work would be easy to use in hospitals, polyclinics and even at home. In future, the proposed framework can be extended to other healthcare diagnostic applications for detecting diabetes, eye diseases, and neural diseases etc.

ACKNOWLEDGMENT

We acknowledge the financial support received from (a) NIT Goa, Seed money project entitled Primary level screening of common heart disorders using non-invasively measured heart sound signals, and (b) Department of Science and Technology (DST) India, Early Career Research project entitled Analysis of cardiovascular disorders using heart sound signals, project no. ECR/2017/000062.

REFERENCES

Alcaraz, R., Abásolo, D., Hornero, R., & Rieta, J. J. (2010). Optimal parameters study for sample entropy-based atrial fibrillation organization analysis. *Computer Methods and Programs in Biomedicine*, *99*(1), 124–132. doi:10.1016/j.cmpb.2010.02.009 PMID:20392514

Bandt, C., & Pompe, B. (2002). Permutation entropy: A natural complexity measure for time series. *Physical Review Letters*, *88*(17), 174102. doi:10.1103/PhysRevLett.88.174102 PMID:12005759

Breiman, L. (1996). Bagging predictors. *Machine Learning*, *24*(2), 123–140. doi:10.1007/BF00058655

Camm, A. J., Lip, G. Y., De Caterina, R., Savelieva, I., Atar, D., & Hohnloser, S. H. (2012). 2012 focused update of the ESC Guidelines for the management of atrial fibrillation: an update of the 2010 ESC Guidelines for the management of atrial fibrillation. Developed with the special contribution of the European Heart Rhythm association. *European Heart Journal, 33*(21), 2719.

Carrara, M., Carozzi, L., Moss, T. J., De Pasquale, M., Cerutti, S., Ferrario, M., ... Moorman, J. R. (2015). Heart rate dynamics distinguish among atrial fibrillation, normal sinus rhythm and sinus rhythm with frequent ectopy. *Physiological Measurement*, *36*(9), 1873–1888. doi:10.1088/0967-3334/36/9/1873 PMID:26246162

Chugh, S. S., Havmoeller, R., Narayanan, K., Singh, D., Rienstra, M., Benjamin, E. J., ... Forouzanfar, M. H. (2014). Worldwide epidemiology of atrial fibrillation. *Circulation*, *129*(8), 837–847. doi:10.1161/CIRCULATIONAHA.113.005119 PMID:24345399

Clifford, G. D., Liu, C., Moody, B., Lehman, L. W. H., Silva, I., Li, Q., ... & Mark, R. G. (2017). *AF Classification from a short single lead ECG recording: the PhysioNet/Computing in Cardiology Challenge 2017*. Academic Press.

Colloca, R. (2013). *Implementation and testing of atrial fibrillation detectors for a mobile phone application*. Academic Press.

DeMazumder, D., Lake, D. E., Cheng, A., Moss, T. J., Guallar, E., Weiss, R. G., ... Moorman, J. R. (2013). Dynamic analysis of cardiac rhythms for discriminating atrial fibrillation from lethal ventricular arrhythmias. *Circulation: Arrhythmia and Electrophysiology*. PMID:23685539

Du, X., Rao, N., Qian, M., Liu, D., Li, J., Feng, W., ... Chen, X. (2014). A Novel Method for Real-Time Atrial Fibrillation Detection in Electrocardiograms Using Multiple Parameters. *Annals of Noninvasive Electrocardiology*, *19*(3), 217–225. doi:10.1111/anec.12111 PMID:24252119

Fell, J., Röschke, J., Mann, K., & Schäffner, C. (1996). Discrimination of sleep stages: A comparison between spectral and nonlinear EEG measures. *Electroencephalography and Clinical Neurophysiology*, *98*(5), 401–410. doi:10.1016/0013-4694(96)95636-9 PMID:8647043

Fuster, V., Rydén, L. E., Asinger, R. W., Cannom, D. S., Crijns, H. J., Frye, R. L., ... McNamara, R. L. (2001). ACC/AHA/ESC guidelines for the management of patients with atrial fibrillation: Executive summary a report of the American College of Cardiology/American Heart Association task force on practice guidelines and the European Society of Cardiology committee for practice guidelines and policy conferences (committee to develop guidelines for the management of patients with atrial fibrillation) developed in collaboration with the North American Society of Pacing and Electrophysiology. *Circulation*, *104*(17), 2118–2150. PMID:11673357

García, M., Ródenas, J., Alcaraz, R., & Rieta, J. J. (2016). Application of the relative wavelet energy to heart rate independent detection of atrial fibrillation. *Computer Methods and Programs in Biomedicine*, *131*, 157–168. doi:10.1016/j.cmpb.2016.04.009 PMID:27265056

Huang, C., Ye, S., Chen, H., Li, D., He, F., & Tu, Y. (2011). A novel method for detection of the transition between atrial fibrillation and sinus rhythm. *IEEE Transactions on Biomedical Engineering*, *58*(4), 1113–1119. doi:10.1109/TBME.2010.2096506 PMID:21134807

Issa, Z. F., Miller, J. M., & Zipes, D. P. (2012). *Clinical arrhythmology and electrophysiology: a companion to Braunwald's heart disease*. Elsevier Health Sciences.

January, C. T., Wann, L. S., Alpert, J. S., Calkins, H., Cigarroa, J. E., Conti, J. B., ... Sacco, R. L. (2014). 2014 AHA/ACC/HRS guideline for the management of patients with atrial fibrillation: A report of the American College of Cardiology/American Heart Association Task Force on Practice Guidelines and the Heart Rhythm Society. *Journal of the American College of Cardiology*, *64*(21), e1–e76. doi:10.1016/j.jacc.2014.03.022 PMID:24685669

Kaiser, J. F. (1990, April). On a simple algorithm to calculate the'energy'of a signal. In *Acoustics, Speech, and Signal Processing, 1990. ICASSP-90., 1990 International Conference on* (pp. 381-384). IEEE.

Kaiser, J. F. (1993, April). Some useful properties of Teager's energy operators. In *Acoustics, Speech, and Signal Processing, 1993. ICASSP-93., 1993 IEEE International Conference on* (Vol. 3, pp. 149-152). IEEE. 10.1109/ICASSP.1993.319457

Keller, K., Unakafov, A. M., & Unakafova, V. A. (2014). Ordinal patterns, entropy, and EEG. *Entropy (Basel, Switzerland)*, *16*(12), 6212–6239. doi:10.3390/e16126212

Ladavich, S., & Ghoraani, B. (2015). Rate-independent detection of atrial fibrillation by statistical modeling of atrial activity. *Biomedical Signal Processing and Control*, *18*, 274–281. doi:10.1016/j.bspc.2015.01.007

Lake, D. E., & Moorman, J. R. (2011). Accurate estimation of entropy in very short physiological time series: The problem of atrial fibrillation detection in implanted ventricular devices. *American Journal of Physiology. Heart and Circulatory Physiology*, *300*(1), H319–H325. doi:10.1152/ajpheart.00561.2010 PMID:21037227

Nabar, A., & Pathan, I. (2016). Pathophysiology of Atrial Fibrillation-current Concepts. *The Journal of the Association of Physicians of India*, *64*(8), 11–15. PMID:28812335

Park, J., Lee, S., & Jeon, M. (2009). Atrial fibrillation detection by heart rate variability in Poincare plot. *Biomedical Engineering Online*, *8*(1), 38. doi:10.1186/1475-925X-8-38 PMID:20003345

Patidar, S., Pachori, R. B., & Acharya, U. R. (2015). Automated diagnosis of coronary artery disease using tunable-Q wavelet transform applied on heart rate signals. *Knowledge-Based Systems*, *82*, 1–10. doi:10.1016/j.knosys.2015.02.011

Petrenas, A., Marozas, V., Sornmo, L., & Lukosevicius, A. (2012). An echo state neural network for QRST cancellation during atrial fibrillation. *IEEE Transactions on Biomedical Engineering*, *59*(10), 2950–2957. doi:10.1109/TBME.2012.2212895 PMID:22929362

Polikar, R. (2006). Ensemble based systems in decision making. *IEEE Circuits and Systems Magazine*, *6*(3), 21–45. doi:10.1109/MCAS.2006.1688199

Potter, B. J., & Le Lorier, J. (2015). Taking the pulse of atrial fibrillation. *Lancet*, *386*(9989), 113–115. doi:10.1016/S0140-6736(14)61991-7 PMID:25960109

Richman, J. S., & Moorman, J. R. (2000). Physiological time-series analysis using approximate entropy and sample entropy. *American Journal of Physiology. Heart and Circulatory Physiology*, *278*(6), H2039–H2049. doi:10.1152/ajpheart.2000.278.6.H2039 PMID:10843903

Rieta, J. J., Ravelli, F., & Sornmo, L. E. I. F. (2013). Advances in modeling and characterization of atrial arrhythmias. *Biomedical Signal Processing and Control*, *8*(6), 956–957. doi:10.1016/j.bspc.2013.10.008

Ródenas, J., García, M., Alcaraz, R., & Rieta, J. J. (2015). Wavelet entropy automatically detects episodes of atrial fibrillation from single-lead electrocardiograms. *Entropy (Basel, Switzerland)*, *17*(9), 6179–6199. doi:10.3390/e17096179

San Roman, J. A., Vilacosta, I., Castillo, J. A., Rollan, M. J., Hernández, M., Peral, V., ... Fernández-Avilés, F. (1998). Selection of the optimal stress test for the diagnosis of coronary artery disease. *Heart (British Cardiac Society)*, *80*(4), 370–376. doi:10.1136/hrt.80.4.370 PMID:9875115

Sarkar, S., Ritscher, D., & Mehra, R. (2008). A detector for a chronic implantable atrial tachyarrhythmia monitor. *IEEE Transactions on Biomedical Engineering*, *55*(3), 1219–1224. doi:10.1109/TBME.2007.903707 PMID:18334416

Savelieva, I., & Camm, A. J. (2000). Clinical relevance of silent atrial fibrillation: Prevalence, prognosis, quality of life, and management. *Journal of Interventional Cardiac Electrophysiology*, *4*(2), 369–382. doi:10.1023/A:1009823001707 PMID:10936003

Schroeder, J. (1994). Signal Processing via Fourier-Bessel Series Expansion. *Digital Signal Processing*, *3*(2), 112–124. doi:10.1006/dspr.1993.1016

Shannon, C. (1948). A mathematical theory of communication. *The Bell System Technical Journal, 27*, 379-423.

Silber, E. N., & Katz, L. N. (1982). *Heart Disease*. New York: MacMillan Publishing Co.

Tateno, K., & Glass, L. (2001). Automatic detection of atrial fibrillation using the coefficient of variation and density histograms of RR and ΔRR intervals. *Medical & Biological Engineering & Computing*, *39*(6), 664–671. doi:10.1007/BF02345439 PMID:11804173

Vos De, C. B., Pisters, R., Nieuwlaat, R., Prins, M. H., Tieleman, R. G., Coelen, R. J. S., ... Crijns, H. J. (2010). Progression from paroxysmal to persistent atrial fibrillation: Clinical correlates and prognosis. *Journal of the American College of Cardiology*, *55*(8), 725–731. doi:10.1016/j.jacc.2009.11.040 PMID:20170808

Zhou, X., Ding, H., Ung, B., Pickwell-MacPherson, E., & Zhang, Y. (2014). Automatic online detection of atrial fibrillation based on symbolic dynamics and Shannon entropy. *Biomedical Engineering Online*, *13*(1), 18. doi:10.1186/1475-925X-13-18 PMID:24533474

Chapter 10
Applications of Machine Learning in Disease Pre-screening

Upendra Kumar
Institute of Engineering and Technology Lucknow, India

ABSTRACT

Computers in disease prescreening are utilized to interpret medical information. This is known as computer-aided pre-screening tool (CAPST). CAPST helps in improving the accuracy of diagnosis in medicine. The medical experts usually take the outcome of the CAPST as a second opinion to make the final diagnostic decisions. Fast and accurate prediction of disease risk and diagnosis is crucial step for the successful treatment of an individual. The AI-based machine learning technology has undergone significant developments over the past few years and is successfully used in many intelligent applications covering problems of variety of domains. One of the most stimulating questions is whether these techniques can be successfully applied to medicine in disease pre-screening and diagnosis and what kind of data it requires to be trained and learned. There are so many real-time examples of the problems where machine learning methods are applied successfully, especially in medicine. Many of them showed significant improvement in classification accuracy.

DOI: 10.4018/978-1-5225-7131-5.ch010

INTRODUCTION

It has been already observed that machine learning has revolutionized the field of computer vision. Hardly a few years ago, It has transformed this field into practically true, in-your-pocket technologies out of those technologies which were usually considered like science fiction. If nearly human-level accuracy can be achieved through modern computer vision system in identifying dog breeds or cars, why not the current disease diagnostic system might not be as much capable of learning to identify the disease (disease pre-screening) using medical data (medical images or biomedical signal)? For the past few years, the researchers have been working in collaboration with clinicians and doctors to explore it and trying to resolve this problem. Their research has shown that the solution to this problem is indeed possible, not in the future but today itself. The current state of arts has been established in two of the research areas, ophthalmology, and digital pathology, where the researchers are highly excited about what and where the significant progress in research to date has been made. The implementation of pre-screening diagnostic systems in both the fields has encouraged doctors to perform decisions in doing better diagnosis with higher efficiency. For example, one of the crucial diseases like diabetic retinopathy has emerged as one of the applications for disease pre-screening and diagnosis in the area of ophthalmology. Researchers have started to explore developing the computer-aided pre-screening diagnostic tools for a variety of diseases; one of those is a pre-screening tool for diabetic retinopathy. This disease is caused by high-intensity blood sugar levels which in turn damage to blood vessels of the retina. These blood vessels may lead to problems of swelling and leak. They may also stop blood flow from passing through the vessels. Sometimes abnormal new blood vessels may also grow on the retina. This may cause heavy damage to the eyesight of a human being. Nowadays, this problem has become common globally in the world and its' count is increasing exponentially day by day. In general, highly trained experts are required to diagnose the condition in examining the abnormality present in individual's organs. It is well known that effective treatments are available until and unless it is caught at its earlier stage. Any delay in disease detection may lead to progression of the disease to the irreversible stage, such as blindness in case of diabetic retinopathy. Considering a large amount of screening (pre-screening before diagnosis and treatment) required to protect the population from a variety of severe diseases, healthcare sector do not have sufficient number of diagnostic experts throughout the world. Similarly, in another field such as pathology, a microscope is used to look and observe the tissue slides by trained pathologists. The analysis only based on the microscope is subjected to enhance the contrast of microscopic images. Once, these microscopic images are digitized, can be shared among various experts, throughout the world (called telepathology). It can also be numerically analyzed with better accuracy using computer algorithms such as machine learning methods. Computer-aided technology can be used to automate the process of physical counting the structures present in slides and can also be used in the classification of tissues with varying conditions in order to grade tumors (tumor grades are described by four degrees of severity: 1, 2, 3, and 4.), which in turn make it easy to perform disease pre-screening for better diagnosis and prognosis.

MACHINE LEARNING METHODS APPLIED IN DISEASE RISK PREDICTION AND PROGNOSIS

Before starting with a thorough analysis of which machine learning methods work best for what kinds of problems, it is necessary to make a decent understanding of what machine learning and training is and what it isn't. Machine learning is the branch of research study comes under artificial intelligence which tries to learn from past experience by employing variety of tools from different fields such as statistics, probabilistic and optimization algorithms and then after training it can classify the newly input data, determine new patterns as well as predict novel trends (Mitchell, 1997). Machine learning method, like statistics, is employed to investigate and interpret knowledge from the dataset. Along with statistical parameters (unlike statistics based traditional methods), machine learning methods utilize other parameters also, such as Boolean logic (AND, OR, NOT), conditional probabilities (the likelihood of event A given event B), absolute restrictions (IF, THEN, ELSE), and unconventional optimization methods for classification purpose. It is also used in modeling the data or extracting useful pattern information. The approaches used by these techniques for pattern-based learning and classification resembles with a human being. Although, most of the machine learning methods utilize the techniques which are largely borrowed from statistics and probability, but has become primarily more powerful classification technique because it can make a decision or inference from the dataset that otherwise traditional statistical techniques could not be able to achieve (Duda et al., 2001).

In general, most of the statistical approaches though are powerful by employing the techniques of multivariate regression or correlation analysis, but they presume variable independence. They also try to build the model by doing linear combination of the concerned variables. Therefore, in the case of possessing nonlinear relationships and interdependence or conditionally dependence among variables of any biological system which are the fundamental inherent features of many complex biological systems, traditional statistical techniques usually stuck into the critical issues and find hard enough to get it resolved. Whereas, only a few systems like simple physical systems are linear in nature and usually they have conditionally dependent variables.

Machine learning techniques are well known to apply in these situations for better performance.

The machine learning based applications do not give assurance of success every time. Though, the success of any method to solve a given problem depends on its good understanding and also the importance of appreciation of the limitation of the available dataset. Therefore, well-understood assumptions, as well as limitations of given algorithms, usually help in making progress. The good chance of success heavily depends on how properly the experimental setup of machine learning is designed. It also depends on how the correct implementation of learners (training tool) and robust validation of results are done. It is usually observed that poor quality data produces poor worth results (garbage-in is equal to garbage-out). A series of redundant learners are also possible to be evolved if a number of variables are much larger than a number of events to be predicted. Therefore, these learning algorithms tempt to down performance regardless of the variety in choice of the input dataset. This situation refers to "curse of dimensionality" which is not only restricted to the study of machine learning but to many statistical methods also. Further to overcome from this problem, either number of variables (features) is required to be reduced or a number of training examples to be increased. Somorjai et al. (2003) showed that the ratio of sample-per-feature should always more than 5:1. The success of machine learning not only depends on a number of training examples but also based on a variety of the training dataset (a set of labeled input and output dataset) equipped with different intrinsic feature elements. The training examples are prepared by the developer as per the expectation of learner to encounter to cover almost all meaningful representative portion of the data required for dimensionality reduction. These techniques suffer from over-training or noisy training phenomenon if the model is trained many times using very few examples equipped with less variety of inherent features (Rodvold et al., 2001). As a result, over-trained learning model behaves just like an overtired student. Usually, this type of student fails in writing good answers. Similarly, the over-trained learner also performs poor in classifying the novel input data.

Sometimes, standard statistics is proved to be additional powerful or additional accurate than machine learning. In these cases, the user's initial assumptions of considering the reciprocity and nonlinearity of the information could be wrong. This cannot be essentially a weakness to machine learning. It is simply a matter of selecting the proper tool for the proper job. All the machine learning methods are not designed and created equally, but they are designed differently in a variety of problems, may be better for some problems and worse for other kinds of problems. For example, some machine learning algorithms scale adequately and fitted to the size of the biological domains, while others do not. Likewise, the prior assumptions and data requirements employed by some machine learning methods may lead to irrelevant situations to handle the given problem. Commonly, it is very difficult to know which method is best applicable to solve a given problem. Therefore, it becomes important to employ more than one machine learning methods on any given training dataset of a particular problem. Most of the people have a misunderstanding about machine learning techniques that the pattern and trends obtained from it are naturally non-obvious and cannot be detected intrinsically. On the other hand, it is fact that a human being can recognize many patterns or trends if the detailed description is obtained from the data by observing it deeply enough. Machine learning techniques help in saving and reducing the time as well as the effort required to discover the intrinsic pattern feature and hence able to perform better classification. It is the fact that any attractive discovery tends to often obvious to the casual observer – notably when the invention has been discovered.

In general, machine learning algorithms can be classified into three classes: i) supervised learning; ii) unsupervised learning and iii) reinforcement learning. This classification is essentially done based on the desired outcome of the algorithm (Duda et al., 2001). Training of supervised learning tools requires a "perceptive provider" or teacher who is responsible to provide a sufficient number of labeled training data or examples. These labeled training datasets are exploited to learn the mapping of input data to the desired output. For example in Figure 1, the labeled training data set has corrupted images of number "8" as labeled input data assigned for the number "8", whereas labeled output image is an uncorrupted image of the number "8". Further, the learner tries to learn under the supervision of trainer (teacher) who tells what it is supposed to find as output, just like the most school students learn. On the other hand, unsupervised learning has an unlabeled dataset in which learner has to find the pattern or discover the classes itself similar to the process of how most of the graduate students learn. The examples of unsupervised learning algorithms are K-means clustering, hierarchical clustering and self-organizing feature maps (SOMs) etc. These algorithms always try to exploit the inherent features in order to create groups or clusters from unlabeled, raw or unclassified data which can be further used to develop the classification model such as disease pre-screening tool.

The approach used in Self Organizing Map (SOM) (Kohonen, 1982) is a specialized form of an Artificial Neural Network (ANN). In this method, the weights of a grid of artificial neurons adapt itself to find similarity and dissimilarity criterion among input data for training purpose. The origin of SOM model is inherently inspired from biological brain function which starts from a set of artificial neurons. Each neuron has its own physical location on the output map of SOM. All the nodes take part in a competition of winner-take-all process inside a competitive network in which a winner node is declared having weight vector closest to the vector of inputs. Further, their weights are adjusted in such a way that winner node becomes closer to the input vector and thereafter the weights of nearest neighboring nodes

Figure 1. The process of training of machine learner to recognize images of number "8" using a training set (comprises a set of corrupted images (number "8")) to map with uncorrupted output image of number "8"

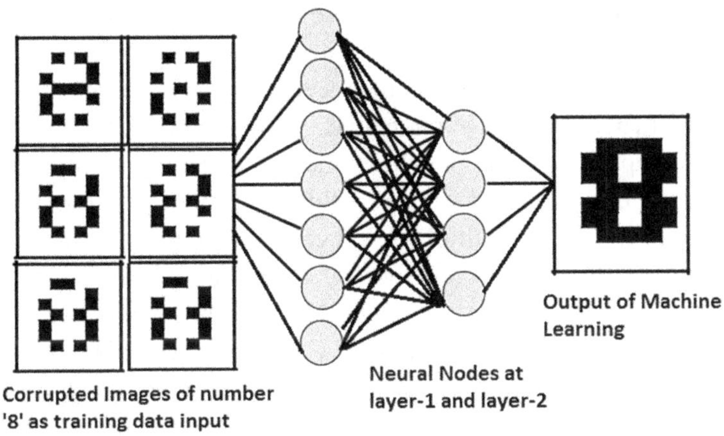

are updated with comparatively larger changes for fine-tuning. On the other hand, the weights of distant neighboring nodes have smaller changes and the complete process is repeated for all input vectors separately one by one for a sufficient number of iterations. As a result, different winning nodes are obtained for a set of input vectors. Finally, in this method, a self-organizing map is obtained as a net result which comprises associations among output nodes with corresponding specific patterns present in the input dataset.

Furthermore, most of the researchers have used supervised learning approaches for almost all machine learning methods in the model of disease pre-screening, risk prediction, and prognosis system. The concept utilized by most of these supervised learning algorithms underlies a specific category of classifiers which rely on the principle of conditional decisions or conditional probabilities. The conditional algorithms are mainly classified into i) Artificial Neural Network (ANN) ii) Genetic Algorithm (GA) iii) Decision Tree (DT) iv) Support Vector Machine (SVM) v) k- nearest neighbor algorithms (k-NN) vi) Linear Discriminant Analysis (LDA) methods. Many researchers have used ANN as a conditional algorithm in various classification based literature.

A wide range of the problems of classification or pattern recognition can be handled by ANN based conditional algorithms. ANN-based classifiers can perform a range of operations as a part of classification process such as statistical operations (linear, logistic and nonlinear regression analysis) as well as logical inferences or operations (AND, OR, NOT, XOR, IF-THEN). Consequently, they are efficient enough to solve or classify a wide range of classification problems (Rodvold et al.,

2001). The architecture of ANN is borrowed from the biological brain network where multiple neurons are interconnected to each other and their junctions are known as axons. It tries to mimic the operations of the human brain by mathematical modeling of its neuro-physiological structure. Likewise, biological learning, the strength of neural network connections are increased or decreased through repeated training on given labeled training dataset. The interconnections of neurons are mathematically represented as a matrix, called weight matrix. This weight matrix corresponds to a layer of ANN computational architecture which is an analogy to the cortical layers inside the human brain network. In classification model as shown in Figure 2, ANN architecture may have multiple layers called hidden layers for multi-layered learning to process their inputs to generate an outputs. Generally, the input and output data is prepared in the form of vectors, or strings or in numbers in order to comply with the mathematical structure of each layer of ANN. The crucial part of classification such as the process of mapping the real world input/output (such as a physical feature, characteristics, an image, a signal, a prognosis, and a list of diseased data, etc.) to a numeric vector, is a big challenge in employing ANNs. In general, a back-propagation optimization technique is used to adjust the strengths of neural connection (by updating weight matrix of each layer). This process follows the derivative-based gradient descent method to compare the output of one layer to the preceding layer. In other words, the numeric weight values in weight matrices of ANN architecture are progressively modified by utilizing the labeled training dataset. A differentiable transfer function (usually a sigmoid curve) is used for learning in back-propagation. In general, multi-layered feed-forward architecture is used in most of the ANN models which do not have any feedback connection or loop. Each application has different design and architecture of ANN model and can be customized or optimized as per application requirements. ANN may suffer from poor performance or even very slow training if ANN has its generic or naive structure of input/output scheme. Another shortcoming of ANNs is that it follows a "black-box" technology, means it is almost impossible to discern when somebody tries to figure out how the classification is performed by an ANN model or why it did not perform well for a particular case. In other words, it is very difficult to decipher the logic of a trained network of an ANN.

Another conditional algorithm is Decision Tree (DT), in comparison to ANNs logic of decision trees can be easily discerned. In general, the structure of a decision tree follows the structure of graph or tree or flow chart, in which nodes represent decisions and leaves or branches represent their possible consequences (Quinlan, 1986). Decision trees have been used for the past many years (especially in taxonomy) and are being generally used as a common component of classification or categorization process to many medical diagnostic based systems such as disease pre-screening process. For example, the process of breast cancer diagnosis can be shown as a decision tree having nodes decisions and leaves as their consequences, as shown in Figure 2. The design of decision trees are formulated through consultation with medical experts and further refined or tuned through years of experience of medical practice. It can also be modified as per their limitations of resources or risk. On the other hand, decision trees can also be constructed automatically using labeled training dataset by decision tree learners if they have real time existance. While classifying the dataset using a decision tree, leaves in the tree represent classifications and branches represent combinations of feature vectors that lead to corresponding classifications. The learning process of a decision tree is achieved by progressively splitting the labeled training dataset into subsets following numerical or logical test and this process of splitting is repeated on each newly derived subset in a recursive manner until further splitting is either a singular classification or no splitting is possible. Although decision trees have many advantages than other conditional algorithms, they need very less data preparation, they are easy to understand and interpret, a variety of data type can be handled by them such as numerical data, nominal (named or alphabetical) and categorical data, etc. They can also generate robust classifiers, quick to learn and can be validated using statistical tests. Moreover, decision trees have poor performance similar to ANNs for more complex kind of classification problems (Atlas et al., 1990).

Somehow a support vector machine (SVM) has emerged as a newer machine learning method nowadays (Duda et al., 2001). Although they are well-known machine learning technique, still it has more scope left in the field of disease pre-screening, risk prediction, diagnosis, and prognosis. The working principle of SVM can be better understood with the help of given scatter plot of points of a specific problem. For example, in Figure 3, a scatter-plot (of breast cancer pre-screening problem) in between tumor masses and number of axillary metastases among individuals with two categories: poor prognoses and excellent prognoses. Obviously, scatter plot has formed two distinct clusters, and SVM machine learner can find out the equation of a line that tries to separate these two clusters up to maximum extent. Furthermore, if the scatter plot is drawn among more than two variables (such as metastases, volume, and content of estrogen receptor), then SVM will have a planer separation line and if a number of variables are increased the separation would be defined as a hyperplane. This hyperplane is formulated by a subset of the points underlying in two classes, called support vectors.

Formally, a hyperplane is constructed by SVM algorithm in such a way that dataset is separated into two classes with maximum margin, such that it tries to maximize the distance between the hyperplane and the closest examples (data of any class nearest to the hyperplane). Furthermore, non-linear classification can also be handled by SVM algorithm by employing a non-linear mathematical kernel function. This kernel function can transform the data from a linear feature vector

Figure 2. A flow depicting decision tree (generally used in disease pre-screening, diagnosis, and treatment of breast cancer). A tree is formulated via expert assessment. Decision tree learners can also generate similar decision tree structures.

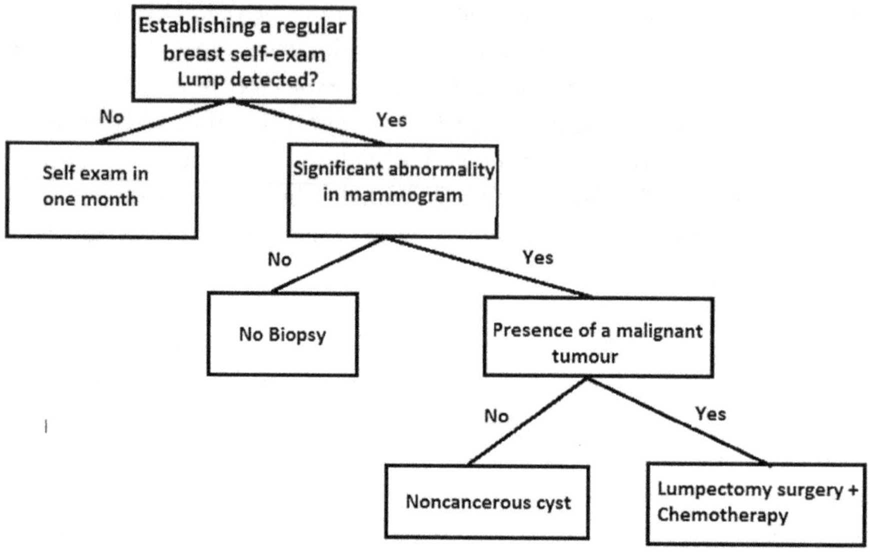

space into a non-linear feature vector space. The performance of an SVM classifier can be dramatically improved by applying different kernels to different datasets. Likewise, ANNs, a wide range of classification and pattern recognition problems can also be handled by SVMs such as text and speech recognition, handwriting analysis, protein function prediction and medical disease pre-screening, diagnosis and prognosis (Duda et al., 2001). Like k-nearest neighbor methods, SVM algorithms suite well and are also very efficient especially to non-linear classification problems (discussed in Table 1).

REGRESSION ANALYSIS IN DEVELOPING BMI VALUES BASED PRE-SCREENING TOOL

Regression Analysis is the mathematical measurement of the average relationship between a response variable and one or more predictor variables in terms of original units of data. It is a set of statistical processes for estimating the relationships among variables and can be used for predicting the unknown value of a variable provided known values of two or more variables, called as predictors. The graph is shown in Figure 4 reflects the relationship between the percentage of fat and BMI (Body

Figure 3. An illustration of classification process by SVM between weightlifters and basketball players based on height/weight support vectors. A hyperplane (actually a separation line) is identified by SVM which maximizes the separation up to an extent between the two clusters.

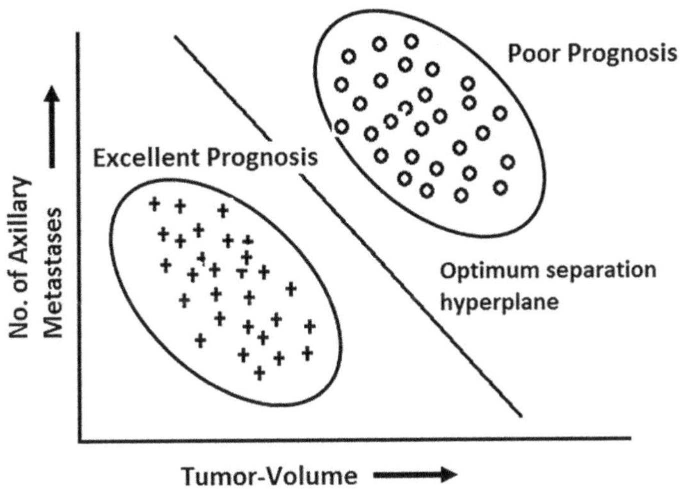

Mass Index) and represented by regression line which can predict fat percentage corresponding to any value of the variable: BMI (predictor variable).

PREDICTIVE MODELS AND PRECISION MEDICINE IN DISEASE PRE-SCREENING

Appropriate disease pre-screening and diagnosis is a fundamental step in medical science because it sets the background for the prediction of actual disease at individual patient level (called prognosis) and making decisions accordingly to apply the most appropriate therapy. However, availability of large series of social, clinical and biological factors responsible to determine the likelihood of an individual's future outcomes, prognosis only partially depends on diagnosis and etiology and further treatment is not followed solely based on underlying disease pre-screening details and diagnosis. Predictive models with deep analytics of big medical data are facilitating clinicians to move towards high precision medicine with more confidence and reliability in this modern age (basics are shown in Figure 5). Approaches that take due account of prognosis based limitations lead to the lingering risk of over diagnosis and maximize the content information value of prognostic information in the clinical decision process.

Table 1. A set of machine learning algorithms with their possible advantages, pre-assumptions, and limitations in developing disease pre-screening tool

S. No.	Machine Learning Algorithms	Advantages	Pre-Assumptions and Limitations
1	Decision Tree (DT) (discussed by Quinlan, 1986)	• Simple to understand & interpret and efficient training & learning algorithm • Require little data preparation • Order of training & learning instances has no impact on training • Quick to learn • The over-fitting problem can be well handled by pruning	• Classes must satisfy the mutually exclusive principle • Final decision tree dependents on as we select the order of attribute • Overly complex decision trees would be formed if training set comprises errors • Testing of an attribute becomes ambiguous about which branch of decision tree should be taken in case attribute has missing values
2	k-Nearest Neighbour (NN) (discussed by Patrick & Fischer 1970)	• Fast classification of data • Robust algorithm towards novel or irrelevant attributes • Useful for non-linear and complex classification problems • Can be used for both regression analysis and classification • Has tolerance to noisy instances or missing attribute values instances	• Able to update concept description very slowly • Assumes about classification that data having similar attributes will have similar classifications • Assumes that all attributes have equal relevance • As the number of attributes increases computational complexity of algorithm also increases
3	Naïve Bayes (discussed by Langley et al., 1992)	• The foundation of the algorithm is based on statistical modeling • Simple to understand & interpret and efficient training & learning algorithm • Order of training & learning instances has no impact on training • Applicable across multiple area and domains	• Assumes statistical independence of attributes, though it may or may not be the case • Assumes normal or Gaussian distribution on numeric data or attributes • Redundant attributes may lead to the wrong classification • Classes must follow the mutually exclusive principle • The accuracy of the algorithm is dependent on attribute and class frequencies
4	Artificial Neural Network (ANN) (discussed by Rummelhart et al., 1986)	• able to handle a wide range of classification or pattern recognition problems • can be used for regression analysis or classification • high tolerance to noisy inputs • Boolean functions (AND, OR, NOT) can be represented by this algorithm • data input can be classified and represented by more than one output symbols	• difficult to understand the structure of Algorithm and also how it performs classification task. • too many attributes may lead tooover-fitting of training architecture and may produce wrong classification results • optimal network structure can only be obtained through repeated experimentation
5	Support Vector Machine (SVM) (discussed by Vapnik, 1982)	• Able to make models for nonlinear class boundaries • In contrast to ANNs, overfitting is unlikely to occur in SVM algorithm • Able to reduce high computational complex problems to quadratic optimization problems • Can easily handle complex decision rules and frequency of errors	• The training process is slow in comparison to Naïve Bayes and Decision Trees • Optimal parameters are difficult to be determined in case of training data is not linearly separable • Not easy to understand the structure of algorithm
6	Genetic Algorithm (GA) (discussed by Holland, 1975)	• A simple algorithm, easy to implement based on selection, mutation, and crossover as follows the biological evolution • Can be used in feature selection and feature classification • Primarily used in optimization problems • Always tries to find a good solution but may lead to getting the optimal solution (not always the best solution)	• Development of scoring or fitness function is computationally non-trivial • May not be able to find the optimal solution, tries to find local optima rather than global • Training input/output data is not easily represented or formed

Figure 4. Regression analysis to predict the percentage of fat from BMI value

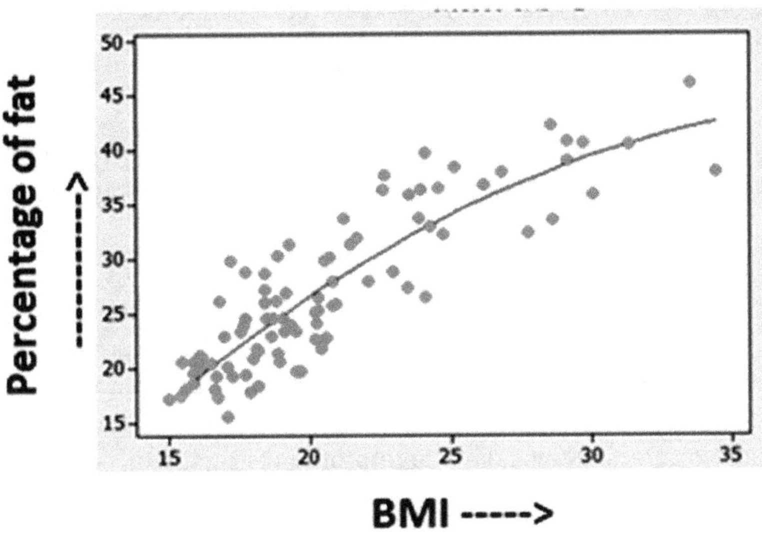

Figure 5. Modeling using big medical data to assist clinicians in high precision medicine (Menon, 2016)

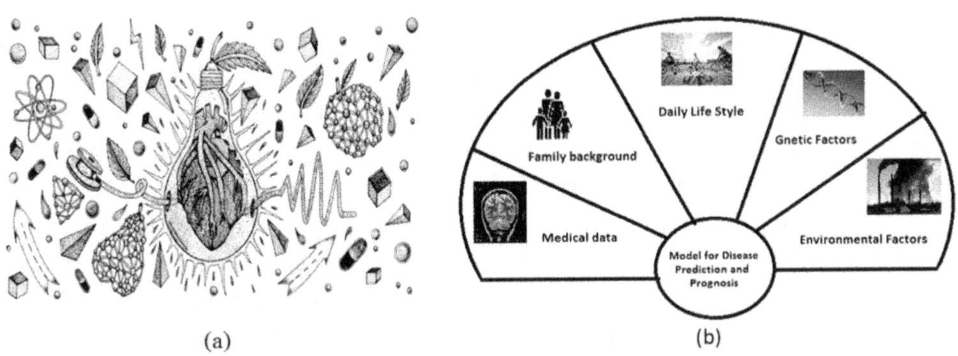

Predictive analytics basically acts as a fuel for transformation from a focus on the volume of procedures to the value of outcomes. Predictive tools are ready to help providers both doctors' groups and hospitals assess patients' risk of contracting a whole host of diseases and conditions. They can come up with individualized regimens by tapping into electronic medical records to identify the types of patients who are most likely to respond to a particular type of therapy. They can pinpoint treatments that try to sustain health in a more precise way than ever before it was. Furthermore, they can identify individuals who are likely to stop getting benefits from a specific regimen at a given time. Honoring the paradigm of volume-to-value shifting in healthcare and medical informatics, predictive analytics of different kind of possible diseases, though rarely visible in the current traditional environment, is the essential enabler and may act as a valuable propeller.

IMPROVING DISEASE DIAGNOSIS AND RISK PREDICTION USING MACHINE LEARNING BASED PRE-SCREENING TOOL

Driven by the vast and ever-increasing day to day availability of huge amount of medical or clinical data such as X-rays, CT scans, MRI scans, biopsy results, blood tests, and epidemiological data – new branch of study, machine learning is becoming a new role player in the doctor's weapon store, helping in disease pre-screening, risk prediction and diagnosis of variety of diseases and disorders with higher reliability and accuracy. Now a days, high-profile research projects in the field so far such as IBM Watson Health, which has promised to develop a predictive and analysis model for disease pre-screening to produce tumor based disease treatment recommendations with higher accuracy, and Google's DeepMind Health organization has recently signed a contract with Britain's National Health Service (BNHC) to incorporate high-end research in order to increase the speed and accuracy of disease pre-screening, care and treatment (better recommendations) provided by the system (https://verneglobal.com, 2018). Moreover, the rapid development in the growth of innovation in a variety of application domains of machine learning especially in the field of disease pre-screening, risk prediction, diagnosis, and prognosis has produced an opportunity to work on it with great excitement, and may potentially lead to revolutionary and remarkable breakthroughs in medicine.

Take, for example, the fast-growing improvement is being achieved in the detection of skin cancer (by using a pre-screening tool) using machine learning algorithms at Stanford University, California such as accuracy of disease pre-screening, risk prediction and diagnostic system which includes machine learning methods, is capable to challenge even to medical dermatology expert also. To achieve this milestone, the Stanford University team created a database of digital images of skin lesions with varying kind of diseases, comprised of 130,000 images of 2,000 different diseases. Thereafter, training of the formerly labeled dataset was done using Google-based machine learning algorithm, initially which was developed for the ImageNet Large Scale Visual Recognition Challenge (ILSVRC) based on skin cancer database. The algorithm performed certain kinds of tasks such as keratinocyte carcinoma classification, melanoma classification. While looking into their results obtained by a pre-screening system including dermoscopy and machine learning application, it was observed that the resultant accuracy matched with the performance of a medical dermatology expert. Therefore, the current skin cancer-based pre-screening tool has been proven up to the mark, as detection at early or premature stage leads to a larger reduction in the mortality rate. The skin cancer-based pre-screening and diagnostic system developers are confident enough about their application or model, which could be launched to run on a standard mobile phone. It has a great potential to have a positive impact on the lives of over the 15 million new skin cancerous people that are being diagnosed every year by a dermatologist. It can also fill the gap of non-availability of enough dermatologists to handle a skin cancer-based large population of patients.

Similarly, remarkable breakthroughs have also been achieved in breast cancer-based pre-screening and diagnostics. In a recent research (Liu et al., 2017), Google team announced that their machine learning based diagnostic system is robust enough and can locate breast cancer that had metastasized to lymph nodes near to the breasts. It has achieved a remarkable milestone in producing improved diagnostic efficiency. The field of study is in high and urgent demand for developing screening tools to handle a large population of breast cancer patients. While screening and diagnosing this disease using current traditional technology-based tools, generally needs huge and rigorous analysis of concerned disease data collected from a variety of patients in very limited time, and also may generate a huge number of false positive predictions. In a survey done in the United States (Fernandez, 2011), it has been found that every year approx. half of the 12.1 million captured mammograms are false positive, consequently causing high stress on patients. It also makes it necessary to follow invasive diagnostic procedures, which in turn incurs high healthcare costs. Other researchers and pre-screening diagnostic system developers have also made significant progress in technological enhancement and improvement on the methods of traditional mammography in combination with machine learning techniques. For example, similar research is also being carried out at the Houston Methodist Research Institute, and IBM research center, where they have started an open forum in order to take initiative to improve the results of diagnosis by their breast cancer screening tool based predictive and prognosis models.

Machine learning has emerged to have a high impact on disease pre-screening and diagnosing ability of medical experts for a wide range of genetic disorder diseases as well, which is very difficult for even experienced physicians to detect (pre-screening) for prognosis. Most of the conditions and causes of these genetic disorders generally possess a group of identical facial characteristics that could provide hints and facilitate in pre-screening and diagnosing to medical experts. But the task to identify human congenital malformations (birth defects) is based on the practice of noticing and observing these facial patterns which in turn is a rarefied skill that naturally comes after learning through decades of practice and experience.

Face2Gene is a mobile application tool that is built on machine learning techniques and can be used to fill thatgap. This application tries to analyze the facial image of an individual and provide predictive decisions to medical experts (maybe less-experienced)in order to identify the presence of the genetic disorder problem with the help of their facial characteristic and feature configurations. The developers of Face2Gene app claim that currently, this software can recognize around 2000 different kind of genetic disorder diseases. Though, this software was designed in such a way that it can improve the prediction accuracy of diseases as the number of scanned patient's facial images increases and can be better analyzed from corresponding databases. Therefore, hopefully, the capability of Face2Gene can be improved in the future by applying machine learning algorithms.

In the field of research of Alzheimer's disease, the people also experience remarkable achievements with the help of machine learning technology. Machine learning techniques based recognition system can be developed not only to analyze the patient's brain MRI scans in order to locate Alzheimer's disease, but the training of the system can also be done to detect the trivial cognitive impairments which often act as a precursor for full-scale Alzheimer's disease. Some of the recent machine learning models claims that they can screen out and diagnose the symptoms of Alzheimer's disease caused around ten years before also. Similar to other types of cancerous diseases such as breast and skin cancer, the early age detection of symptoms of Alzheimer's disease (by using the pre-screening tool) can help in improving treatment process of a genetic disorder, and further can lead to better clinical outcomes and cure operations.

Obviously, it is very exciting and enthusiastic time to work on the development of machine learning based applications. Some researchers in the medical science and community, even some doctors also, have started envisioning a world where machine learning has completely captured all the diagnosing ability to screen out and diagnosing a disease that has surpassed the ability of human pathologists and anyhow cannot be handled by them. Probably, it is really the best time for machine learning developers to begin signing the Hippocratic Oath in the field of disease pre-screening and medical diagnostic. Not only, researchers are investigating the effects of the application of machine learning techniques on the healthcare and pharmaceutical industry but also, focus on the application of these algorithms in the process of drug discovery and development. In Table 2, different architectures of Machine learning models have been discussed with their corresponding advantages and disadvantages.

Table 2. Comparison of the different architecture of Machine learning models

Type of Machine Learning Network	Architecture of Network	Advantages	Disadvantages
Deep Neural Networks (DNNs)	Its architecture has more than two layers, which allows coping with a complex non-linear relationship. It is heavily used in classification as well as regression analysis.	It has wide application and produces high accuracy	The training process is complex because it has more hidden layers and the error is propagated back to the previous layer and becomes very small. The learning process is also very slow.
Convolutional Neural Networks (CNNs)	They have good performance for 2-D data. They use Convolution filters to transform 2-D data into 3-D data.	Produce high efficiency and having a faster learning	The classification has a prerequisite that all data should be labeled.
Recurrent Neural Networks (RNNs)	They have the capability of learning large sequences. The weights associated with layers are shared across all other layers and nodes	Sequential events are learned efficiently, time dependency can be modeled. A variant of RNNs are used such as LSTM, BLSTM, HLSTM MDL-STM. They have produced state of art accuracies in speech recognition, character recognition, and many other natural language processing related applications	Requires big databases and falls into issues because of gradient vanishing

MACHINE LEARNING IN MEDICAL IMAGING BASED PRE-SCREENING TOOL

Many tasks of disease pre-screening, diagnosis, and prognosis of medical images require an initial search to identify abnormalities present in images, then quantify the measurement and changes occurred over time. Automatic image processing based diagnostic systems including machine learning algorithms are the key enablers to make it capable to improve the quality of pre-screening, diagnosis and interpretation process of medical images by facilitating through efficient recognition and learning techniques. Machine and deep learning is one Artificial Intelligence (AI) based technique extensively applied in a variety of real-world problems that may provide state of the art level accuracy. Nowadays, it has become more demanding in the field of medical image analysis that was not been possible before. Applications of the machine and deep learning techniques in healthcare science largely cover a broad range of problems ranging from a screening of different diseases and their monitoring in order to achieve personalized treatment suggestions and prognosis. Today, a variety of sources of medical data available such as radiological imaging (X-Ray, CT scans and MRI scans), pathology-based imaging data and very recently, genomic sequences (components are A, T, G, C) have brought an huge amount of data that can be utilized for implementing disease pre-screening tool, which can be used for better analysis and prediction by the medical experts. However, the researchers are unable to model such a tool that may convert all these kind of raw medical data into useful information for disease pre-screening. In many kinds of literature, state of the art applications of the machine and deep learning methods have been discussed in medical image analysis and furthermore obtained improved screening and diagnostic results.

MACHINE LEARNING IN DIABETIC RETINOPATHY BASED PRE-SCREENING TOOL

Diabetes Mellitus (DM) is a kind of metabolic disorder disease in which pancreases cannot produce proper insulin (Type-1 diabetes) or in another category of diabetes, and body tissues are not able to give a proper response to the insulin (Type-2 diabetes), which in turn results in high blood sugar. Diabetic Retinopathy (DR) is a kind of retinal disease caused by diabetes which may lead to eye blindness in an individual with the passage of time of diabetes. According to the survey (https://everylifecounts.ndtv.com, 17 October 2016), 69.1 million people are suffering from the diabetic disease in India and 15% of those patients have a high probability of risk of vision loss, impairment or blindness. This risk of this disease can be controlled and cured easily if it is detected prematurely on time (pre-screening) and in fact at an early stage by using retinal image based pre-screening tool.

The process of manual detection of DR is a difficult and time-consuming method at present due to non-availability of good equipment and expert physicians. The dark part of this disease is it hardly shows any symptoms at the pre-mature stage and the medical experts need to examine the colored retinal images of the patients which causes the treatment process to be delayed, the prescription may lead to the wrong direction due to miscommunication and hence follow up may be loosed. Machine learning models based automated detection of DR has been proved to perform at their optimized and better accuracy by many researchers.

Gulshan et al., (2016) applied Deep Convolutional Neural Network (DCNN) based machine learning method on retinal images of Archive Communication System (EyePACS-1) database and Messidor-2 dataset for detection and classification of moderate and even worse kind of diseased images. The EyePACS-1 pre-screening tool comprises approximately 10,000 retinal fundus images and the Messidor-2 image database comprises 1,700 retinal fundus images corresponding to 874 different patients. They claimed classification results as 97.5% sensitivity and 93.4% specificity on the EyePACS-1 dataset; and also similar results as 96.1% sensitivity and 93.9% specificity on the Messidor-1 dataset, respectively. Kathirvel (2016) used DCNN with dropout layer techniques for training the model and applied to test on publically available databases such as DRIVE, Kaggle fundus and STARE for classification and detection of retinal fundus images. The accuracy of their pre-screening model was reported in the range of 94-96%. Pratt et al. (2016) applied NVIDIA CUDA DCNN (cu-DCNN) library based classification model on Kaggle database comprising above 80,000 digital retinal fundus images for a variety of cases. They also performed the task of validation of the network having around 5,000 retinal images with a sufficient number of subjects. In image pre-processing task, they resized the image into a 512X512 set of pixels and then passed through the sharpening process resulting in the feature vector. Finally, these feature vectors were fed into Cu-DCNN (a variant of DCNN) classifier based pre-screening tool to get desired output (actual class of retinal disease). They trained the classifier for 5 different classes and used a variant of a feature part of the image such as hemorrhages, exudates, and micro-aneurysms and finally obtained up to 95% specificity, 30% sensitivity, and 75% accuracy. Haloi et al. (2015) also implemented machine learning based five layers CNN with drop-out mechanism to detect pre-mature stage of DR on a web-based database Retinopathy Online Challenge (ROC) and Messidor database of retinal images and they claimed the accuracy, sensitivity, specificity, and area under the curve (AUC) up to 96%, 97%, 96% and 0.988 respectively on Maddissor database and AUC up to 0.98 on ROC retinal image database. Table 3 shows different Machine Learning methods (MLS) used in the development of disease pre-screening models for Diabetic Retinopathy.

MACHINE LEARNING IN HISTOLOGICAL AND MICROSCOPICAL ELEMENTS DETECTION BASED PRE-SCREENING TOOL

Histological analysis is the branch of study which mainly focuses on cell, group of cells and tissues of human body. When different natural changes occur at cellular and tissue level of human body then microscopic changes, their corresponding morphological characteristics and features can be detected using microscopic image technology-based tool and stains information (colorful chemicals: is a discoloration process that can be clearly distinguished and easily identified from the surface, material, or medium) (Shirazi et al., 2015). This process includes a number of

Table 3. Summary of Machine Learning methods (MLS) used for pre-screening and detection of Diabetic Retinopathy (DR)

Authors	Machine learning model	Database	Accuracy (%)	Sensitivity (%)	Specificity (%)
Gulshan et al., 2016	Deep Convolutional Neural Network (DCNN)	EyePACS-1	---	97.5	93.4
		Messidor-2	---	96.1	93.9
Chandrakumar & Kathirvel, 2016	Convolutional Neural Network with dropout layer	Kaggle-fundus, DRIVE, and STARE	Range 94-96%	---	---
Pratt et al., 2016	Convolutional Neural Network library	Kaggle database	75%	---	---
Haloi et al., 2015	Convolutional Neural Network with five layers	Messidor and ROC database	98% and 97%(AUC)	---	---
Alban et al., 2016	Deep Convolution Neural Network	EyePACS	45%	---	---

steps such as fixation, sectioning, staining and the finally it goes through optical microscopic imaging technology. Different kinds of skin diseases can be analyzed and predicted by microscopic image technology and machine learning based pre-diagnostic tool especially includes Squamous cell carcinoma (SCC) disease caused by uncontrolled growth of abnormal cells, melanoma (is most dangerous skin cancer disease caused by unrepaired DNA damage in the cell)and other diseases also such as gastric carcinoma, breast carcinoma, gastric epithelial metaplasia (GEM), malaria (mosquito-borne infectious disease), intestinal parasites and TB (Tuberculosis) etc. Genus Plasmodium parasite (uses the host's resources to fuel and complete its life cycle) is the main cause of Malaria disease through human body interface. Microscopic imaging technology is the standard method primarily used for identification of parasites in stained blood smear sample. Mycobacteria (a type of germs, are immobile, slow in growing and rod-shaped) in sputum (a mixture of saliva and mucus in coughing through the respiratory tract) is the main cause of Tuberculosis disease (TB). Smear microscopy and Auramine-Rhodamine fluorescence stain or Ziehl-Neelsen (ZN) stain are golden standards for detection of Tuberculosis disease.

Recently, a research has been published by Sirinukunwattana et al., (2016) on the Histo-Phenotypes database where they applied DCNN classifier for pre-screening and diagnosing the nuclei of cells of colon cancer disease using stained histological digital images. The researchers Bayramoglu and Heikkil (2016) performed two studies for two different problems such as detection of interstitial lung disease (pre-screening) (ILD: affects the human's ability to breathe and reduces flow of oxygen into bloodstream) and thoraco abdominal lymph node (TAL: causes calcification and vascularity) and used transfer learning (fine tuning) based training approach with CNN classification model to implement disease pre-screening tool. In the work of Quinn et al., (2016), authors also included some shape features such as moment (in general calculated by weighted average (moment) of the image pixels' intensity values) and morphological features (geometrical characteristics) to the class of problems that predict diseases such as malaria, hookworm from blood, tuberculosis, sputum and stool samples. They performed an automatic microscopic image analysis using DCNN model as a classification tool and performance was reported as AUC (area under the curve- mean to compare the performance of classifiers) 100% for Malaria disease and 99% for tuberculosis and hookworm. Fully CNN based deep learning approach has been used in the work of Sirinukunwattana et al., (2016) for automatic cell counting. Quin et al. (2016) also conducted an experiment using DCNN for pre-screening and detection of leukemia in metaphase and malaria disease in a thick blood smear. The study on malaria detection is a crucial and important research area (Malaria is a well-known life-threatening disease caused by parasites to make their life cycles that are transmitted or spread to people through the bites of infected female mosquitoes). In a recent survey done by World Health Organization in 2015, it was observed that around 438,000 people were died due to malaria (URL is given reference section). Dong et al. (2018) developed four automated pre-screening and detection systems for identification of infected and non-infected cells by malaria disease using a combination of CNN models and SVM classification models. The architectures of three of them using CNN model were named as LeNet-5, GoogLeNet, and AlexNet. They involved automatic features extraction and then classification process in developing pre-screening tool. After classification, they reported a pre-screening efficiency of these diagnostic models 96.18%, 98.13% and 95.79% respectively. Their SVM based pre-screening and the diagnostic system got the lowest accuracy among them up to 91.66%.

MACHINE LEARNING IN GASTROINTESTINAL (GI) DISEASES DETECTION BASED PRE-SCREENING TOOL

Gastrointestinal (GI) comprised of all body organs which are involved in digestion of food and absorption of nutrients extracted from it and then excretion of the waste residue material outside the body. The digestion process follows a specified path from mouth to anus. These organs include stomach, esophagus, small intestine (small bowel) and large intestine (large bowel). Based on functionality, the Gastrointestinal may also be divided into two tracts such as upper GI tract and lower GI tract. The upper GI tract comprises stomach, esophagus, and duodenum (part of small bowel) and on the other side lower GI tract comprises most of the small intestine (jejunum and Lilium) and a major part of large intestine. The complete process of food digestion and absorption is majorly affected because of different ailments and diseases such as bleeding, inflammation, a variety of infections and even cancer disease in the GI tract (Quinn et al., 2016). Stomach ulcers (are a type of peptic ulcer disease that heavily affects both the stomach and small intestines) is a severe disease causes bleeding in upper GI tract. Polyps' disease, cancer or diverticulitis kind of stomach disease causes bleeding from colon or large bowl. Small intestine may suffer from the diseases such as Crohn, Celiac, malignant and benign tumor, duodenal ulcer, intestinal obstruction, Irritable bowel syndrome and serious issue of bleeding due to abnormal blood vessels, generally called as Arteriovenous Malformations (AM).

A combined, medical image processing and machine learning based analysis play a key role in screening out, diagnosing and analyzing these severe diseases and provide help as pre-screening diagnostic and prognosis tool to the doctors or medical experts in making quick decisions for better treatment of the patients with high accuracy. Due to the availability of more and more advanced computer-aided pre-screening tools (CAPST) with cutting-edge technology, the experts are involved in practicing a variety of medical imaging tests for digestive systems of a human being in order to screen out and detecting them into its actual class of disease. These tests for digestive systems include various technologies such as endoscopy and enteroscopy, wireless capsule endoscopy, Radioopaque dyes and X-ray studies, colonoscopy or sigmoidoscopy, deep small bowel enteroscopy (DSBE), intraoperative enteroscopy (IOE), Computed tomography (CT scan) and magnetic resonance imaging (MRI scan). These cutting-edge technology based datasets in combination with machine learning methods can provide a platform to develop disease pre-screening tool with better accuracy.

Jia and Meng (2016) employed DCNN based machine learning model for pre-screening and detection of bleeding in gastrointestinal dataset consist of around 10,000 wireless capsule endoscopy (WCE) images. The WCE method is a non-invasive image video capturing technology for the small intestine to identify or examine its disease as a pre-screening tool. The author Pei et al., (2017) mainly concerned about evaluating contraction frequency of bowel by exploration of different features such as diameter patterns and length of the bowel by measuring temporal information both the small and large bowl. Thereafter, they implemented hybrid classification model (FCN-LSTM) using Fully Convolutional Networks (FCN) and stacked FCN with LSTM (Long short-term memory based learning model) and applied on both kinds of datasets such as small and massive datasets. FCN-LSTM hybrid classifier was applied and trained on a small dataset comprised of 5 cine-MRI sequence data without labeling whereas FCN classifier system was employed on a large dataset comprised of fifty raw cine-MRI sequence data with the labeling of input/output. The author (Wimmer et al., 2016) extracted and learned features from ImageNet database comprising duodenums endoscopic digital images and thereafter these learned feature vector were fed to CNN SoftMax based classifier for screening, detection, and classification of celiac disease (a serious autoimmune disorder).

A popular approach of extracting automatic feature in the form of a vector and learning from endoscopy digital images was discussed by Zhu et al., (2015) and thereafter they applied CNN based classifier for classification. Furthermore, these feature vectors were also tested on SVM classifier for screening, detection, and classification of gastrointestinal lesions (iron deficiency based anemia and hookworm infection). This proposed model was applied and learned on around 180 digital images for lesions detection and classification and reported 80% accuracy. Similar kind of work using hybrid approach was also used by the authors (Spiros et al., 2016). The authors (Shirazi et al., 2016) used fast features extraction approach using CNN feature extraction architecture on wireless capsule endoscopy videos dataset and then the extracted features were passed to SVM classifier for screening, detection, and classification of inflammatory gastrointestinal disease (IGD-disorder disease that involves chronic inflammation of our digestive tract). The similar experiment was also conducted on around 337 annotated and labeled inflammatory digital images and 599 non-inflammatory digital images of the gastrointestinal tract of KID by Shirazi et al., (2015). In this work, training set comprised 200 normal and 200 abnormal inflammatory digital image data while test set containing 27 normal and 27 abnormal digital images data and finally reported accuracy up to 90%.

MACHINE LEARNING IN CARDIAC IMAGING BASED HEART DISEASES PRE-SCREENING AND DETECTION TOOL

For the past few years, cardiovascular disease (CVD- related to heart and blockade of blood vessel disease) has become the global leading cause of premature death. The amount of deposition of coronary artery calcification (CAC) can be utilized as a strong and independent predictor of CVD causing events which are generally screened out and quantified from cardiac CT scans by cardiac-based medical experts (Wolterink et al., 2016).Though less availability of good cardiac experts, the recent research on machine learning technology has provided opportunity to produce extremely promising pre-screening based diagnostic and prognostic results for cardiac imaging using digital cardiac images especially for quantification of calcium score (calcium score is the amount of calcium deposited in the walls of the arteries, used to calculate risk of developing Coronary Artery Disease (CAD) by CT scan method) to identify the disease risk. Till now, a number of diverse applications including machine learning methods have been developed for disease pre-screening using CT scans and MRI scans which are the most used imaging modality nowadays. Though, it requires a common and important task of image segmentation of left ventricle before detection and quantification process. On the other hand, manual identification and observation of these diseases in the cardiac digital image based CT scans require significant medical expert interactions, which in turn makes it very time-consuming, infeasible and even more costly for large-scale or epidemiological cardiac disease research-based studies. To overcome these shortcomings, semi-automatic calcium scoring methods have been proposed by Wolterink et al., (2016) for CT scan images called CSCT (CT image based Calcium Scoring method). Now a days, the researchers are mainly focusing on using CT scan angiographic images (imaging technology used to visualize the inside region or lumen of blood vessels and also detailed view of organs especially the arteries, veins and the left and right chambers of heart) in combination with advanced machine learning methods for CAC computation. For example, deep conventional neural network (DCNN) was applied on CT scan images by Wolterink et al., (2016). Their overall architecture of pre-screening tool is discussed as shown in Figure 6.

MACHINE LEARNING IN ECG BASED HEART DISEASE PRE-SCREENING AND DETECTION TOOL

Cardiovascular disease, especially, Coronary Artery Blockade is a major cause of premature dying (Kochanek et al., 2011). If any patient is diagnosed at an early stage of cardiovascular disease (especially myocardial infarction (MI) disease), it may be possible to reverse a disease process (Ferrari, 1998). An easy way of regular monitoring of the cardiac events is possible via home care, self-care, or emergency recording with the help of ECG based pre-screening diagnostic tool mainly. A similar study has been done by Lahiri et al.(2009). They worked on standard 12-lead ECG data (downloaded from www.physionet.org). This study investigates embedded diagnostic information related to MI disease within chaos profile of a quasi-periodic ECG by extracting Phase Space Fractal Dimension (PSFD) feature. This PSFD was taken as a feature vector, to input into classification model, to get the class information of the data being inputted. A Discriminant function based technique, i.e. Neuro-GA classifier (which utilizes the concept of both ANN and Genetic Algorithm) was proposed and utilized for identification of MI disease patient from other subjects. In this work, 12-lead ECG based model was studied to implement the system and results are shown in Table 4.

Figure 6. Classification of calcium score from CT scan cardiac Image used in pre-screening tool (Wolterink et al., 2016)

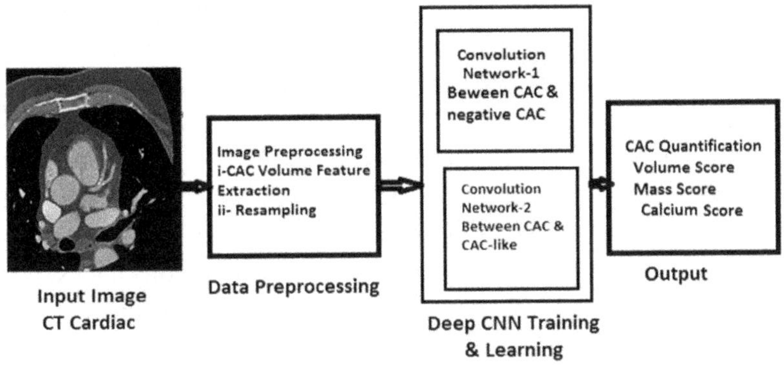

Table 4. Comparative Results of Classification Efficiency for various cases of pre-screening tool on ECG models using Neuro-GA classifier and chaos protocol (Lahiri et al., 2009)

ECG Model	Classes	Total data set	The correctly classified data set	Sensitivity (%)	Specificity (%)	False positive %	False negative %	Overall Accuracy (%)
12-lead ECG (standard data)	MI subject	53	51	96.22	94.59	5.41	3.78	95.55%
	Non-MI subject	37	35	94.59	96.22			

MACHINE LEARNING IN TUMOR DETECTION BASED PRE-SCREENING TOOL

Development of tumor detection based pre-screening tools is also not far away from being applied on machine learning methods in order to produce the efficient and robust system. Abnormal growth of the cells of any part of the body which makes a mass (cell material deposition) then it is called Tumor or Neoplasm. The tumor can be of two types such as one is non-cancerous tumor called Benign tumor and another type is cancerous tumor called a Malignant tumor. A benign tumor does not possess a serious issue as does not have high disease risk because it remains in one part of the body where it is originated and does not spread through other parts of the body. On the other side, a malignant tumor is very dangerous and harmful in nature and can be spread through other parts of the body that can potentially result in death. The issue with a malignant tumor is that the abnormal cells that play roles in forming it, successively multiply at a faster rate and spread over the parts of the body, consequently makes the treatment and prognosis process very difficult.

Wang et al. (2014) worked on making solutions to these problems. They used around 482 mammographic images (a specific type of breast imaging technique that utilizes low-dose x-rays to identify cancer at the early or pre-mature stage) of women having an age range from 32 years to 70 years. This database consists of mammographic images of 246 women affected by the tumor. In this work, firstly the images were de-noised using median filter technique and then segmentation of the breast tumor was achieved using a combined approach of region growth method, morphological operations (such as erosion, dilation, and some sort of simple set-theoretic operations) and modified wavelet transformation (MWT). Thereafter these combinations of morphological and textural features were passed to a combination of extreme learning machine (ELM) model and SVM for detection and classification of breast tumor as a pre-mature level diagnosis. The reported accuracy was approximately 83% using ELM and 82% using SVM (Support Vector Machines). This research work demonstrated that computer-aided pre-screening tool based diagnosis model built for breast tumor detection in digital mammographic images provides a conformational support to the radiologists in performing better detection and prediction of suspicious regions (tumor regions) in corresponding images with improved accuracy and efficiency which in turn leads to better treatment and cure accordingly. Authors (Wolterink et al., 2015) worked on a limited dataset of malignant tumor mass and benign tumor solitary cysts. CNN based classification and a prediction model was applied but it requires a large amount of image dataset for better and more accurate finding of cysts and mass present as a tumor in the body part. However, in this work CNN based model in combination with different variations of mammographic images reported Area under the curve (AUC) based efficiency up to 87%.

Arevalo et al. (2016) conducted an experiment for tumor detection for benchmarking purpose on a database having around 736 mediolateral oblique and craniocaudal mammographic digital images of 344 cancer suffering patients. Firstly, they segmented the tumor images manually into two classes such as 310 images as a malignant tumor and 426 as benign tumor or lesions. First, pre-processing was applied on the images to enhance their relevant features then fed to CNN model for screening and classification of benign and malignant tumors or lesions. They reported 82.6% AUC (accuracy as the area under the curve). In another study, Huynh et al. (2016) used CNN based classification model for features extraction and then learning on breast ultrasound digital images having around 2393 different regions of interests (ROIs) form 1125 different patients. Further two experiments were performed such as in the first experiment, SVM model was trained to classify the extracted features into three classes such as malignant, benign and cystic (classes of the type of tumor) and got satisfactory classification results. In the second, SVM model was used for classification on handcrafted features (like traditional feature extraction methods as SIFT, SURF etc.). They obtained 88% AUC on CNN features based model and 85% AUC on handcrafted features based SVM classification model. Antropova et al. (2017) worked on CNN model for transfer learning of features extracted from ImageNet database (of non-medical type) and applied SVM classifier on around 4,096 extracted features for classification of breast tumors or lesions into two classes such as malignant tumor and benign tumor. They used 551 MRI scan digital images consists of 194 images of benign tumor class and 357 of malignant tumor class. Pre-screening based classification results were reported up to 85% as AUC. The author (Haloi, 2015) used SVM model for classification and CNN model for features extraction. They applied this hybrid model on a database consisting of 219 lesions of 607 breast images of different patients and obtained 86% AUC based accuracy.

MACHINE LEARNING IN ALZHEIMER'S (AD) AND PARKINSON'SDISEASES (PD) DETECTION BASED PRE-SCREENING TOOL

Alzheimer's disease (AD) causes memory loss and other losses also such as cognitive abilities which are very essential and serious enough to interfere with our daily routine life. Parkinson's disease (PD) is a long-term degenerative disorder (loss of function) of the central nervous system that largely affects the motor system of the body. In general, symptoms are looked slowly over time passes away. It is one of the most painful, dangerous and incurable diseases which generally occurs at older ages (above around 50 years) in humans. Sriram et al., (2015) used the database for the Parkinson's disease retrieved from UCI (UC Irvine Machine Learning) repository. Many researchers worked relatively on analysis of the importance of extracted feature and the accuracy of their models by applying different classification methods on a certain number of standard Parkinson databases in order to build pre-screening tool. Two different techniques such as Sieve multigram data (Sieve multigram technology shows how features are correlated to each other) and Survey graph provide the platform for statistical analysis on the human's voice data so that both classes of data such as healthy subject and Parkinson patients could be correctly classified (pre-screening) with better accuracy. They also used other two classification methods such as KStar and NNge, which produce good pre-screening performance.

In general, speech or voice tests can be used to identify and monitor Parkinson's disease because vocal impairment (any symptoms that cause a human experiencing difficulty with vocal communication) being a common symptom and may act as an early stage disease indicator. Using an at-home recording device, for example one device developed by Intel organization for telemonitoring the Parkinson's disease patients, which in turn useful for doctors in monitoring health of the patients remotely. A study was done by Tsanas et al., (2010) in which certain part of voice recordings of a patient was passed through signal processing algorithms and thereafter a classification and regression tree based prediction models were used to predict (act as pre-screening tool) a rating of quantification of disease on the unified PD rating scale Another study by Das et al., (2012) discussed a weakly supervised multiple instance learning (WSMIL) classification and prediction based pre-screening tool to detect and identify symptoms of Parkinson's Disease. This approach has shortcomings addressing the issue of self-reporting which in turn produce inaccurate or incomplete pre-screening based classification results. Their proposed algorithm tried to learn localize symptoms to approximate one not to exact one, and also to time ranges, so that the proposed algorithm would make it suitable for the sparse kind of data that is generated and originated from incomplete reporting. The authors Gil and Johnson (2009) used a multi-layered neural network model that consists of one hidden layer and an output layer. The output layer of this system is responsible to produce pre-screening based prediction results as either healthy or PD subject. In this pre-screening tool, sigmoidal activation function was used for inputs to be passed through, and gradient descent based back-propagation learning algorithm was used to adjust and modify the weights. They achieved a classification and prediction accuracy of 92.31% as pre-screening. Training of SVM classifier was also done using the sequential minimal optimization (SMO) algorithm. Application of SMO speeds up training of SVMs using a divide and conquer approach, especially a certain kind of problems those with non-linear kernel functions (Platt, 1998). Gil and Johnson (2009) used a linear kernel function and reported 91.79% accuracy, and for Pearson VII kernel function, accuracy was reported 93.33%. The authors, Mandal and Sairam (2013) also used an artificial neural network based classifier with a sigmoidal activation function. But, they used back-propagation method with dynamic learning rate and momentum to modify ANN layers-weights and reported a pre-screening accuracy of 94.71%. They also used SVM model with a linear kernel function and reported an accuracy of 97.65%.

MACHINE LEARNING FOR HEMATOLOGICAL DIAGNOSISBASED PRE-SCREENING TOOL

Hematology is the branch of medicine which study and analyzes blood in health and disease. Fast and accurate disease diagnosis and the prognosis is a crucial step for the successful treatment and cure of a disease. The AI technique of machine learning has undergone through significant development over the past few decades and it is observed that it has already been used in many intelligent applications successfully, covering a wide range of problem domains. One of the most stimulating and curious questions is whether these techniques can be successfully applied to the field of medical diagnosis and prognosis (disease risk prediction at an early stage) and what kind of data it requires to be trained and learned. There are so many real-time examples of the problems where machine learning methods are applied successfully, especially in medical fields, for example, most recently, a cancer detection model has been developed which is capable of classifying skin cancer data using skin cancer digital images, with a competent level of performance comparable to that of an expert dermatologist (branch of medical science dealing with the problems related to nails, skin, hair and its associated diseases). However, there is not good enough research which has such competent successful machine learning applications that would tackle with broader and more complex fields of pre-screening based medical diagnosis and prognosis, such as hematology.

The authors (Gunčar et al., 2018) worked on the implementation of pre-screening and diagnostic tool for hematological diagnosis. They built two predictive models in order to predict a hematologic blood disease by applying machine learning algorithms to laboratory-based blood test results of the concerned patient. In one model, all the available parameters of the blood test were used for training and in another model a reduced set of parameters, which are generally captured and measured during the admittance of patient in the hospital. After training and learning while considering the five most probable class of diseases, both models produced significant pre-screening based classification results as prediction accuracy of 88% and 86% respectively. On the other hand, while considering only one most probable class of disease, the prediction accuracy of 59% and 57% were obtained respectively. There is no significant difference between accuracies of both the models which in turn indicates that a reduced set of parameters also keeps the almost all significant information about a disease. These characteristics expand the power of utilizing the model for general practitioner's use and also indicate the possibility of availability of more information in the blood test results than physicians, would help to recognize. In the clinical test and examination, they showed that the accuracy of their pre-screening based predictive and classification models have performed on a par with the ability of hematology experts. They claimed that their study is the first to show that a machine learning based predictive model applying only on blood tests reports alone can be successfully used to screen out and predict hematologic diseases with better accuracy and also can open a door of unparalleled possibilities in the field of pre-screening tool based medical diagnosis and prognosis.

Medical diagnosis and prognosis is the process of determining the type of disease based on a person's symptoms and signs observed either by a medical expert or by an automated system. The ability of a medical expert or physician to observe the feature points in order to get an efficient differential diagnosis and accordingly to plan quickly, majorly depends on a variety of factors such as depth of medical knowledge, skills, analytical ability, repeated experience and so on. During the process of diagnosis and prognosis, available clinical information is supplemented and enriched by an additional collection of other relevant medical data, which can be retrieved from a certain kind of data such as medical history of the relevant patient, a set of all available physical examination data or tests and also from different kinds of diagnostic tests, including clinical laboratory based pathological tests etc.

Obviously, the laboratory-based tests are either being used to confirm or classify or exclude or to monitor or control the diseases and thereafter being used to take help by a medical expert in providing appropriate treatment. However, most of the time the actual power and usability of laboratory test results is being underestimated because test results reports prepared by clinical laboratories just consist of individual numerical or categorical values with the limitation that physicians mainly focus on those values that fall outside a given threshold or range of values. The process of clinical based diagnosis and prognosis of hematological blood diseases is primarily based on laboratory blood tests alone and even the most skilled experts of hematological diseases overlook and analyze the patterns, its deviations, and close relations is measured between the blood parameters which are successively increasing in numbers in a modern and day to day advanced laboratory for diagnosis purpose. Alternatively, looking into complex nature of the manual analysis, machine learning algorithms are capable to handle set of hundreds of attributes (blood test related parameters) and are efficient enough to detect and utilize their inter-relationship behavior, which encourages this field of medicine particularly interesting for the applications of machine learning algorithms. This study claimed that the hypothesis of considering the findings of blood test results values as "fingerprint" of certain hematological diseases that are sufficient enough for development of an efficient machine learning based pre-screening and predictive model to suggest a reasonable diagnosis seems to be reasonable enough. But its prior condition is it has to be learned and trained to screen out disease from a sufficiently large amount of dataset. This dataset of different medical cases is prepared by standard clinical laboratory blood tests by performing correct screening results determined and recommended by a hematology specialist or experts who have sufficient relevant experience to utilize all kinds of the diagnostic procedures necessary and sufficient to confirm it. In this work, the authors discussed and tried to evaluate two Smart Blood Analytics (SBA) based hematological predictive models (SBA-HPM) applied on two different sets of clinical laboratory-based blood test results (with a variety of blood parameters) and performed coding corresponding to diseases, and also performed their evaluation. Both these models were evaluated using stratified ten-fold cross-validation of 8233 different cases of blood disease, along with them 20 additional randomly selected hematological cases of blood disease were also evaluated and their performance was compared against an evaluation done by a hematological expert and internal medicine expert and they got much better classification results.

OPEN RESEARCH ISSUES AND FUTURE DIRECTIONS OF APPLICATION OF MACHINE LEARNING IN MEDICINE BASED PRE-SCREENING TOOL

There are three trends that drive and encourage the researchers to apply machine learning methods in implementing healthcare based pre-screening tool, first is the availability of big medical data, second, most of the recent machine or deep learning methods are modeled based on human brain and third is the availability of computing devices of high processing capability to handle complex real-time problems. Obviously, the machine and deep learning based outcome and its potential benefits are extremely very significant and henceforth the initial effort and costs are also within the proper limit in the development of disease pre-screening and diagnostic systems.

Today's machine learning (ML) algorithms try to identify statistical regularities present in complex datasets (inherent feature) and are regularly being used across a wide range of application areas (especially in medical imaging based pre-screening and diagnostic system). But most of them are lacking behind human learning capability in terms of robustness and generalizability. If machine learning techniques could enable computers to learn or train from fewer annotated examples (due to constraints of unavailability of large amount of data), can transfer the knowledge between tasks, and could have nature of flexibility and can adapt itself towards changing environments and their contexts, then classification and prediction results would have very large scientific as well as societal impacts. Although increased processing power and o enormous memory resources have encouraged and enabled larger and more capable for even complex learning models, but it has been observed that even large number of computing resources would not be sufficient enough to yield such kind of training algorithms, which can learn from a fewer examples and can generalize beyond initial training sets. There are few key areas which are essential to be looked after in order to enhance the ML algorithms capability such as feature selection, transfer learning, representation as well as interpretability schemes, continuous learning, and learning & adaptation process in time-varying contexts as well as environments. Any learning task that requires all these capabilities may be an appropriate example that could demonstrate the power of novel machine learning approaches that could address these challenges faced by traditional ML algorithms.

Recently, most of the large solution provider companies such as Google DeepMind, IBS Watson, medical research labs as well as leading hospitals and vendors are encouraged to come and sit together and start working towards finding the optimal solutions of the challenges which are largely faced by big medical imaging research. There are some organizations like Philips, Siemens, Hitachi and GE Healthcare etc. have already done significant investments in research for building efficient automatic pre-screening and diagnostic tool. Similarly research lab such as Google, TCS and IBM are also investing huge amount towards the development of effcient medical imaging applications. For example IBM Watson is currently working with more than 15 healthcare providers (group of experts) to learn how machine or deep learning technology could work in real-world medical applications in disease pre-screening tool. Similarly, Google-based DeepMind health company is working in collaboration with National Health Service (NHS), UK to apply these methods on variety of healthcare problems and applications (i.e., analysis of anonymized eye scans digital images could help to identify its sign or remark of diseases that could lead to eye blindness- task of pre-screening of patient) on a database of digital images of around 1.6 million patient. The medical research-based company GE Healthcare in the partnership of Boston's Children Hospital (395-licensed-bed children's hospital in the college of Longwood Medical and Academic Area of Boston, Massachusetts) is working towards creating smart medical imaging technology in order to screen out pediatric brain disorders patient. Furthermore, recently GE Healthcare in collaboration with University of California, San Francisco (UCSF) has also announced a 3-year research-based partnership to develop a set of such algorithms which can differentiate between the healthy subject result and one that has suspects and needs further attention by a medical expert to develop disease pre-screening tool.

THE REQUIREMENT OF EXTENSIVE INTER-ORGANIZATION COLLABORATION FOR THE DEVELOPMENT OF EFFICIENT AND ROBUST DISEASE PRE-SCREENING TOOL

Though, in spite of great effort done by many big stakeholders and their future based predictions about the growth of Machine learning algorithms and medical digital imaging technology, still, it is a matter of debate how the replacement of human can be done with a machine. However, machine and deep learning based technology has sufficient potential benefits towards disease pre-screening, risk diagnosis, and prognosis, provided the arising possible issues and problems need to be sorted out at an earlier stage to make it possible to have. This challenge requires collaboration between hospital service providers, medical vendors and machine learning based scientists, which is extremely required to bring to a most interesting end in order to exploit this beneficial solution for improving the quality of healthcare and diagnosis. This collaboration will definitely fruitful in resolving the issues of data unavailability (help in providing data in large amount) to fulfill the essential requirements of machine learning experts (need a large dataset for learning and testing). Another major challenge with healthcare solution is more sophisticated techniques are increasingly required in order to deal with large amount of healthcare data for better disease pre-screening, diagnosis and prognosis, especially in forthcoming years, when data would be more of from the healthcare industry, largely based on body sensor network based capturing devices. The healthcare industry will have to face great challenges in forthcoming years that could be solved by a collaborative work by reputed medical research organizations and hospitals equipped with modern healthcare and medical devices.

NEED TO CAPITALIZE BIG IMAGE DATA FOR DEVELOPMENT OF DISEASE PRE-SCREENING TOOL

Machine learning techniques and its different applications heavily rely on the availability of large dataset of any application area. However, availability of dataset in the form of annotated data (labeled dataset which is required by machine learning algorithms to learn) is not easily possible especially in the field of medical imaging in comparison to another imaging area. In some real-world imaging area, annotation of the real world data is a very simple process such as annotation of two different gender-based classes of human as men and woman in the crowd by annotating of different objects present in given real-world images. However, annotation of medical-related data (digital medical images) is very expensive, tiresome and time-consuming process because it requires extensive time for involvement of medical expert (especially due the sensitivity of medical data domain and its annotation (may be based on variety of disease types) requires opinions of different medical experts on same class of data or field). Furthermore, it may not be always possible that given medical data could be annotated because of some rare or unknown cases. Therefore this problem can be resolved somehow up to some extent if the medical data resources are shared among several healthcare service providers to get proper annotation and hence better pre-screening, classification, and prediction.

ADVANCEMENTS REQUIRED IN MACHINE AND DEEP LEARNING TECHNOLOGY IN MEDICINE TO DEVELOP DISEASE PRE-SCREENING TOOL

Most of the machine learning algorithms mainly focus on supervised machine learning approach which in turn requires labeled dataset (annotations) for learning. However, the process of annotations of medical data especially medical imaging data is very difficult even sometimes not possible i.e. in case of rare disease (characteristics are unknown) or unavailability of a qualified medical expert. Therefore, many researchers have proposed to shift from supervised machine learning field to unsupervised or semi-supervised learning in order to overcome the challenge of big data unavailability (mostly a common issue). Furthermore it also becomes a challenge that how much efficient and accurate will be unsupervised and semi-supervised learning & training approaches in the area of medical imaging and how one can move from supervised to unsupervised transform learning without affecting the systems' performance by keeping in view that healthcare systems are very sensitive and very small difference in outcome can lead to dangerous situation (i.e. wrong prediction), even may lead to death. Despite current best efforts and outcomes, machine & deep learning based technology is not yet able to provide complete solutions to the problems (especially complex medical problems) and correspondingly many questions are still not answerable, in turn, however, provides unlimited scope and opportunity to work on building improved machine & deep learning models.

BLACK-BOX TECHNOLOGY AND ITS ACCEPTANCE BY HEALTH PROFESSIONAL

Health professional is still worried about the challenges as many questions are still left unanswered and machine learning theories are not even can provide a complete solution for those problems till now. In contrast to the conception of a health professional, machine learning based researchers argue that the ability of a computer or software-based system to share or exchange and then make use of information is less of an issue than a reality. As it is well known that humans do not much care about all parameters and them not able to perform complicated decisions, it can be just called as mater of trust of a human being. Acceptance of machine & deep learning in the healthcare field (disease pre-screening and diagnosis) need a real-time proof from the other kind of areas. Medical expert and doctors are hoping and waiting to see its success on some other real-world kind of critical application areas such as autonomous vehicles, self-decision making, and following robots etc. Though researchers have great success of machine & deep learning based methods, the decent and standard theory of machine and deep learning algorithms is still missing in most of the real world kind of applications. This kind of embarrassment of the absence of decent theory is well accepted and recognized by the machine learning based research community people. Another challenge of black-box processing while training and learning in machine learning model, legal implications of black box functionality and behavior could act as a barrier in accepting the outcomes of the learning models, medical experts would not rely on it. The main issue arises when the outcome or prediction went wrong who will be responsible. Due to the high sensitivity of processing and outcome of models of this field, hospital service providers may not be comfortable with black-box processing i.e. how particular processing and outcome could be traced that it has come from the ophthalmologist. Hence, unlocking of black box processing (clear internal structure of processing) is big research challenge to deal with and machine and deep learning researchers are continuously working toward unlocking this black box which is in the limelight of many healthcare professionals nowadays (shown in Figure 7).

PRIVACY AND LEAGUE BASED CHALLENGES IN HEALTHCARE DISEASE PRE-SCREENING AND DETECTION

Data privacy is very important and crucial for all in real time development of any system. It is affected by both kind of challenges such as sociological and technical issues and it is highly required to be well addressed and clarified jointly from both sociological and technical perspectives. The well-known medical related act, HIPAA (Health Insurance Portability and Accountability Act of 1996) comes into picture

Figure 7. Machine and deep learning process: A Black Box (absence of decent theory)

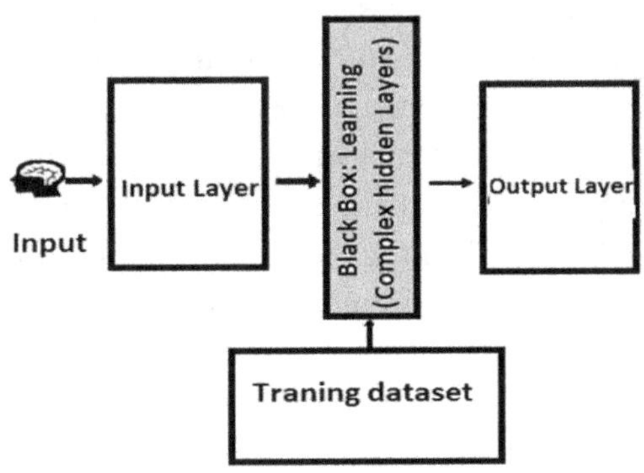

during a discussion of privacy is being done in healthcare or medical sector. The former act mainly provides the possible legal rights to patients regarding making privacy of their personal information (for identification) and also provide certain rules and regulations to establish obligations for healthcare service providers in order to protect and also to restrict its wrong use or unauthorized disclosure. Though the size of healthcare data is rapidly increasing day by day using advanced and current age technologies, researchers are facing another huge challenge that how to remove identifying particulars or details of the patient to prevent its misuse or unauthorized disclosure. Unfortunately, the restriction imposed for accessing the data in limit produce the reduction of information content that might be very useful and important for diagnosis and prognosis. Furthermore, real-world data especially medical data is not static in nature but its size and number are increasing and changing day by day, thus currently available methods are not sufficient to handle such complex kind of real-world dataset.

CONCLUSION

During the past few years, the study of machine learning has earned remarkable milestones towards the automation of disease pre-screening, diagnosis, and prognosis and rather delivered significant improvements in performance as compared to other traditional algorithms. It has a wide range of applications for the problems existing in real world especially in medical science. Owing to their tremendous performance in building classification and detection systems, most of the researchers started to believe that within next few years, machine learning and deep learning based applications will take over human being at par and the automated machine would help to perform most of the daily routine tasks. However, application of machine and deep learning in the field of healthcare and medical science especially in developing robust and more accurate disease pre-screening tools and medical image analysis is quite slow in comparison to the other kind of real-world problems. In this chapter, the state of the art applications of machine learning techniques in medical data analysis were highlighted for better disease risk prediction and prognosis. The obstacles against the application of these techniques were also discussed that leads to a reduction of growth in the healthcare sector. Though, the discussed list is by no means complete for all the cases in medical diagnosis and prognosis however it provides an indication of the wide range of impact of machine learning techniques in growing pre-diagnostic tool based medical research industry today. Finally, open research issues and challenges were also discussed to make enriched the current research work especially implementing the pre-screening diagnostic tools.

Identification of most of the rare diseases especially at its early stage (pre-mature level) is very difficult and challenging task among a large number of other possible diagnoses. Better availability of patient data (patient record) and continuous improvement in machine learning algorithms empower us to build efficient disease pre-screening and diagnostic models to tackle the problems computationally. Many big medical research and development organizations are rigorously working on machine learning based solutions that encourage the developers to employ machine learning techniques on medical data to implement various disease pre-screening diagnostic tools. Looking towards the futuristic scope and brighter side of machine learning approaches, hopefully, very soon human will be replaced by automated diagnostic systems in most of the medical based applications especially disease pre-screening, diagnosis, and prognosis. However, this approach cannot be considered as the only solution as it comes across several issues and challenges that very often becomes a bottleneck in its growth. One of such challenges is the unavailability of labeled or annotated dataset. Also, training of machine learning tool requires a large set of data and most of the cases they do not have sufficient dataset as much as it is required for proper training. Although, the question is still unanswered whether the sufficient training dataset is made available that will not compromise with the performance of the machine and deep learning algorithms. Recent research and development on other kinds of application areas showed that bigger the dataset, better the classification and analysis results. However, this situation creates another challenge that how big data could be used in medicine especially in disease pre-screening, diagnosis, and prognosis.

So far, in the study of disease pre-screening and diagnostic system based research, machine learning applications and solutions provided positive feedback and proved to be very effective approaches. However, though healthcare data and its challenges are very sensitive to small error, more sophisticated kind of machine learning or even deep learning methods are required that can efficiently deal with very complex healthcare data. Finally, looking into recent trends and achievements of the current pre-screening and diagnostic based research works indicate that there is an unlimited number of possible opportunities available to improve the healthcare system. Not only, researchers are investigating and analyzing the impact of the application of machine learning algorithms in the research field of healthcare and pharmaceutical industry but also, started focusing on their application in the field of drug discovery and development.

ACKNOWLEDGMENT

I would like to kindly acknowledge those authors whose references have been taken in this book chapter. I would like to give sincere thanks to my head of the department, CSED, IET Lucknow, India, Prof. S. P. Tripathi and my Ph. D. supervisor, Prof. Tapobrata Lahiri, IIIT Allahabad, India for continuous guidance and encouragement. I would like to give thanks to all those who were involved directly or indirectly in preparation of this book chapter.

REFERENCES

Antropova, N., Huynh, B. Q., & Giger, M. L. (2017). A deep feature fusion methodology for breast cancer diagnosis demonstrated on three imaging modality datasets. *Medical Physics Online*, *44*(10), 5162–5171. doi:10.1002/mp.12453 PMID:28681390

Arevalo, J., González, F. A., Ramos-Pollán, R., Oliveira, J. L., & Guevara Lopez, M. A. (2016). Representation learning for mammography mass lesion classification with convolutional neural networks. *Computer Methods and Programs in Biomedicine*, *127*, 248–257. doi:10.1016/j.cmpb.2015.12.014 PMID:26826901

Atlas, L., Cole, R., Connor, J. T., El-Sharkawi, M. A., Marks, R. J. II, ... Barnard, E. (1990). Performance comparisons betweenbackpropagation networks and classification trees on three real world applications. *Advances in Neural Information Processing Systems*, *2*, 622–629.

Baldus, S. E., Engelmann, K., & Hanisch, F. G. (2004). MUC1 and the MUCs: A family of human mucins with impact in cancer biology. *Critical Reviews in Clinical Laboratory Sciences*, *41*(2), 189–231. doi:10.1080/10408360490452040 PMID:15270554

Bayramoglu, N., & Heikkila, J. (2016). Transfer learning for cell nuclei classification in histopathology images. In Computer Vision–ECCV 2016 Workshops (pp. 532–539). Springer.

Burke, H. B., Bostwick, D. G., & Meiers, I. (2005). Prostate cancer outcome: Epidemiology and biostatistics. *Analytical and Quantitative Cytology and Histology*, *27*, 211–217. PMID:16220832

Capriotti, E., & Altman, R. B. (2011). A new disease-specific machine learning approach for the prediction of cancer-causing missense variants. *Genomics*, *98*(4), 310–317. doi:10.1016/j.ygeno.2011.06.010 PMID:21763417

Case Western Reserve University. (2017). *New Machine-learning program shows promise for early Alzheimer's diagnosis*. Retrieved from http://thedaily.case.edu/new-machine-learning-program-shows-promise-early-alzheimers-diagnosis/

Chanrakumar, T., & Kathirvel, R. (2016). Classifying Diabetic Retinopathy using Deep Learning Architecture. *International Journal of Engineering Research Technology, 5*(6).

Colozza, M., Cardoso, F., Sotiriou, C., Larsimont, D., & Piccart, M. J. (2005). Bringing molecular prognosis and prediction to the clinic. *Clinical Breast Cancer*, *6*(1), 61–76. doi:10.3816/CBC.2005.n.010 PMID:15899074

Das, S., Amoedo, B., De la Torre, F., & Hodgins, J. (2012). Detecting parkinsons' symptoms in uncontrolled home environments: A multiple instance learning approach. *Annual International Conference of the IEEE*, 3688-3691.

Domchek, S. M., Eisen, A., Calzone, K., Stopfer, J., Blackwood, A., & Weber, B. L. (2003). Application of breast cancer risk prediction models in clinical practice. *Journal of Clinical Oncology*, *21*(4), 593–601. doi:10.1200/JCO.2003.07.007 PMID:12586794

Dong, Y., Simões, M. L., Marois, E., & Dimopoulos, G. (2018). CRISPR/Cas9 -mediated gene knockout of Anopheles gambiae FREP1 suppresses malaria parasite infection. *PLoS Pathogens*, *14*(3), e1006898. doi:10.1371/journal.ppat.1006898 PMID:29518156

Duda, R. O., Hart, P. E., & Stork, D. G. (2001). *Pattern classification* (2nd ed.). New York: Wiley.

Fernandez, E. (2011, October 17). High Rate of False-Positives with Annual Mammogram. UCFS news article, University of California San Francisco.

Georgakopoulos, S. V., Iakovidis, D. K., Vasilakakis, M., Plagianakos, V. P., & Koulaouzidis, A. (2016). Weakly-supervised convolutional learning for detection of inflammatory gastrointestinal lesions. In *Imaging Systems and Techniques (IST), 2016 IEEE International Conference on* (pp. 510–514). IEEE. 10.1109/IST.2016.7738279

Gil, D., & Manuel, D. J. (2009). *Diagnosing Parkinson by using artificial neural networks and support vector machines* (Vol. 9). Global Journal of Computer Science and Technology.

Gulshan, V., Peng, L., Coram, M., Stumpe, M. C., Wu, D., Narayanaswamy, A., ... Webster, D. R. (2016). Development and validation of a deep learning algorithm for detection of diabetic retinopathy in retinal fundus photographs. *Journal of the American Medical Association*, *316*(22), 2402–2410. doi:10.1001/jama.2016.17216 PMID:27898976

Gunčar, G., Kukar, M., Notar, M., Brvar, M., Černelč, P., Notar, M., & Notar, M. (2018). An application of machine learning to hematological diagnosis. *Scientific Reports*, *8*(1), 411. doi:10.103841598-017-18564-8 PMID:29323142

Hagerty, R. G., Butow, P. N., Ellis, P. M., Dimitry, S., & Tattersall, M. H. (2005). Communicating prognosis in cancer care: A systematic review of the literature. *Annals of Oncology: Official Journal of the European Society for Medical Oncology*, *16*(7), 1005–1053. doi:10.1093/annonc/mdi211 PMID:15939716

Haloi, M. (2016). *Improved microaneurysm detection using deep neural networks*. arXiv preprint arXiv: 1505.04424v2

Holland, J. H. (1975). *Adaptation in Natural and Artificial Systems*. Ann Arbor, MI: University of Michigan Press.

Huynh, B. Q., Li, H., & Giger, M. L. (2016). Digital mammographic tumor classification using transfer learning from deep convolutional neural networks. *Journal of Medical Imaging (Bellingham, Wash.)*, *3*(3), 034501. doi:10.1117/1.JMI.3.3.034501 PMID:27610399

Indo-Asian News Service. (2016). *In India, Deaths due to Diabetes increased by 50% in Last Decade Study*. Retrieved from https://everylifecounts.ndtv.com/india-deaths-due-diabetes-increased-50-last-decade-study-5934

Jia, X., & Meng, M. Q.-H. (2016). A deep convolutional neural network for bleeding detection in wireless capsule endoscopy images, *38th Annual International Conference of the IEEE Engineering in Medicine and Biology Society (EMBC)*, pp. 639–642. IEEE.

Joshi, S., Shenoy, D., Vibhudendra Simha, G. G., Rashmi, P. L., ... Patnaik, L. M. (2010). Classification of Alzheimer's Disease and Parkinson's Disease by Using MachineLearning and Neural Network Methods. *2010 Second International Conference on Machine Learning and Computing*, 219-222.

Kamnitsas, K., Ledig, C., Newcombe, V. F. J., Simpson, J. P., Kane, A. D., Menon, D. K., ... Glocker, B. (2017). Efficient multiscale 3d cnn with fully connected crf for accurate brain lesion segmentation. *Medical Image Analysis*, *36*, 61–78. doi:10.1016/j.media.2016.10.004 PMID:27865153

Kohonen, T. (1982). Self-organized formation of topologically correct featuremaps. *Biological Cybernetics*, *43*(1), 59–69. doi:10.1007/BF00337288

Kourou, K., Exarchos, T. P., Exarchos, K. P., Karamouzis, M. V., & Fotiadis, D. I. (2015). Machine learning applications in cancer prognosis and prediction. *Computational and Structural Biotechnology Journal*, *13*, 8–17. doi:10.1016/j.csbj.2014.11.005 PMID:25750696

Lahiri, T., Kumar, U., Mishra, H., Sarkar, S., & Das, R. A. (2009). Analysis of ECG signals by chaos principle to help automatic diagnosis of myocardial infarction. *Journal of Scientific and Industrial Research*, *68*, 866–870.

Lamb, S. (2017). *Improving Disease Diagnosis with Machine Learning*. Retrieved on march 15, 2018 from https://verneglobal.com/blog/improving-disease-diagnosis-with-machine-learning

Langley, P., Iba, W., & Thompson, K. (1992). An analysis of Bayesian classifiers. *Proceedings of the Tenth National Conference on Artificial Intelligence*, 223-228.

Liu Y., Gadepalli K., Norouzi M., Dahl, G.E., & Stumpe, M.C. (2017). *Detecting cancer metastases on gigapixel pathology images*. CoRRabs/1703.02442

Maclin, P. S., Dempsey, J., Brooks, J., & Rand, J. (1991). Using neural networks to diagnose cancer. *Journal of Medical Systems*, *15*(1), 11–19. doi:10.1007/BF00993877 PMID:1748845

Mandal, I., & Sairam, N. (2012). Accurate telemonitoring of parkinson's disease diagnosis using robust inference system. *International Journal of Medical Informatics*. PMID:23182747

McCarthy, J. F., Marx, K. A., Hoffman, P. E., Gee, A. G., O'Neil, P., Ujwal, M. L., & Hotchkiss, J. (2004). Applications of machine learning and high-dimensional visualization in cancer detection, diagnosis, and management. *Annals of the New York Academy of Sciences*, *1020*(1), 239–262. doi:10.1196/annals.1310.020 PMID:15208196

Menon. (2016, February). *What is the Relationship between Precision Medicine & Predictive Analytics?* Editor's Note.

Mitchell, T. (1997). *Machine Learning*. New York: McGraw Hill.

Patrick, E. A., & Fischer, F. P. III. (1970). A generalized k-nearest neighbor rule. *Information and Control*, *16*(2), 128–152. doi:10.1016/S0019-9958(70)90081-1

Pei, M., Wu, X., Guo, Y., & Fujita, H. (2017). Small bowel motility assessment based on fully convolutional networks and long short-term memory. *Knowledge-Based Systems*, *121*, 163–172. doi:10.1016/j.knosys.2017.01.023

Piccart, M., Lohrisch, C., Di Leo, A., & Larsimont, D. (2001). The predictive value of HER2 in breast cancer. *Oncology*, *61*(Suppl 2), 73–82. doi:10.1159/000055405 PMID:11694791

Pratt, H., Coenen, F., Broadbent, D., Harding, S. P., & Zheng, Y. (2016). Convolutional neural networks for diabetic retinopathy. *Procedia Computer Science*, *90*, 200–205. doi:10.1016/j.procs.2016.07.014

Quinlan, J. R. (1986). Induction of decision trees. *Machine Learning*, *1*(1), 81–106. doi:10.1007/BF00116251

Quinn, J. A., Nakasi, R., Mugagga, P., Byanyima, P., . . . Andama, A. (2016). *Deep convolutional neural networks for microscopy-based point of care diagnostics*. arXiv preprint arXiv:1608.02989

Rodvold, D. M., McLeod, D. G., Brandt, J. M., Snow, P. B., & Murphy, G. P. (2001). Introduction to artificial neural networks for physicians: Taking the lid off the blackbox. *The Prostate*, *46*(1), 39–44. doi:10.1002/1097-0045(200101)46:1<39::AID-PROS1006>3.0.CO;2-M PMID:11170130

Shirazi, S. H., Umar, A. I., Haq, N., Naz, S., & Razzak, M. I. (2015). Accurate microscopic red blood cell image enhancement and segmentation. In *International Conference on Bioinformatics and Biomedical Engineering* (pp. 183–192). Springer International Publishing. 10.1007/978-3-319-16483-0_18

Shirazi, S. H., Umar, A. I., Naz, S., & Razzak, M. I. (2016). Efficient leukocyte segmentation and recognition in peripheral blood image. *Technology and Health Care*, *24*(3), 335–347. doi:10.3233/THC-161133 PMID:26835726

Simes, R. J. (1985). Treatment selection for cancer patients: Application of statistical decision theory to the treatment of advanced ovarian cancer. *Journal of Chronic Diseases*, *38*(2), 171–186. doi:10.1016/0021-9681(85)90090-6 PMID:3882734

Sirinukunwattana, K., Raza, S. E. A., Tsang, Y. W., Snead, D. R., Cree, I. A., & Rajpoot, N. M. (2016). Locality sensitive deep learning for detection and classification of nuclei in routine colon cancer histology images. *IEEE Transactions on Medical Imaging*, *35*(5), 1196–1206. doi:10.1109/TMI.2016.2525803 PMID:26863654

Somorjai, R. L., Dolenko, B., & Baumgartner, R. (2003). Class prediction and discovery using gene microarray and proteomics mass spectroscopy data: Curses, caveats, cautions. *Bioinformatics (Oxford, England)*, *19*(12), 1484–1491. doi:10.1093/bioinformatics/btg182 PMID:12912828

Sriram, T. V. S., Rao, M. V., Narayana, G. V. S., & Kaladhar, D. S. V. G. K. (2014). Diagnosis of Parkinson Disease Using Machine Learning and Data Mining Systems from Voice Dataset. In *Proceedings of the 3rd International Conference on Frontiers of Intelligent Computing: Theory and Applications (FICTA)*. Springer.

Tsanas, A., Little, M. A., McSharry, P. E., & Ramig, L. O. (2010). Accurate telemonitoring of parkinsons diseaseprogression by noninvasive speech tests. *IEEE Transactions on Biomedical Engineering*, *57*(4), 884–893. doi:10.1109/TBME.2009.2036000 PMID:19932995

Upstill-Goddard, R., Eccles, D., Fliege, J., & Collins, A. (2012). Machine learning approaches for the discovery of gene-gene interactions in disease data. *Briefings in Bioinformatics*, *14*(2), 251–260. doi:10.1093/bib/bbs024 PMID:22611119

Vapnik, V. (1982). *Estimation of Dependences Based on Empirical Data*. New York: Springer Verlag.

Vendrell, E., Morales, C., Risques, R. A., Capella, G., & Peinado, M. A. (2005). Genomic determinants of prognosis in colorectal cancer. *Cancer Letters*, *221*(1), 1–9. doi:10.1016/j.canlet.2004.08.023 PMID:15797621

Wang, Z., Kang, Y., Zhao, Y., & Qu, Q. (2014). Breast tumor detection in digital mammography based on extreme learning machine. Neurocomputing, 128, 175-184.

Weston, A. D., & Hood, L. (2004). Systems biology, proteomics, and the future of health care: Toward predictive, preventative, and personalized medicine. *Journal of Proteome Research*, *3*(2), 179–196. doi:10.1021/pr0499693 PMID:15113093

Wimmer, G., Hegenbart, S., Vecsei, A., & Uhl, A. (2016). Convolutional neural network architectures for the automated diagnosis of celiac disease. In *International Workshop on Computer-Assisted and Robotic Endoscopy* (pp. 104–113). Springer.

Wolterink, J. M., Leiner, T., de Vos, B. D., van Hamersvelt, R. W., Viergever, M. A., & Isgum, I. (2016). Automatic coronary artery calcium scoring in cardiac ct angiography using paired convolutional neural networks. *Medical Image Analysis*, *34*, 123–136. doi:10.1016/j.media.2016.04.004 PMID:27138584

Wolterink, J. M., Leiner, T., Viergever, M. A., & Isgum, I. (2015). Automatic coronary calcium scoring in cardiac ct angiography using convolutional neural networks. In *International Conference on Medical Image Computing and Computer-Assisted Intervention* (pp. 589–596). Springer. 10.1007/978-3-319-24553-9_72

World Health Organization (WHO). (2016). *Ten facts on malaria.* Retrieved from http://www.who.int/features/factfiles/malaria/en/

Zhu, R., Zhang, R., & Xue, D. (2015). Lesion detection of endoscopy images based on convolutional neural network features. In *Image and Signal Processing (CISP), 2015 8th International Congress on* (pp. 372–376). IEEE. 10.1109/CISP.2015.7407907

Chapter 11
Safety and Regulatory Aspects of Systems for Disease Pre-Screening

Sagar Mohammad
Philips Research, India

ABSTRACT

Pre-screening solutions for disease prediction fall under medical device regulations because of the intended purpose of diagnosis. The chapter begins with an overview of the medical device regulations focusing on the two major regulations. The definition of a medical device to the guideline of how a medical device is classified is then discussed. The later part of the chapter covers the design control process with stages of user needs translating to requirements, the design process with the design outputs, design verification conforming that the design is right, followed by design validation that proves that a right medical device is made. The risk management, usability engineering, and security and privacy risk management are part of the product realization process. Having a clear regulatory strategy and plan beginning with the list of target countries and intended use followed by identification of all the applicable product standards is vital. The process thus culminates in the design and development file which is a formal document that describes the design history of the medical device.

DOI: 10.4018/978-1-5225-7131-5.ch011

INTRODUCTION

The healthcare delivery models in modern medicine have evolved a lot from the conventional physician auscultating and making clinical judgement to the current practices of evidence based medicine with heavy dependence on medical devices and healthcare solutions. One cannot imagine any segment of the healthcare continuum be it prevention, diagnosis, treatment or rehabilitation without the assistance of devices and solutions. Imagine yourself lying on a surgical table in front of tools of dubious origin; would you feel safe? Let us envisage the scenario of a pacemaker being implanted on our dear one. Do you feel confident that the pacemaker will effectively perform its intended function?

It is clear that as a consumer of devices and solutions used in healthcare practice, we need them to be safe and effective. But, how does one ensure that the systems used in healthcare are safe and effective. How does the user report if he notices, issues related to safety or effectiveness. It is hence essential to have a mechanism by which the devices and solutions for healthcare are controlled and monitored for its safety and effectiveness.

The mechanism of such a system that controls the use of devices and solutions for medical purpose is called Medical Regulatory body. The Food and Drug Administration (FDA) in the United States of America is one such regulatory body. Similarly, European Commission, Health Canada, Pharmaceuticals and Medical Devices Agency (PMDA), China Food and Drug Administration (CFDA) and other agencies have responsibility to ensure that the medical devices are safe for potential users before manufacturers start to market the devices in their respective geographies (eInfochips, 2017). The whole mechanism of the regulation is like a gatekeeper who first ensures that only appropriate devices that show evidences of the product being safe and effective are allowed inside and further continues to keep a watch on the safety and effectiveness of the medical devices.

In order to get into the market, the medical device must comply with regulatory compliances defined by the medical regulatory body, subject to both regional and international standards. Medical device standards are thus helpful and also enforced by law in specifying and evaluating the requirement for design and performance parameters for biomedical materials, tools, and equipment (eInfochips, 2017).

The focus of screening test is mainly to detect the cause of certain symptoms and help in confirmation of presence or absence of the disease. The goal of disease pre-screening however is to detect potential health disorders or diseases in people who do not have clear visible symptoms of disease. This gives an advantage in treating the diseases much earlier which also results in a better health outcome. Non-invasive biomedical sensing devices offer benefits such as early detection and thus prevention of the risk of infection, ease of use and suitability for long-term monitoring. The book in rest of the chapters is covering non-invasive biomedical sensor devices, IoT based solutions, and knowledge database solutions for pre-screening of diseases for reducing the risk of disease, or early detection to improve the treatment effectiveness.

As a researcher or designer trying to develop or use systems for diseases pre-screening it is important to very clearly understand the safety and regulatory aspects. This chapter gives an overview of the safety and regulatory aspects of medical devices followed by practical tips on how to go about taking a product or solution for disease pre-screening through the stages of design control to get the same market ready.

OVERVIEW OF MEDICAL DEVICE REGULATIONS

As explained in the introduction, the mechanism or system that controls the use of medical devices is called Medical Regulatory body and there are many such bodies covering different geographical regions. The European Union's regulatory process and the United States FDA process which are the major two regulations will only be covered here as examples to understand the methodology.

In Europe, until the 1990s, each country had its own approach to device evaluation (Chai, 2000). European Union (EU) directives were laid out then, that outlined requirements under which all commercial goods including medical devices could be marketed across all EU member states after earning a Conformité Européenne (CE) mark in any one member country. Device approval in each EU country is overseen by a governmental body called a Competent Authority like the Medicines and Healthcare Products Regulatory Agency in the United Kingdom and the French Agency for the Safety of Health Products. The approval process is based on the risk. The lowest-risk devices are declared to the Competent Authority, which may conduct inspections to confirm manufacturing standards and review the technical file for the device. Approval for more complex devices is directly handled by Notified Bodies. Notified bodies are independent companies that specialize in evaluating many products, including medical devices, for CE marking. The notified bodies are designated by Competent Authorities to cover certain types of devices. First, a manufacturer of a device selects a properly designated Notified Body in a country of the manufacturer's choosing. For approval by a Notified Body, devices are subject to performance and reliability testing linked to the risks of their intended use. For most devices, the standard is met if the device successfully performs as intended in a manner in which benefits outweigh expected risks (Kramer, Xu & Kesselheim, 2012b).

In the post marketing phase, manufacturers are required to report all serious adverse events to the Competent Authorities. Since 1998, each Competent Authority has had access to the European Databank on Medical Devices (EUDAMED).

However the public do not have access to the same. This database stores information on manufacturers, data related to approvals and clinical studies, and details on post market events. Manufacturers are required to directly report events to EUDAMED since May 2011. In 2004, the guidelines published by the European Commission urged manufacturers to include both general and device-specific follow-up as part of their quality-assurance programs (Kramer et al., 2012b). There has been however reports of lapse in the overall system due to which safety of some of the released products were clearly not acceptable.

There are changes being brought about to further improve the regulatory process. According to Ruthanne Vendy (2017), the Council of the European Union has adopted the European Medical Device Regulations: MDR 2017/745, which were published in the Official Journal of the European Union and entered into force on May 26, 2017. The official date of application for the MDR will be May 26, 2020. The new EU MDR is replacing the Medical Device Directive: Council Directive 93/42/EEC and the Active Implantable Medical Device Directive: Council Directive 90/385/EEC (European Commission. Medical Devices Regulatory framework, 2018). The major change with this transition from directive to regulation is the new requirements surrounding clinical evidence. The key objectives of the new EU MDR is to ensure a high level of health and safety protection for EU citizens. Making clinical investigation and evaluation requirements more stringent is aimed at improving health and safety through transparency and traceability. If someone had difficulty in getting the clinical portion of technical documentation ready in the past, it would most likely lead to some additional hurdles; however, Under the new regulation, EUDAMED will integrate information regarding devices and the relevant economic operators, certain aspects of conformity assessment, notified bodies, certificates, clinical investigations, vigilance and market surveillance. This web-based portal will enhance information-sharing between Member States, economic operators, notified bodies, sponsors, and the Commission. Use of the EUDAMED database will not be optional anymore. For Class III devices and implantable, the mandatory summary of safety and clinical performance will be made available to the public via EUDAMED post-notified body validation.

FDA's Center for Devices and Radiological Health (CDRH) is responsible for regulating firms who manufacture, repackage, relabel, and/or import medical devices sold in the United States. In addition, CDRH regulates radiation-emitting electronic products (medical and non-medical) such as lasers, x-ray systems, ultrasound equipment, microwave ovens and color televisions (FDA, 2018c).

According to Kramer et al. (2012b) the Medical Device Amendments of 1976 gave the FDA primary authority to regulate medical devices and required the FDA to obtain "reasonable assurance of safety and effectiveness" before marketing. This legislation has been updated several times, including the Medical Device User Fee and Modernization Act of 2002, which established sponsor user fees for application reviews and set performance targets for review times. The review and approval process is different and based on the safety classification of the medical device. The process is explained in the section Medical Device Classification.

According to the Safe Medical Devices Act of 1990 (as cited in Kramer et al., 2012b) sites where cleared or approved devices are used must report related serious adverse events to the FDA and the manufacturer. These reports are stored in a searchable, publicly available database called Manufacturer and User Facility Device Experience (MAUDE). In addition, the FDA may conduct inspections, require manufacturers of high-risk devices to conduct post approval studies, and initiate recalls. Central coordination in the United States allows post market phenomena in one generation of devices to inform later applications and study designs. For example, specific criteria for trial design and end points have been developed to standardize the development of artificial heart valves and devices to treat congenital heart disease. These criteria also informed novel methods and statistical approaches to studying devices. A central registration system also provides publicly searchable listings and databases of adverse events.

The difference between the medical device regulation in United States and that in the European Union is summarized in Table 1.

One important factor that can be observed is that the regulations are still not harmonized to a level that can facilitate global release of medical devices under one unified process. However there are efforts being carried out by the Global Harmonization Task Force to find common elements and ways to unify the different national standards and regulatory practices (Cheng et al., World Health Organization, 2003). The GHTF is now known as International Medical Device Regulators Forum (IMDRF).

In Africa, the South African Department of Health has taken lead and issued new regulatory requirements covering both medical devices and in vitro diagnostic (IVD) devices by means of the Medicines and Related Substances Amendment Act 14 of 2015. Prior to this South Africa did not have a comprehensive regulatory framework that governed medical devices (T Saidi, T S Douglas, 2018).

In India, rules with regard to drugs were applied to medical devices, which led to burdensome regulations that delayed the development of the medical device industry. The new Medical Device Rules of 2017, separate the regulations for medical devices from those designed for the pharmaceutical sector. The rules are supposed to come into force with effect from 1st day of January, 2018.

Many of the proposed pre-screening solutions described in other chapters come under the broad scope of digital health which includes categories such as mobile health (mHealth), health information technology (IT), wearable devices, telehealth

Table 1. Differences in the device regulation in United States and European Union

Factor	United States	European Union
Purpose /structure	The FDA is a government agency mandated to protect the public's health.	Notified bodies regulate device approval as private companies. Competent authorities are government agencies that regulate postmarket surveillance of safety and facilitate trade among countries of the European Union.
Centralization	The FDA regulates device approval and surveillance under one umbrella.	More than 70 notified bodies regulate device approval separately. A competent authority in each of the countries of the European Union is tasked with device safety and surveillance.
Funding	Federal appropriations provide 80% of funding. User fees provide approximately 20% of funding.	Notified bodies are completely funded by contracts with device manufacturers. Funding of competent authorities varies by country.
Data requirement for approval	A device must prove to be safe and efficacious through premarket authorization approval or prove to be substantially equivalent to a predicate device through 510(k) clearance.	Proof is required that the device can perform its intended function
Premarket transparency	Proprietary limits exist on the sharing of information, but safety and approval data are shared through the FDA.	Approval decisions of the notified bodies are not made public.
Device surveillance	Reporting by manufacturers and healthcare institutions to the FDA is mandatory. Reporting by healthcare professionals and consumers is voluntary. The FDA can issue public health advisories, safety alerts, and product suspensions or withdrawals.	Manufacturers must submit adverse events to competent authorities. All adverse events have been required to be submitted to the European Databank on Medical Devices since 2011. Postmarket data are shared among competent authorities but not with the public. Competent authorities can issue adverse-event reports and field safety notices or device recalls.

Source: *Travis G. Maak, James D Wylie. (2016, May). Medical Device Regulation: A comparison of the United States and the European Union. The Journal of the American Academy of Orthopaedic Surgeons,* 24(8), 537-543

and telemedicine, and personalized medicine. According to FDA (2018d) Providers and other stakeholders are using digital health in their efforts to:

- Reduce inefficiencies
- Improve access
- Reduce costs
- Increase quality
- Make medicine more personalized for patients.

The FDA (2018d) reports that patients and consumers can use digital health to better manage and track their health and wellness related activities. The use of technologies such as smart phones, social networks and internet applications is not only changing the way we communicate, but is also providing innovative ways for us to monitor our health and well-being and giving us greater access to information. Together these advancements are leading to a convergence of people, information, technology and connectivity to improve health care and health outcomes. In case you are developing a mobile health app that collects, creates, or shares consumer information, check in the Mobile Health Apps Interactive Tool on Federal Trade Commission's website to find out whether FDA, Federal Trade Commission (FTC) or Office of Civil Rights (OCR) laws apply to your App. The tool asks 10 questions one of which is about the intended use;

Is your app intended for use in the diagnosis of disease or other conditions, or in the cure, mitigation, treatment or prevention of disease?

If the answer is yes, the tool clearly says that your app is a medical device subject to the Federal Food, Drug, and Cosmetic Act. It further asks to answer below question no. 6 to see if the FDA intends to apply its regulatory oversight for your type of app.

Does your app pose "minimal risk" to a user?

According to the FDA, "minimal risk" apps are those that are **only** intended for one or more of the following:

- helping users self-manage their disease or condition without providing specific treatment suggestions;
- providing users with simple tools to organize and track their health information;
- providing easy access to information related to health conditions or treatments;
- helping users document, show or communicate potential medical conditions to health care providers;
- automating simple tasks for health care providers;
- enabling users or providers to interact with Personal Health Records (PHR) or Electronic Health Record (EHR) systems; and
- transferring, storing, converting format or displaying medical device data, as defined by the FDA's Medical Device Data Systems regulations.

In case your app is intended for only one of the above and hence falls under a minimal risk app category, the FDA does not intend to enforce compliance with its regulatory requirements (Federal Trade Commission, 2016).

The 21st Century Cures Act released on 13 Dec 2016 clarified FDA's regulation of medical software. The new law amended the definition of "device" in the Food, Drug and Cosmetic Act to exclude certain software functions. There are three guidance documents related to Digital Health now available to clarify the FDA's position on digital health in relation to the 21st Century Cures Act and the regulation of digital health products internationally (FDA, 2018d).

What Is a Medical Device?

When we are discussing about a pre-screening solution being considered a medical device and hence comes under the purview of medical device regulations, it is important to first understand the definition of a medical device. Though the definitions may slightly vary between FDA (2018a) and MDD, it is in general similar to the one defined by the Global Harmonization Task Force (GHTF).

According to the World Health Organization (WHO, 2003) the GHTF has proposed the following harmonized definition for medical devices:

"Medical device" means any instrument, apparatus, implement, machine, appliance, implant, in vitro reagent or calibrator, software, material or other similar or related article, intended by the manufacturer to be used, alone or in combination, for human beings for one or more of the specific purposes of:

- diagnosis, prevention, monitoring, treatment or alleviation of disease
- diagnosis, monitoring, treatment, alleviation of or compensation for an injury
- investigation, replacement, modification, or support of the anatomy or of a physiological process
- supporting or sustaining life
- control of conception
- disinfection of medical devices
- providing information for medical purposes by means of in vitro examination of specimens derived from the human body and which does not achieve its primary intended action in or on the human body by pharmacological, immunological or metabolic means, but which may be assisted in its function by such means.

An accessory is generally not considered to be a medical device. However, where an accessory is intended specifically by its manufacturer to be used together with the 'parent' medical device to enable the medical device to achieve its intended purpose, it should be subjected to the same procedures and the GHTF guidance applicable to the medical device itself. The definition of a device for in vitro examination includes, for example, reagents, calibrators, sample collection devices, control materials, and related instruments or apparatus. The information provided by such an in vitro diagnostic device may be for diagnostic, monitoring or compatibility purposes. In some jurisdictions, reagents and the like may be covered by separate regulations. Products, which are considered to be medical devices in some jurisdictions but for which there is not yet a harmonized approach, are:

- aids for disabled/handicapped people
- devices for the treatment/diagnosis of diseases and injuries in animals
- spare parts for medical devices
- devices incorporating animal and human tissues which may meet the requirements of the above definition but be subject to different controls.

If you think about it, the purpose of all disease pre-screening is diagnosis and hence will fall under the first purpose "diagnosis, prevention, monitoring, treatment or alleviation of disease". Do all pre-screening systems fall under the classification of medical device? In general yes, but not always. To understand this better let us look at an important term called intended use or intended purpose which has far reaching consequence in medical device regulation. The intended purpose defined by a manufacturer for the pre-screening solution will define whether it will become a medical device or not. It will also further drive what device classification applies for the device.

As per the European Commission (2010), Intended purpose means the use for which the device is intended according to the data supplied by the manufacturer on the labelling, in the instructions and/or in promotional materials. The "intended use" of a device is critical for determining its safety classification, and is usually defined during the initial regulatory stages. However, the "intended use" is often misunderstood. Its purpose is not to describe what all the device is intended to be used for. Instead, it should clearly lay out the claims of what your device is meant to do. This is precisely why the device safety classification will be based on the intended use which in turn is, based on the manufacturer's claims. It is always recommended to keep the intended use statement concise, as long as it details all the fundamental claims appropriately. So if the manufacturer wants to keep the intended purpose to be limited to making user aware of the wellbeing and do not claim disease detection or diagnosis, the solution can potentially not be a medical device. But one should remember that by underplaying on the claims and intended purpose, you will also loose on the marketing advantage for the product.

It is also important to understand if your solution is a mobile medical app. A "mobile medical app" is one that is intended for any of the following:

- use as an accessory to a regulated medical device (for example, an app that alters the function or settings of an infusion pump)
- transforming a mobile platform into a regulated medical device (for example, an app that uses an attachment to the mobile platform to measure blood glucose levels)
- performing sophisticated analysis or interpreting data from another medical device (for example, an app that uses consumer-specific parameters and creates a dosage plan for radiation therapy)

Please note that many of the pre-screening mobile app based solutions could be using sophisticated analysis based on data from other vital signs devices. Hence some of these solutions could fall under the category of mobile medical app. The FDA is focusing its regulatory oversight on a small subset of mobile apps that may impact the performance or functionality of currently regulated medical devices or may independently pose a greater risk to consumers if they don't work as intended. Mobile medical apps that undergo FDA review will be evaluated according to the same regulatory standards and risk-based approach that the agency applies to other medical devices.

Medical Device Classification

Once you have defined the intended use based on the claims the next step is to complete the device classification. The safety classification of medical devices is always according to the perceived potential hazards.

According to the FDA (2018b) medical devices are generally classified based on the risks associated with the device and by evaluating the amount of regulation that provides a reasonable assurance of the device's safety and effectiveness. Devices are classified into one of three regulatory classes: Class I, Class II, or Class III. Class I devices include low-risk devices, such as stethoscopes, arm sling and mechanical wheel chair. They are assumed to be safe and effective if the tenets of good manufacturing practices, proper labeling, and adequate packaging and storage are followed. Class II devices are medium-risk devices, such as electrocardiographs, computed tomographic scanners, sutures and automated cell counter. They are more complex and must be proved to perform as expected. These moderate-risk devices generally pass through the 510(k) review pathway, which refers to the section of the Food, Drug, and Cosmetic Act dealing with premarket notification. In this process, the FDA and the manufacturer rely on similarities between the device at issue and a previously cleared device. If a manufacturer can show that its device is "substantially equivalent," additional clinical data are usually not required, although requirements for performance standards and post marketing surveillance may be imposed.

Class III devices are high-risk devices that require stringent safety and efficacy data for FDA approval unless they can be proved to be substantially equivalent to a predicate device (i.e., a device in use before 1976 or with proved safety and efficacy). Examples of class III devices include deep brain stimulators, implantable cardioverter– defibrillators, joint arthroplasty implants and spinal implants . Class III products require clinical studies evaluating the safety and effectiveness of the device, called a Premarket Approval (PMA) application. However, class III devices that arise from changes to previously PMA-approved devices may not need additional clinical studies. In addition, some older class III devices for which the FDA has not specifically called for PMAs can receive clearance through the 510(k) pathway (Travis G. Maak, James D Wylie., 2016).

According to Kramer et al. (2012b) devices that treat rare disorders (fewer than 4000 patients annually) may receive a Humanitarian Device Exemption and be approved on the basis of "probable" benefits, a more flexible standard that recognizes the difficulty of studying patient populations with small numbers and limited treatment options.

The European Union assigns three classes Class I, Class II and Class III with class II being further sub-divided into IIa and IIb (effectively four classes). Factors like the degree of invasiveness, duration of contact, the body system affected, and local versus systemic effects have to be taken in to account while assessing potential areas of hazard for classifying devices. This is because an invasive device is usually considered to have higher potential hazard than an equivalent non-invasive device. Similarly, devices that have a long duration of contact that affect vital organs such the heart or the great arteries, or that have systemic effects are assigned higher classes of potential hazard or risk. The degree of regulation imposed on any device is proportional to its potential hazard (Cheng et al., 2003).

GETTING YOUR DISEASE SCREENING SOLUTION MARKET READY

Design Controls

As explained in the previous section the medical regulations mandate the Medical device manufacturers to follow Design Control guidelines to ensure that the medical devices are safe for potential users before manufacturers start to market the devices. As a responsible owner of the disease screening solution, it is important to follow the design control process and steer through the regulatory compliance stages and get the solution ready for market release. Design controls are an interrelated set of practices and procedures that are incorporated into the design and development process, i.e., a system of checks and balances. Design control process is like a relay race with a baton being exchanged at every process stage. Design controls make systematic assessment of the design an integral part of development. As a result, deficiencies in design input requirements, and discrepancies between the proposed designs and requirements, are made evident and corrected earlier in the development process. Design controls increase the likelihood that the design transferred to production will translate into a device that is appropriate for its intended use. Design controls are supposed to be a component of a comprehensive quality system that covers the life of a device. The assurance process is a total systems approach that extends from the development of device requirements through design, production, distribution, use, maintenance, and eventually, obsolescence. Design control begins with development and approval of design inputs, and includes the design of a device and the associated manufacturing processes.

In case of the EU regulations, the design control process is part of the ISO13485. ISO 13485 specifies requirements for a quality management system where an organization needs to demonstrate its ability to provide medical devices and related services that consistently meet customer and applicable regulatory requirements. Such organizations can be involved in one or more stages of the life-cycle, including design and development, production, storage and distribution, installation, or servicing of a medical device and design and development or provision of associated activities (e.g. technical support). This International Standard can also be used by suppliers or external parties that provide product, including quality management system-related services to such organizations. Requirements of this International Standard are applicable to organizations regardless of their size and regardless of their type except where explicitly stated. Wherever requirements are specified as applying to medical devices, the requirements apply equally to associated services as supplied by the organization. The processes required by the International Standard that are applicable to the organization, but are not performed by the organization, are the responsibility of the organization and are accounted for in the organization's quality management system by monitoring, maintaining, and controlling the processes.

If applicable regulatory requirements permit exclusions of design and development controls, this can be used as a justification for their exclusion from the quality management system. These regulatory requirements can provide alternative approaches that are to be addressed in the quality management system. It is the responsibility of the organization to ensure that claims of conformity to the International Standard reflect any exclusion of design and development controls. For the EU directives, compliance with all the normative clauses in EN ISO 13485 will ensure that a process is in place to address quality system aspects related to medical devices, which are included in the conformity assessment annexes of the Directive. However, because the process standard is an adoption of an international standard, intended to be applicable in jurisdictions all over the world, the standard does not cover exactly the European quality system requirements. Therefore, for all of the quality system requirements, conformity is not entirely achieved by complying only with the requirements specified in the ISO13485 standard. Manufacturers and conformity assessment bodies need to also look at quality system requirements in the applicable Annex of the Directive and apply the same into the processes provided by the ISO13485 standard.

The FDA doesn't follow the ISO 13485 as it has different requirements for quality management. The quality management is defined in FDA QSR 21CFR part 820. Design controls in particular are defined under FDA 21CFR part 820.30 which has a similar intent to section 7.3 Design and Development described under the guidelines for ISO 13485. Additionally, FDA incorporates Current Good Manufacturing Practice (CGMP) requirements into the quality system regulation with an aim to follow good quality practices for medical devices designs. Design controls guideline is a quality system approach that covers the entire life of medical device starting from design, production, distribution, use, maintenance, and obsolescence.

The design and development process depicted below in Figure 1 is a traditional model in which design and development proceeds in a logical sequence of phases or stages. Basically, requirements are first developed, and then a medical device is created to meet those requirements. The medical device is then verified and validated, transferred to production, and the medical device is manufactured. In practice, feedback paths are necessary between each phase of the process and previous phases, representing the iterative nature of design and development. However, this detail has been omitted from Figure 1 to make the influence of design control on the design and development process more distinct.

The importance of the design and development inputs and verification of design and development outputs is illustrated by this example. When the input has been reviewed and determined to be acceptable, an iterative process of translating those inputs into a medical device begins. The first step is conversion of the inputs into system or high-level specifications. Thus, these specifications are a design and development output. Upon verification that the high-level specifications conform to the inputs, they become the design and development input for the next step in the design and development process, and so on. This basic technique is used repeatedly throughout the design and development process. Each input is converted into an output; each output is verified as conforming to its input; and it then becomes the input for another step in the process. In this manner, the inputs are translated into a medical device conforming to requirements. The importance of design and development reviews is also illustrated by the example. The reviews are conducted at strategic points in the design and development process. For example, a review is conducted to assure that the inputs are adequate before they are converted into outputs. Another review is used to assure that the outputs are adequate before prototypes are produced for simulated use testing or clinical evaluation. Another review is conducted prior to transfer of the medical device to production. Generally, reviews are used to provide assurance that an activity or phase has been completed in an acceptable manner, and that the next activity or phase can begin. As Figure 1 illustrates, design and development validation extends the assessment to address whether medical devices produced in accordance with the design and development process actually satisfy user needs and intended uses.

The Design Control guidance for Medical Device Manufacturers by FDA (1997) discusses an analogy from automobile design and development to help clarify these concepts. Fuel efficiency is a common requirement in automobile industry. This could be expressed as the number of kilometers-per-liter of a particular grade of fuel for a specified set of driving conditions. As the design and development of the automobile proceeds, requirements are converted into system and subsystem specifications needed for the automobile, including the fuel efficiency requirement. As these various systems and subsystems evolve, verification methods are used to establish conformance to specifications. Because several factors directly affect fuel efficiency, many of the verification activities help to provide confirmation that the overall output will meet the fuel efficiency requirement. This might include simulated road testing of prototypes or actual road testing. This establishes that

Figure 1. Application of Design Control to the Design and Development Process
Source: US FDA, Design Control Guidance for Medical Device Manufacturers, 1997

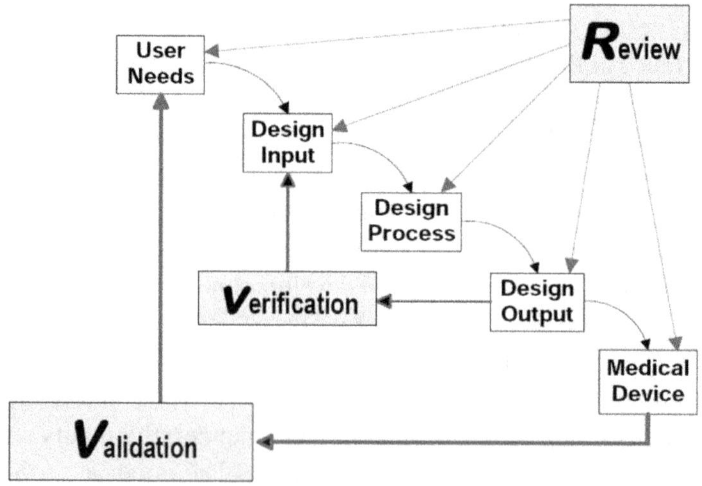

the output conforms to the fuel efficiency requirement using objective evidence. However, these verification activities alone are not sufficient to validate the fuel efficiency. The fuel efficiency could be validated when representative users have driven automobiles representative of production cars, under a specified range of driving conditions and judged the fuel efficiency to be adequate. This provides objective evidence that the particular requirement for a specific intended use can be consistently fulfilled.

Although the model in Figure 1 is a useful tool for introducing design control and the model does apply to the design and development of some simpler medical devices, its usefulness in practice is limited. This is because for more complex medical devices, above model does not directly apply and concurrent engineering model is more appropriate of the design and development processes in use in the medical device industry. In a traditional design and development scenario, the engineering department completes the design and development process and formally transfers the product specification to production. Subsequently, other groups or functions develop processes to manufacture and service the product. Historically, there has frequently been a divergence between the intent of the designer and the reality of the factory floor, resulting in such undesirable outcomes as low manufacturing yields, rework or redesign of product, or unexpectedly high cost to service the product.

One benefit of concurrent engineering is the involvement of production and service personnel throughout the design and development process, assuring the mutual optimization of the characteristics of a medical device and its related processes. While the primary motivations of concurrent engineering are shorter development time and reduced production cost, the practical result is often improved product quality. Concurrent engineering encompasses a range of practices and techniques. From a design control standpoint, it is sufficient to note that concurrent engineering can blur the line between design and development and production. On the one hand, the concurrent engineering model properly emphasizes that the development of production processes is a design and development rather than a manufacturing activity. On the other hand, various components of a medical device could enter production before the specification of the medical device as a whole has been approved. Thus, concurrent engineering and other more complex models of design and development usually require a comprehensive matrix of design and development reviews and approvals to ensure that each component and process is validated prior to entering production and the medical device as a whole is validated prior to release (FDA, Design Control guidance for Medical Device Manufacturers, 1997).

Software is often an integral part of medical devices and solutions and the proportion of software in medical devices is increasing day by day. Establishing the safety and effectiveness of a medical device containing software requires knowledge of what the software is intended to do and demonstration that the use of the software fulfils those intentions without causing any unacceptable risks. The IEC 62304: Medical device software – Software life cycle processes standard provides a framework of life cycle processes with activities and tasks necessary for the safe design and maintenance of medical device software. This standard provides requirements for each life cycle process and identifies two additional processes considered essential for developing safe medical device software; software configuration management process and software problem resolution process. The software risk management process required in the standard has to be embedded in the device risk management process.

Risk Management

Risk management is the systematic application of management policies, procedures, and practices to the tasks of identifying, analyzing, controlling, and monitoring risk. It is intended to be a framework within which experience, insight, and judgment are applied to successfully manage risk. Risk management begins with the identification of the design and development inputs. As the medical device proceeds through the design and development process, new risks could become evident. An organization's system has to identify and, when necessary, reduce these risks. The risk management process is integrated into the design and development process. In this way, risks can be identified and managed earlier in the design and development process when changes are easier to make and less costly. An example of this could be an exposure control system for a general-purpose x-ray system. The control function was intended to be achieved through software. If the risk management system discovered several failure modes that could not be controlled by the software until late in the design and development process, risk analysis of the system uncovered several failure modes that could not be controlled by the software and an expensive design change to add a back-up timer would have to be implemented to mitigate a potential overexposure to the patient to an acceptable level.

ISO 14971 is a standard that specifies a process for a manufacturer to identify the hazards associated with medical devices, including in vitro diagnostic (IVD) medical devices, to estimate and evaluate the associated risks, to control these risks, and to monitor the effectiveness of the controls. The requirements of ISO 14971 are applicable to all stages of the life-cycle of a medical device. Hazards traditionally considered in risk analysis include:

- Physical hazards (e.g., sharp corners or edges),
- Mechanical hazards (e.g., kinetic or potential energy from a moving object),
- Thermal hazards (e.g., high-temperature components),

- Electrical hazards (e.g., electrical current, electromagnetic interference (EMI)),
- Chemical hazards (e.g., toxic chemicals),
- Radiation hazards (e.g., ionizing and non-ionizing), and
- Biological hazards (e.g., allergens, bio-incompatible agents and infectious agents).

These hazards are generally associated with instances of device or component failure that are not dependent on how the user interacts with the device.

Human Factors Engineering or Usability Engineering

Manufacturers should follow human factors or usability engineering processes during the development of new medical devices, focusing specifically on the user interface, where the user interface includes all points of interaction between the product and the user(s) including elements such as displays, controls, packaging, product labels, instructions for use, etc. It is clear that these processes can be beneficial for optimizing user interfaces in other respects (e.g., maximizing ease of use, efficiency, and user satisfaction), but the main purpose of these processes is to ensure that devices are safe and effective for the intended users, uses, and use environments. The goal is to ensure that the device user interface has been designed such that use errors that occur during use of the device that could cause harm or degrade medical treatment are either eliminated or reduced to the extent possible. As explained in previous section as part of design controls, manufacturers conduct a risk analysis that includes the risks associated with device use and the measures implemented to reduce those risks (FDA, 2016).

ISO 14971, Medical Devices – Application of risk management to medical devices, defines risk as the combination of the probability of occurrence of harm and the severity of the potential harm. However, because probability is very difficult to determine for use errors, and in fact many use errors cannot be anticipated until device use is simulated and observed, the severity of the potential harm is more meaningful for determining the need to eliminate (design out) or reduce resulting harm. If the results of risk analysis indicate that use errors could cause serious harm to the patient or the device user, then the manufacturer should apply appropriate human factors or usability engineering processes.

Human factors testing is a valuable component of product development for medical devices and it is recommended that manufacturers consider human factors testing for medical devices as a part of a robust design control subsystem. In case of PMA or 510(k) submissions, for those devices where an analysis of risk indicates that users performing tasks incorrectly or failing to perform tasks could result in serious harm, manufacturers should submit human factors data as part of the premarket submissions (FDA, 2016).

Similar to the guidance issued by CDRH of FDA, for the European Union, the standard IEC 62366-1: Medical devices: Part 1: Application of usability engineering to medical devices specifies a Process for a manufacturer to analyze, specify, develop and evaluate the usability of a medical device as it relates to safety. IEC62366-2: Medical devices. Part 2: Guidance on the application of usability engineering to medical devices further shares background information and provides guidance that addresses specific areas that experience suggests can be helpful for those implementing a Usability Engineering (Human Factors Engineering) Process. This process permits the manufacturer to assess and mitigate risks associated with correct use and use errors i.e., normal use. It can be used to identify but does not assess or mitigate risks associated with abnormal use. The standard has been updated to include contemporary concepts of usability engineering, while also streamlining the process. It now strengthens links to ISO 14971 and the related methods of risk management as applied to safety related aspects of medical device user interfaces.

Security and Privacy Risk Management

I would urge all the readers to give a special focus on this topic which typically goes off the mind of the system designer or developer purely because the threats posed due to security and privacy are typically latent and not very explicit. Off late one of the key concerns of all the regulatory bodies is the lack of adequate security and privacy threat management in medical devices and solutions. Kramer, Baker, and Ransford (2012a), brings out that to detect a security or privacy problem that could harm patients, a more effective information sharing system for medical device cybersecurity should be established.

The need for effective cybersecurity to assure medical device functionality and safety has become more important with the increasing use of wireless, Internet- and network- connected devices, and the frequent electronic exchange of medical device-related health information. The FDA has issued guidance in 2014 to assist industry in identifying issues related to cybersecurity that manufacturers should consider in the design and development of their medical devices as well as in preparing premarket submissions for those devices. The new guidelines mandate the manufacturer to address cybersecurity during the “design and development” of the medical device. The FDA expects that the following are covered in the pre-market approval submissions (FDA, 2014)

- A specific list of all cybersecurity risks (both intentional and unintentional) that were considered in the design of the device and a list, and justification for all cybersecurity controls that were established for the device;
- A "traceability matrix" that links the actual cybersecurity controls to the cybersecurity risks that were considered;
- A summary describing the plan for providing validated software updates and patches as needed throughout the lifecycle of the medical device to continue to assure its safety and effectiveness;
- A summary describing controls that are in place to assure that the medical device software will remain free of malware from the point of origin to the point at which that device leaves the control of the manufacturer; and
- Device instructions for use and product specifications related to recommended cybersecurity controls appropriate for the intended use environment.

Data security and privacy is an important aspect. Many of the pre-screening solutions discussed in other chapters proposed use of artificial intelligence, be it machine learning or deep learning using big data to arrive at early prediction of diseases as tool for pre-screening. One should realize that there are strict policies to be adhered to when patient data is being handled. The Health Insurance Portability and Accountability Act (HIPAA) have clearly defined rules and are applicable to all covered entities and business associates. Depending on the services provided with the medical devices, manufacturers or the subcontractors can be in the scope of business associates. For example, if the device is used within a health plan, manufacturers are indirectly impacted by the physical and technical safeguards of the HIPAA. These safeguards affect the design of medical devices with additional rules that add new requirements like:

- Unique user identification,
- Automatic logoff,
- Backup and restore,
- Export of a copy of health data of a person.

The latest GDPR, or General Data Protection Regulation, is a regulation from the European Union that is intended to strengthen and further harmonize data protection laws across EU, while at the same time addressing new technological developments. Not only EU based companies but organizations outside the EU who target consumers inside Europe, will be subject to the rules and requirements of the GDPR. This regulation comes into force from 25 May 2018, and has broad implications for companies who process personal data. The GDPR is a significant step-up of the privacy rules as they apply in Europe (and often also outside of Europe).

Regulatory Strategy and Plan

One of the important aspect of the medical device design and development is to have a clear regulatory strategy and plan from the beginning. The strategy is linked with the business marketing plan for the product. The first and foremost input here is the list of countries for which the solution is targeted for release and the plan. The plan could have a phased approach with few countries requiring additional controls, country regulations, or localization being targeted later to the initial release. It is important to understand that apart from the product compliance and getting the CE mark, there is a need to get the country registration for the product. Based on the target countries it would be clear if only a CE marking or FDA approval is required or both. In case of other geographies outside of the purview of European Union directives or the FDA the relevant regulatory compliance should be targeted. The intended use gets defined in the customer requirement specification or user needs document. Based on the intended use and other guidelines the device classification is arrived at. As part of defining the design inputs, remember that there are following sources for the design inputs.

- User Needs including the customer requirements gathered from clinical specialists and product marketing specialists
- Requirements coming out of risk management including the usability engineering inputs
- Requirements coming out of security and privacy risk assessments
- Requirements coming out of IEC standards; performance, safety and electromagnetic compatibility (EMC) standards

Let us briefly understand the last point, performance, safety and EMC standards in little more detail. IEC 60601 is a series of technical standards for the safety and essential performance of medical electrical equipment, published by the International Electrotechnical Commission. It consists of a general standard, about 10 collateral standards, and about 60 particular standards. The general standard IEC 60601-1 - Medical electrical equipment - Part 1: General requirements for basic safety and essential performance - gives general requirements of the series of standards. IEC 60601 is a widely accepted benchmark for medical electrical equipment and compliance with IEC60601-1 has become a requirement for the commercialization of electrical medical equipment in many countries. The IEC 60601-1 has undergone many revisions time to time over the years in order to remain adaptive and up-to-date with newer medical technologies. The latest set of changes was introduced with the 2012 publication of Amendment 1 to IEC 60601-1. This standard includes the requirements for essential performance, commands usability engineering evaluations and human factor consideration, and mandates the adoption of a formal development life cycle process for software. The general standard applies for all medical devices, the collateral standards and particular standards only apply depending on the specific device. For example, the IEC60601-1-11 will only apply if the device is intended to be used outside of the clinical setting in a home use environment. One of the key input to be covered in regulatory plan is to identify all the applicable standards for the product.

Once the system requirements (design inputs) are derived from all the sources listed above, apply the design control process to review and develop the design outputs. That is followed by the design verification to evidence that device is designed right. The verification is then followed by the design validation to conform that the right product is designed.

Design and Development File

The design and development file is a formal document that is prepared for each medical device or family of medical devices and describes the design history of a medical device. As this file provides history of the product, it is important that it is controlled and maintained. The file can be either a collection of the actual documents generated in the design and development process or an index of documents and their storage location. The compilation of the design and development records is also known as the Design History File (DHF). The design and development file contains references in the records necessary to demonstrate that the medical device was developed in accordance with the approved plan, that it performs as intended and that the appropriate requirements for the medical device have been met. The file is necessary so that your organization can exercise control over and be accountable for the design and development process, thereby increasing the probability that the medical device conforms to the design and development requirements. This file can include, but is not limited to:

- Results of engineering, laboratory, simulated use, animal tests and evaluation of published literature applicable to the medical device or substantially similar medical devices regarding the safety of the medical device and its conformity with its specifications;
- Detailed information regarding test design, complete test or study protocols, methods of data analysis, in addition to data summaries and test results and conclusions regarding:
    - Biocompatibility (identifying all materials in direct or indirect contact with the patient or user);
    - Physical, chemical and microbiological characteristics;

 - Electrical safety and electromagnetic compatibility;
 - Stability/shelf life;
- Software verification and validation describing the software design and development process and evidence of the validation of the software, including the summary results of all verification, validation and testing performed both in-house and in a simulated or actual user environment prior to final release, addressing all of the different hardware configurations and, where applicable, operating systems identified in the information supplied by the manufacturer;
- Evidence of application of the principles of good laboratory practice and the verification of their applications for tests on chemical substances;
- The report on the clinical evaluation;
- Post market clinical follow-up plan and post market clinical follow-up evaluation report;
- Regulatory strategy and submission documentation.

DISCUSSION

The goal of disease pre-screening is to detect potential health disorders or diseases in people who do not have clear visible symptoms of disease. Because of the intended purpose of doing a diagnosis, pre-screening solutions fall under the category of medical device. Safety and regulatory aspects are critical component in the design, development and sustenance of a medical device. In order to get into the market, the medical device needs to comply with regulatory compliances defined by the medical regulatory body, subject to both regional and international standards. For system designers or researchers developing systems for diseases pre-screening it is important to very clearly understand the safety and regulatory aspects. Understanding the intent and reasoning behind the medical device regulations enables us to bring in the right rigor in our approach towards setting up and enforcing the design control process requirements and the design documentation. Conceptualizing a disease pre-screening solution and creating a proof of concept or a laboratory model is a great achievement, but remember that it is just the beginning of the challenging transformation journey required to make a market ready solution.

REFERENCES

Chai, J. Y. (2000). Medical device regulation in the United States and the European Union: A comparative study. *Food and Drug Law Journal*, *55*(1), 57–80. PMID:12296349

Cheng, D. M. (2003). *Medical Device Regulations: Global overview and guiding principles*. WHO.

eInfochips (2017). *A Definitive Guide to Medical Device Design and Development*. Retrieved from https://www.einfochips.com/resources/publications/a-definitive-guide-to-medical-device-design-and-development/

European Commission. (2018, April). *The new Regulations on medical devices*. https://ec.europa.eu/growth/sectors/medical-devices/regulatory-framework_en

European Commission. (2010, June). *DG Health and Consumer. Guidelines Relating to the Application of the Council Directive 93/42/EEC on Medical Devices*. Guidance document - Classification of medical devices. MEDDEV 2. 4/1 Rev. 9.

FDA - U.S. Department of Health and Human Services, Food and Drug Administration. (2014). *Content of Premarket Submissions for Management of Cybersecurity in Medical Devices*. FDA.

FDA - U.S. Department of Health and Human Services, Food and Drug Administration. (2016). *Applying Human Factors and Usability Engineering to Medical Devices*. FDA.

Federal Trade Commission (2016). *Mobile Health Apps Interactive Tool*. Author.

FDA - US Food and Drug Administration, Center for Devices and Radiological Health. (1997, March). *Design Control Guidance for Medical Device Manufacturers*. FDA.

FDA- US Food and Drug Administration. (2018a). *Is The Product A Medical Device?* FDA.

FDA - US Food and Drug Administration. (2018b). *Reclassification*. FDA.

FDA- US Food and Drug Administration. (2018c). *Overview of Device Regulation*. FDA.

FDA -US Food and Drug Administration. (2018d). *Digital Health*. FDA.

Kramer, D. B., Baker, M., Ransford, B., Molina-Markham, A., Stewart, Q., Fu, K., & Reynolds, M. R. (2012a). *Security and Privacy Qualities of Medical Devices: An Analysis of FDA Postmarket Surveillance*. Public Library of Science.

Kramer, D. B., Xu, S., & Kesselheim, A. S. (2012b). Regulation of medical devices in the United States and European Union. *The New England Journal of Medicine*, *366*(9), 848–855. doi:10.1056/NEJMhle1113918 PMID:22332952

Saidi, T., & Douglas, T. S. (2018). Medical device regulation in South Africa: The Medicines and Related Substances Amendment Act 14 of 2015. *South African Medical Journal, 108*(3), 168–170. doi:10.7196/SAMJ.2018.v108i3.12820

Travis, G. (2016, May). Medical Device Regulation: A comparison of the United States and the European Union. *The Journal of the American Academy of Orthopaedic Surgeons, 24*(8), 537–543. doi:10.5435/JAAOS-D-15-00403 PMID:27195383

Vendy, R. (2017, November). *EU MDR and Clinical Evidence: What You Need to Know.* Retrieved from https://www.meddeviceonline.com/doc/eu-mdr-and-clinical-evidence-what-you-need-to-know-0001

ADDITIONAL READING

International Organization for Standardization. (2017). *ISO13485 (2016) Medical Devices: A Practical Guide.*

International Organization for Standardization. (2007). *ISO 14971:2007 Medical Devices: Application of risk management to medical devices.* ISO.

Study Group 1 of the Global Harmonization Task Force. (2007, March). *Summary Technical Documentation for Demonstrating Conformity to the Essential Principles of Safety and Performance of Medical Devices (STED).* Retrieved from http://www.imdrf.org/docs/ghtf/archived/sg1/technical-docs/ghtf-sg1-n011r20-essential-principles-safety-performance-medical-devices-sted.pdf

The International Electrotechnical Commission. (2015). *IEC 62304: Medical device software – Software life cycle processes.*

Compilation of References

Abdollah, F., Dalela, D., Dalela, D., Haffner, M. C., Culig, Z., & Schalken, J. (2015). *The Role of Biomarkers and Genetics in the Diagnosis of Prostate Cancer*. doi:10.1016/j.euf.2015.08.001

Abed, A., Alkhatib, A., & Baicher, G. S. (2012). Wireless Sensor Network Architecture. *International Conference on Computer Networks and Communication Systems, 35*, 11–15.

Abiodun, O. A., Olu-Abiodun, O. O., Sotunsa, J. O., & Oluwole, F. A. (2014). Impact of health education intervention on knowledge and perception of cervical cancer and cervical screening uptake among adult women in rural communities in Nigeria. *BMC Public Health, 14*(814), 1–9. doi:10.1186/1471-2458-14-814 PMID:25103189

Acharya, A. S., Prakash, A., Saxena, P., & Nigam, A. (2013). *Sampling: Why and How of it?* Academic Press.

Ahmed, W., Shaikh, Z. N., Soomro, J. A., Qazi, H. A., & Soomro, A. K. (2018). Assessment of health literacy in adult population of Karachi: A preliminary investigation for concept-based evidence. *International Journal of Health Promotion and Education, 56*(2), 95–104. doi:10.1080/14635240.2017.1421866

Akande, K. O., Owolabi, T. O., Twaha, S., & Olatunji, S. O. (2014). Performance comparison of SVM and ANN in predicting compressive strength of concrete. *IOSR Journal of Computer Engineering, 16*(5), 88–94. doi:10.9790/0661-16518894

Albinati, J., Meira, W., & Pappa, G. L. (2016). An Accurate Gaussian Process-Based Early Warning System for Dengue Fever. In Intelligent Systems (BRACIS) (pp. 43-48). IEEE.

Alcaraz, R., Abásolo, D., Hornero, R., & Rieta, J. J. (2010). Optimal parameters study for sample entropy-based atrial fibrillation organization analysis. *Computer Methods and Programs in Biomedicine, 99*(1), 124–132. doi:10.1016/j.cmpb.2010.02.009 PMID:20392514

Alemdar, H. (2015). *Human activity recognition with wireless sensor networks using machine learning* (Doctoral dissertation). Bogaziçi University.

Ali, F., Islam, S. R., Kwak, D., Khan, P., Ullah, N., Yoo, S. J., & Kwak, K. S. (2017). Type-2 fuzzy ontology–aided recommendation systems for IoT–based healthcare. *Computer Communications*.

Aljumah, Ahamad, & Siddiqui. (2012). Application of data mining: Diabetes health care in young and old patients. *Journal of King Saud University – Computer and Information Sciences, 25*, 127–136.

Althouse, B. M., Ng, Y. Y., & Cummings, D. A. (2011). Prediction of dengue incidence using search query surveillance. *PLoS Neglected Tropical Diseases, 5*(8), e1258. doi:10.1371/journal.pntd.0001258 PMID:21829744

Ancker, J. S., Brenner, S., Richardson, J. E., Silver, M., & Kaushal, R. (2015). Trends in Public Perceptions of Electronic Health Records During Early Years of Meaningful Use. *The American Journal of Managed Care, 21*(8), e487–e493. PMID:26625503

Andreeva, P. (2006). Data modelling and specific rule generation via data mining techniques, *Proc. International Conference on Computer Systems and Technologies,* 17–23.

Anguita, D., Ghio, A., Oneto, L., Parra, X., & Reyes-Ortiz, J. L. (2013, April). A Public Domain Dataset for Human Activity Recognition using Smartphones. ESANN.

Antropova, N., Huynh, B. Q., & Giger, M. L. (2017). A deep feature fusion methodology for breast cancer diagnosis demonstrated on three imaging modality datasets. *Medical Physics Online, 44*(10), 5162–5171. doi:10.1002/mp.12453 PMID:28681390

Arevalo, J., González, F. A., Ramos-Pollán, R., Oliveira, J. L., & Guevara Lopez, M. A. (2016). Representation learning for mammography mass lesion classification with convolutional neural networks. *Computer Methods and Programs in Biomedicine, 127*, 248–257. doi:10.1016/j.cmpb.2015.12.014 PMID:26826901

Aribarg, T., Supratid, S., & Lursinsap, C. (2012). Optimizing the modified fuzzy ant-miner for efficient medical diagnosis. *Applied Intelligence, 37*(3), 357–376. doi:10.100710489-011-0332-x

Asuncion, A., & Newman, D. (2007). *UCI machine learning repository*. Academic Press.

Athanasios, T., Eleazar, G.-H., Ali, Y., & Benjamin, D. (2011). Designing patient-centric applications for chronic disease management. *Proceedings of the Annual International Conference of the IEEE Engineering in Medicine and Biology Society, EMBS*, 3146–3149. 10.1109/IEMBS.2011.6090858

Atlas, L., Cole, R., Connor, J. T., El-Sharkawi, M. A., Marks, R. J. II, ... Barnard, E. (1990). Performance comparisons betweenbackpropagation networks and classification trees on three real world applications. *Advances in Neural Information Processing Systems*, *2*, 622–629.

Attia, S. J., Blackledge, J. M., Abood, Z. M., & Agool, I. R. (2012). *Diagnosis of Breast Cancer by Optical Image Analysis*. ISSC. doi:10.1049/ic.2012.0198

Attié, E., & Meyer-Waarden, L. (2017). *The Impacts of Social Value*. Cognitive Factors and Well-Being on the Use of the Internet of Things and Smart Connected Objects.

Austin, P. C., Lee, D. S., Steyerberg, E. W., & Tu, J. V. (2012). Regression trees for predicting mortality in patients with cardiovascular disease: What improvement is achieved by using ensemble-based methods? *Biometrical Journal. Biometrische Zeitschrift*, *54*(5), 657–673. doi:10.1002/bimj.201100251 PMID:22777999

Australian Institute of Primary Care. (2008). Measuring health promotion impacts : A guide to impact evaluation in integrated health promotion. *Community Health*.

Baig, M. M., GholamHosseini, H., & Linden, M. (2015). Tablet-based patient monitoring and decision support systems in hospital care. *Conference Proceedings: ... Annual International Conference of the IEEE Engineering in Medicine and Biology Society. IEEE Engineering in Medicine and Biology Society. Annual Conference*, *2015*, 1215–8. 10.1109/EMBC.2015.7318585

Bakic, P. R., Ringer, P., Kuo, J., Ng, S., & Maidment, A. D. (2010). Analysis of Geometric Accuracy in Digital Breast Tomosynthesis Reconstruction. *IWDM*, *2010*, 62–69.

Baldus, S. E., Engelmann, K., & Hanisch, F. G. (2004). MUC1 and the MUCs: A family of human mucins with impact in cancer biology. *Critical Reviews in Clinical Laboratory Sciences*, *41*(2), 189–231. doi:10.1080/10408360490452040 PMID:15270554

Balthazar, E. J., Robinson, D. L., Megibow, A. J., & Ranson, J. (1990). Acute pancreatitis: Value of CT in establishing prognosis. *Radiology*, *174*(2), 331–336. doi:10.1148/radiology.174.2.2296641 PMID:2296641

Banaee, H., Ahmed, M. U., & Loutfi, A. (2013). Data mining for wearable sensors in health monitoring systems: A review of recent trends and challenges. *Sensors (Basel)*, *13*(12), 17472–17500. doi:10.3390131217472 PMID:24351646

Bandodkar, A. J., Jia, W., Yardımcı, C., Wang, X., Ramirez, J., & Wang, J. (2015). Tattoo-based noninvasive glucose monitoring: A proof-of-concept study. *Analytical Chemistry*, *87*(1), 394–398. doi:10.1021/ac504300n PMID:25496376

Bandt, C., & Pompe, B. (2002). Permutation entropy: A natural complexity measure for time series. *Physical Review Letters*, *88*(17), 174102. doi:10.1103/PhysRevLett.88.174102 PMID:12005759

Bardhan, I., Oh, J. H., Zheng, Z., & Kirksey, K. (2014). Predictive analytics for readmission of patients with congestive heart failure. *Information Systems Research*, *26*(1), 19–39. doi:10.1287/isre.2014.0553

Barer, M. (2017). *Why are Some People Healthy and Others Not?* (M. Barer, Ed.). New York: Routledge.

Barizuddin, S., Bok, S., & Gangopadhyay, S. (2016). Plasmonic Sensors for Disease Detection - A Review [Abstract]. *Journal of Nanomedicine & Nanotechnology*, *7*, 373. doi:10.4172/2157-7439.1000373

Barua, M., Liang, X., Lu, R., & Shen, X. (2011). ESPAC: Enabling Security and Patient-centric Access Control for eHealth in cloud computing. *International Journal of Security and Networks*, *6*(2/3), 67. doi:10.1504/IJSN.2011.043666

Bates, D. W., & Bitton, A. (2010). The future of health information technology in the patient-centered medical home. *Health Affairs*, *29*(4), 614–621. doi:10.1377/hlthaff.2010.0007 PMID:20368590

Bauer, H., Patel, M., & Veira, J. (2014, December). *The Internet of Things: Sizing up the opportunity*. McKinsey & Company. Retrieved February 21, 2018, from https://www.mckinsey.com/industries/semiconductors/our-insights/the-internet-of-things-sizing-up-the-opportunity

Bayramoglu, N., & Heikkila, J. (2016). Transfer learning for cell nuclei classification in histopathology images. In Computer Vision–ECCV 2016 Workshops (pp. 532–539). Springer.

Behara, S. K., & Das, S. (2017.). Integrated Non-Invasive Biomedical Sensor Module for Measurement of Vital Signs of Human Body for Remote Health Monitoring. *International Journal of Advanced Research in Electrical, Electronics and Instrumentation Engineering, 6*(7). Retrieved July, 2017, from www.ijareeie.com

Bellazzi, R., & Zupan, B. (2008). Predictive data mining in clinical medicine: Current issues and guidelines. *International Journal of Medical Informatics*, *77*(2), 81–97. doi:10.1016/j.ijmedinf.2006.11.006 PMID:17188928

Belle, A., Thiagarajan, R., Soroushmehr, S. M., Navidi, F., Beard, D. A., & Najarian, K. (2015). Big data analytics in healthcare. *BioMed Research International*. PMID:26229957

Beloufa, F., & Chikh, M. (2013). Design of fuzzy classifier for diabetes disease using modified artificial bee colony algorithm. *Computer Methods and Programs in Biomedicine*, *112*(1), 92–103. doi:10.1016/j.cmpb.2013.07.009 PMID:23932385

Bergman, B., Neuhauser, D., & Provost, L. (2011). Five main processes in healthcare: a citizen perspective. *BMJ Quality & Safety, 20*(Suppl_1), i41-2. doi:10.1136/bmjqs.2010.046409

Berkman, N. D., Sheridan, S. L., Donahue, K. E., Halpern, D. J., & Crotty, K. (2011). Low health literacy and health outcomes: An updated systematic review. *Annals of Internal Medicine*, *155*(2), 97–107. doi:10.7326/0003-4819-155-2-201107190-00005 PMID:21768583

Betschart, P., Zumstein, V., Ali, O. H., Schmid, H. P., & Abt, D. (2018). Readability assessment of patient education material published by German-speaking associations of urology. *Urologia Internationalis*, *100*(1), 79–84. doi:10.1159/000480095 PMID:29151111

Bhat, Rao, & Shenoy. (2009). An Efficient Prediction Model for Diabetic Database Using Soft Computing Techniques. In *Architecture*. Springer-Verlag.

Bihani, P., & Patil, S. T. (2014). A comparative study of data analysis techniques. *International Journal of Emerging Trends & Technology in Computer Science, 3*(2), 95-101.

Bluestone, J. A., Herold, K., & Eisenbarth, G. (2010). Genetics, pathogenesis and clinical interventions in type 1 diabetes. *Nature*, *464*(7293), 1293–1300. doi:10.1038/nature08933 PMID:20432533

Bortolotti, D., Mangia, M., Bartolini, A., Rovatti, R., Setti, G., & Benini, L. (2016). Energy-aware bio-signal compressed sensing reconstruction on the WBSN-gateway. *IEEE Transactions on Emerging Topics in Computing*, 1. doi:10.1109/TETC.2016.2564361

Bosse, E., Roy, J., & Grenier, D. (1996, May). *Data fusion concepts applied to a suite of dissimilar sensors*. In *Electrical and Computer Engineering, 1996. Canadian Conference on* (Vol. 2, pp. 692-695). IEEE. 10.1109/CCECE.1996.548247

Boulton, A. J. M., & Vinik, A. J. (2005). AI and Brief Clinical. *Diabetes Care, 28*(4), 956–962.

Bourouis, A., Feham, M., Hossain, M. A., & Zhang, L. (2014). An intelligent mobile based decision support system for retinal disease diagnosis. *Decision Support Systems*, *59*, 341–350. doi:10.1016/j.dss.2014.01.005

Brand, C. S. (2012). Management of retinal vascular diseases: A patient-centric approach. *Eye (Basingstoke)*, *26*(S2), S1–S16. doi:10.1038/eye.2012.32 PMID:22495396

Breiman, L. (1996). Bagging predictors. *Machine Learning*, *24*(2), 123–140. doi:10.1007/BF00058655

Breiman, L., Friedman, J., Stone, C. J., & Olshen, R. A. (1984). *Classification and regression trees*. Chapman and Hall/CRC.

Brentani, H., Paula, C. S., Bordini, D., Rolim, D., Sato, F., Portolese, J., & McCracken, J. T. (2013). Autism spectrum disorders: An overview on diagnosis and treatment. *RevistaBrasileira De Psiquiatria*. doi:. doi:10.1590/1516-4446-2013-S104

Brownstein, J. S., Freifeld, C. C., Reis, B. Y., & Mandl, K. D. (2008). Surveillance sans frontières: Internet-based emerging infectious disease intelligence and the HealthMap project. *PLoS Medicine*, *5*(7), 1019–1024. doi:10.1371/journal.pmed.0050151 PMID:18613747

Broza, Y.Y., & Haick, H. (2013). Nanomaterial-based sensors for detection of disease by volatile organic compounds. *Nanomedicine,* (8), 785-806. doi:10.2217/nnm.13.64

Buckley, Feuring, & Hayashi. (n.d.). Multivariate non-linear fuzzy regression: an evolutionary algorithm approach. *International Journal of Uncertainty*.

Buckley, J. J., & Feuring, T. (2000). Linear and non-linear fuzzy regression: Evolutionary algorithm solutions. *Fuzzy Sets and Systems*, *112*(3), 381–394. doi:10.1016/S0165-0114(98)00154-7

Buckley, J. J., & Jowers, L. J. (2008). *Fuzzy Linear Regression I. Studies in Fuzziness and Soft Computing* (Vol. 22). Springer.

Buechi, R., Faes, L., Bachmann, L. M., Thiel, M. A., Bodmer, N. S., Schmid, M. K., ... Lienhard, K. R. (2017). Evidence assessing the diagnostic performance of medical smartphone apps: A systematic review and exploratory meta-analysis. *BMJ Open*, *7*(12), e018280. doi:10.1136/bmjopen-2017-018280 PMID:29247099

Bujlow, T., Riaz, M. T., & Pedersen, J. M. (2012). A method for classification of network traffic based on C5.0 machine learning algorithm. *Proc. of the International Conference on Computing, Networking and Communications (ICNC)*, 237–241. 10.1109/ICCNC.2012.6167418

Burges, C., Shaked, T., Renshaw, E., Lazier, A., Deeds, M., Hamilton, N., & Hullender, G. (2005, August). Learning to rank using gradient descent. In *Proceedings of the 22nd international conference on Machine learning* (pp. 89-96). ACM.

Burke, H. B., Bostwick, D. G., & Meiers, I. (2005). Prostate cancer outcome: Epidemiology and biostatistics. *Analytical and Quantitative Cytology and Histology*, *27*, 211–217. PMID:16220832

Businessdictionary. (2018). Retrieved from http://www.businessdictionary.com/definition/diagnosis.html

Camm, A. J., Lip, G. Y., De Caterina, R., Savelieva, I., Atar, D., & Hohnloser, S. H. (2012). 2012 focused update of the ESC Guidelines for the management of atrial fibrillation: an update of the 2010 ESC Guidelines for the management of atrial fibrillation. Developed with the special contribution of the European Heart Rhythm association. *European Heart Journal, 33*(21), 2719.

Campbell, J., Gibbons, P., Nath, S., Pillai, P., Seshan, S., & Sukthankar, R. (2005). IrisNet: an internet-scale architecture for multimedia sensors. In *Proceedings of the 13th annual ACM international conference on Multimedia* (pp. 81–88). ACM Digital Library. 10.1145/1101149.1101162

Capriotti, E., & Altman, R. B. (2011). A new disease-specific machine learning approach for the prediction of cancer-causing missense variants. *Genomics*, *98*(4), 310–317. doi:10.1016/j.ygeno.2011.06.010 PMID:21763417

Carrara, M., Carozzi, L., Moss, T. J., De Pasquale, M., Cerutti, S., Ferrario, M., ... Moorman, J. R. (2015). Heart rate dynamics distinguish among atrial fibrillation, normal sinus rhythm and sinus rhythm with frequent ectopy. *Physiological Measurement*, *36*(9), 1873–1888. doi:10.1088/0967-3334/36/9/1873 PMID:26246162

Case Western Reserve University. (2017). *New Machine-learning program shows promise for early Alzheimer's diagnosis*. Retrieved from http://thedaily.case.edu/new-machine-learning-program-shows-promise-early-alzheimers-diagnosis/

Catanuto, G., Spano, A., Pennati, A., Riggio, E., Farinella, G. M., Impoco, G., & Nava, M. B. (2006). *Experimental methodology for digital breast shape analysis and objective surgical outcome evaluation. Journal of Plastic, Reconstructive, & Aesthetic Surgery*. doi:10.1016/j.bjps.2006.11.016

Cavallari, R., Martelli, F., Rosini, R., Buratti, C., & Verdone, R. (2014). A survey on wireless body area networks: Technologies and design challenges. *IEEE Communications Surveys and Tutorials*, *16*(3), 1635–1657. doi:10.1109/SURV.2014.012214.00007

Celmins. (1991). A practical approach to nonlinear fuzzy regression. *SIAM Journal on Scientific and Statistical Computing, 12*, 521–546.

Chai, J. Y. (2000). Medical device regulation in the United States and the European Union: A comparative study. *Food and Drug Law Journal*, *55*(1), 57–80. PMID:12296349

Chandra, S., & Chandra, H. (2011). *Myocardial Infarction Associated with Plasmodium Falciparum Malarial Infection*. Academic Press.

Chanrakumar, T., & Kathirvel, R. (2016). Classifying Diabetic Retinopathy using Deep Learning Architecture. *International Journal of Engineering Research Technology, 5*(6).

Chapman, S. J., & Hill, A. V. S. (2012). Human genetic susceptibility to infectious disease. *Nature Reviews. Genetics, 13*(3), 175–188. doi:10.1038/nrg3114 PMID:22310894

Chauhan, S. (2014). *Confocal laser endomicroscopy*. The American Society for Gastrointestinal Endoscopy; doi:10.1016/j.gie.2014.06.021

Chen, Y.-F., Madan, J., Welton, N., Yahaya, I., Aveyard, P., Bauld, L., … Munafò, M. R. (2012). Effectiveness and cost-effectiveness of computer and other electronic aids for smoking cessation: a systematic review and network meta-analysis. *Health Technology Assessment (Winchester, England), 16*(38), 1–205, iii–v. doi:10.3310/hta16380

Cheng, D. M. (2003). *Medical Device Regulations: Global overview and guiding principles*. WHO.

Chen, H., Chiang, R. H., & Storey, V. C. (2012). Business intelligence and analytics: From big data to big impact. *Management Information Systems Quarterly*, 1165–1188.

Chen, M., Ma, Y., Li, Y., Wu, D., Zhang, Y., & Youn, C. H. (2017). Wearable 2.0: Enabling human-cloud integration in next generation healthcare systems. *IEEE Communications Magazine, 55*(1), 54–61. doi:10.1109/MCOM.2017.1600410CM

Chen, M., Ma, Y., Song, J., Lai, C. F., & Hu, B. (2016). Smart clothing: Connecting human with clouds and big data for sustainable health monitoring. *Mobile Networks and Applications, 21*(5), 825–845. doi:10.100711036-016-0745-1

Chen, M., Zhang, Y., Li, Y., Hassan, M. M., & Alamri, A. (2015). AIWAC: Affective interaction through wearable computing and cloud technology. *IEEE Wireless Communications, 22*(1), 20–27. doi:10.1109/MWC.2015.7054715

Cheong, Y. L., Leitão, P. J., & Lakes, T. (2014). Assessment of land use factors associated with dengue cases in Malaysia using Boosted Regression Trees. *Spatial and Spatio-temporal Epidemiology, 10*, 75–84. doi:10.1016/j.sste.2014.05.002 PMID:25113593

Chesser, A. K., Keene Woods, N., Smothers, K., & Rogers, N. (2016). Health Literacy and Older Adults. *Gerontology and Geriatric Medicine, 2*, 233372141663049. doi:10.1177/2333721416630492 PMID:28138488

Chopra, A., Saluja, M., & Venugopalan, A. (2014). Effectiveness of chloroquine and inflammatory cytokine response in patients with early persistent musculoskeletal pain and arthritis following chikungunya virus infection. *Arthritis & Rheumatology (Hoboken, N.J.), 66*(2), 319–326. doi:10.1002/art.38221 PMID:24504804

Christaki, E. (2015). New technologies in predicting, preventing and controlling emerging infectious diseases. *Virulence, 6*(6), 558–565. doi:10.1080/21505594.2015.1040975 PMID:26068569

Chugh, S. S., Havmoeller, R., Narayanan, K., Singh, D., Rienstra, M., Benjamin, E. J., ... Forouzanfar, M. H. (2014). Worldwide epidemiology of atrial fibrillation. *Circulation*, *129*(8), 837–847. doi:10.1161/CIRCULATIONAHA.113.005119 PMID:24345399

Chu, M., Shirai, T., Takahashi, D., Arakawa, T., Kudo, H., Sano, K., & Mochizuki, M. (2011). Biomedical soft contact-lens sensor for in situ ocular biomonitoring of tear contents. *Biomedical Microdevices*, *13*(4), 603–611. doi:10.100710544-011-9530-x PMID:21475940

Chung-Ho, Lu, Lee, Wen, Min-Huei, & Li. (2011). Novel solutions for an old disease: Diagnosis of acute appendicitis with random forest, support vector machines, and artificial neural networks. *Surgery*, *149*(1). PMID:20466403

Clifford, G. D., Liu, C., Moody, B., Lehman, L. W. H., Silva, I., Li, Q., ... & Mark, R. G. (2017). *AF Classification from a short single lead ECG recording: the PhysioNet/Computing in Cardiology Challenge 2017*. Academic Press.

Colloca, R. (2013). *Implementation and testing of atrial fibrillation detectors for a mobile phone application*. Academic Press.

Colozza, M., Cardoso, F., Sotiriou, C., Larsimont, D., & Piccart, M. J. (2005). Bringing molecular prognosis and prediction to the clinic. *Clinical Breast Cancer*, *6*(1), 61–76. doi:10.3816/CBC.2005.n.010 PMID:15899074

Corcos, J., & Przydacz, M. (2018). Patient education. In *Consultation in Neurourology: A Practical Evidence-Based Guide* (Vol. 17, pp. 285–297). Springer International Publishing AG.

Costanzo, S. (2017). *Non-Invasive Microwave Sensors for Biomedical Applications: New Design Perspectives*. Academic Press. doi:10.13164/re.2017.0406

Covolo, L., Ceretti, E., Moneda, M., Castaldi, S., & Gelatti, U. (2017). Does evidence support the use of mobile phone apps as a driver for promoting healthy lifestyles from a public health perspective? A systematic review of Randomized Control Trials. *Patient Education and Counseling*, *100*(12), 2231–2243. doi:10.1016/j.pec.2017.07.032 PMID:28855063

Coyle, S., Curto, V. F., Benito-Lopez, F., Florea, L., & Diamond, D. (2015). Wearable bio and chemical sensors. In Wearable Sensors (pp. 65-83). Academic Press.

Crowe, C. S., Liao, J. C., & Curtin, C. M. (2015). Optical Biopsy of Peripheral Nerve Using Confocal Laser Endomicroscopy: A New Tool for Nerve Surgeons. *Archives of Plastice Surgery,* 626-629. .2015.42.5.626 doi:10.5999/aps

Cunningham, P., Carney, J., & Jacob, S. (2000). Stability problems with artificial neural networks and the ensemble solution. *Artificial Intelligence in Medicine*, *20*(3), 217–225. doi:10.1016/S0933-3657(00)00065-8 PMID:10998588

Das, S., Amoedo, B., De la Torre, F., & Hodgins, J. (2012). Detecting parkinsons' symptoms in uncontrolled home environments: A multiple instance learning approach. *Annual International Conference of the IEEE*, 3688-3691.

Das, R., Turkoglu, I., & Sengur, A. (2009). Effective diagnosis of heart disease through neural networks ensembles. *Expert Systems with Applications*, *36*(4), 7675–7680. doi:10.1016/j.eswa.2008.09.013

Davidoff, F., Case, K., & Fried, P. W. (1995). Evidence-based medicine: Why all the fuss? *Annals of Internal Medicine*, *122*(9), 727–727. doi:10.7326/0003-4819-122-9-199505010-00012 PMID:7702236

de Veer, A. J. E., Peeters, J. M., Brabers, A. E. M., Schellevis, F. G., Rademakers, J. J. D. J. M., & Francke, A. L. (2015). Determinants of the intention to use e-Health by community dwelling older people. *BMC Health Services Research*, *15*(1), 103. doi:10.118612913-015-0765-8 PMID:25889884

Demarco, J., & Nystrom, M. (2010). The importance of health literacy in patient education. *Journal of Consumer Health on the Internet*, *14*(3), 294–301. doi:10.1080/15398285.2010.502021

DeMazumder, D., Lake, D. E., Cheng, A., Moss, T. J., Guallar, E., Weiss, R. G., ... Moorman, J. R. (2013). Dynamic analysis of cardiac rhythms for discriminating atrial fibrillation from lethal ventricular arrhythmias. *Circulation: Arrhythmia and Electrophysiology*. PMID:23685539

Dengue Guidelines for Diagnosis, Treatment, Prevention, and Control in Subsaharan Africa and 1 Countries in South America. (2009). Geneva: World Health Organization.

Devraj, R., Borrego, M. E., Vilay, A. M., Pailden, J., & Horowitz, B. (2018). Awareness, self-management behaviors, health literacy and kidney function relationships in specialty practice. *World Journal of Nephrology*, *7*(1), 41–50. doi:10.5527/wjn.v7.i1.41 PMID:29359119

Di, L., & Li, Y. (2018). The risk factor of false-negative and false-positive for T-SPOT.TB in active tuberculosis. *Journal of Clinical Laboratory Analysis*, *32*(2), e22273. doi:10.1002/jcla.22273 PMID:28594104

Dimitrov, D. V. (2016). Medical Internet of Things and Big Data in Healthcare. *Healthcare Informatics Research*, *22*(3), 156–163. doi:10.4258/hir.2016.22.3.156 PMID:27525156

Dismantling the NHS National Programme for IT - GOV.UK. (2011, September). Retrieved March 2, 2018, from https://www.gov.uk/government/news/dismantling-the-nhs-national-programme-for-it

Domchek, S. M., Eisen, A., Calzone, K., Stopfer, J., Blackwood, A., & Weber, B. L. (2003). Application of breast cancer risk prediction models in clinical practice. *Journal of Clinical Oncology*, *21*(4), 593–601. doi:10.1200/JCO.2003.07.007 PMID:12586794

Donaldson, M. S., Corrigan, J. M., & Kohn, L. T. (Eds.). (2000). *To err is human: building a safer health system* (Vol. 6). National Academies Press.

Dong, Y., Simões, M. L., Marois, E., & Dimopoulos, G. (2018). CRISPR/Cas9 -mediated gene knockout of Anopheles gambiae FREP1 suppresses malaria parasite infection. *PLoS Pathogens*, *14*(3), e1006898. doi:10.1371/journal.ppat.1006898 PMID:29518156

Duda, R. O., Hart, P. E., & Stork, D. G. (2001). *Pattern classification* (2nd ed.). New York: Wiley.

Du, X., Rao, N., Qian, M., Liu, D., Li, J., Feng, W., ... Chen, X. (2014). A Novel Method for Real-Time Atrial Fibrillation Detection in Electrocardiograms Using Multiple Parameters. *Annals of Noninvasive Electrocardiology*, *19*(3), 217–225. doi:10.1111/anec.12111 PMID:24252119

Edoh, T. O. C., Atchome, A., Alahassa, B. R. U., & Pawar, P. (2016). Evaluation of a Multi-Tier Heterogeneous Sensor Network for Patient Monitoring – The Case of Benin. In *MMHealth '16 Proceedings of the 2016 ACM Workshop on Multimedia for Personal Health and Health Care* (pp. 23–29). Amsterdam, The Netherlands: ACM Digital Library. 10.1145/2985766.2985772

Edoh, T. (2017). Smart medicine transportation and medication monitoring system in EPharmacyNet. In *2017 International Rural and Elderly Health Informatics Conference (IREHI)* (pp. 1–9). Lomé: IEEE. 10.1109/IREEHI.2017.8350381

Edoh, T. (2018). Risk Prevention of Spreading Emerging Infectious Diseases Using a HybridCrowdsensing Paradigm, Optical Sensors, and Smartphone. *Journal of Medical Systems*, *42*(5), 91. doi:10.100710916-018-0937-2 PMID:29633021

Edoh, T. O. C. (2018). *Advanced Systems For Improved Public Healthcare And Disease Prevention Emerging Research And Opportunities* (A. Moumtzoglou, Ed.). IGI Global, Medical Information Science Reference (an imprint of IGI Global). doi:10.4018/978-1-5225-5528-5

Edoh, T. O., Pawar, P. A., Brügge, B., & Teege, G. (2016). A Multidisciplinary Remote Healthcare Delivery System to Increase Health Care Access, Pathology Screening, and Treatment in Developing Countries. *International Journal of Healthcare Information Systems and Informatics*, *11*(4), 1–31. doi:10.4018/IJHISI.2016100101

Edoh, T., Zogbochi, V., Pawar, P., Hounsou, J. T., & Alahassa, B. R. (2017). Impact of the Internet on diseases awareness and patient empowerment — A study in Benin (West Africa). In *2017 Fourth International Conference on Advances in Biomedical Engineering (ICABME)* (pp. 1–4). IEEE. 10.1109/ICABME.2017.8167543

eInfochips (2017). *A Definitive Guide to Medical Device Design and Development*. Retrieved from https://www.einfochips.com/resources/publications/a-definitive-guide-to-medical-device-design-and-development/

Ekpu, V. U., & Brown, A. K. (2015). The Economic Impact of Smoking and of Reducing Smoking Prevalence: Review of Evidence. *Tobacco Use Insights*, *8*, 1–35. doi:10.4137/TUI.S15628 PMID:26242225

Elmenreich, W. (2002). *An introduction to sensor fusion*. Vienna University of Technology.

Elrakshy, Y. M., & Fayed, A. M. (2014, March). Role of biomarkers to identify individuals with silent cardiac disease to help improve primary prevention. *The Egyptian Heart Journal*, *66*(1), 22. doi:10.1016/j.ehj.2013.12.062

Elshorbagy, M. H., Cuadrado, A., & Alda, J. (2017). High-sensitivity integrated devices based on surface plasmon resonance for sensing applications. *Photonics Research*, *5*(6), 654–661. doi:10.1364/PRJ.5.000654

Epstein, R. M., Fiscella, K., Lesser, C. S., & Stange, K. C. (2010). Analysis & commentary: Why the nation needs a policy push on patient-centered health care. *Health Affairs*, *29*(8), 1489–1495. doi:10.1377/hlthaff.2009.0888 PMID:20679652

Er, O., Temurtas, F., & Tanrıkulu, A. Ç. (2010). Tuberculosis disease diagnosis using artificial neural networks. *Journal of Medical Systems*, *34*(3), 299–302. doi:10.100710916-008-9241-x PMID:20503614

Ertl, P., Sticker, D., Charwat, V., Kasper, C., & Lepperdinger, G. (2014). *Lab-on-a-chip technologies for stem cell analysis*. Academic Press.

Esmaeilzadeh, P., & Sambasivan, M. (2017). Patients' support for health information exchange: A literature review and classification of key factors. *BMC Medical Informatics and Decision Making*, *17*(1), 33. doi:10.118612911-017-0436-2 PMID:28376785

Espina, J., Falck, T., Panousopoulou, A., Schmitt, L., Mülhens, O., & Yang, G. Z. (2014). Network topologies, communication protocols, and standards. In *Body sensor networks* (pp. 189–236). London: Springer. doi:10.1007/978-1-4471-6374-9_5

Etzioni, R., Cooperberg, M. R., Penson, D. M., Weiss, N. S., & Thompson, I. M. (2013). *Limitations of basing screening policies on screening trials: The US Preventive Services Task Force and prostate cancer*. Academic Press. doi:10.1109/TMI.2012.2196707.Separate

European Commission. (2010, June). *DG Health and Consumer. Guidelines Relating to the Application of the Council Directive 93/42/EEC on Medical Devices*. Guidance document - Classification of medical devices. MEDDEV 2. 4/1 Rev. 9.

European Commission. (2018, April). *The new Regulations on medical devices*. https://ec.europa.eu/growth/sectors/medical-devices/regulatory-framework_en

Evangelista, L. S., Rasmusson, K. D., Laramee, A. S., Barr, J., Ammon, S. E., Dunbar, S., ... Yancy, C. W. (2010). Health Literacy and the Patient With Heart Failure-Implications for Patient Care and Research: A Consensus Statement of the Heart Failure Society of America. *Journal of Cardiac Failure*, *16*(1), 9–16. doi:10.1016/j.cardfail.2009.10.026 PMID:20123313

Fabbri, M., Yost, K., Finney Rutten, L. J., Manemann, S. M., Boyd, C. M., Jensen, D., ... Roger, V. L. (2018). Health Literacy and Outcomes in Patients With Heart Failure: A Prospective Community Study. *Mayo Clinic Proceedings*, *93*(1), 9–15. doi:10.1016/j.mayocp.2017.09.018 PMID:29217337

Fahlman, S. E., & Lebiere, C. (1990). The cascade-correlation learning architecture. In Advances in neural information processing systems (pp. 524-532). Academic Press.

Faisal, T., Ibrahim, F., & Taib, M. N. (2010). A noninvasive intelligent approach for predicting the risk in dengue patients. *Expert Systems with Applications*, *37*(3), 2175–2181. doi:10.1016/j.eswa.2009.07.060

FDA - U.S. Department of Health and Human Services, Food and Drug Administration. (2014). *Content of Premarket Submissions for Management of Cybersecurity in Medical Devices*. FDA.

FDA - U.S. Department of Health and Human Services, Food and Drug Administration. (2016). *Applying Human Factors and Usability Engineering to Medical Devices.* FDA.

FDA - US Food and Drug Administration, Center for Devices and Radiological Health. (1997, March). *Design Control Guidance for Medical Device Manufacturers.* FDA.

FDA - US Food and Drug Administration. (2018b). *Reclassification.* FDA.

FDA- US Food and Drug Administration. (2018a). *Is The Product A Medical Device?* FDA.

FDA- US Food and Drug Administration. (2018c). *Overview of Device Regulation.* FDA.

FDA -US Food and Drug Administration. (2018d). *Digital Health.* FDA.

Federal Trade Commission (2016). *Mobile Health Apps Interactive Tool.* Author.

Fell, J., Röschke, J., Mann, K., & Schäffner, C. (1996). Discrimination of sleep stages: A comparison between spectral and nonlinear EEG measures. *Electroencephalography and Clinical Neurophysiology, 98*(5), 401–410. doi:10.1016/0013-4694(96)95636-9 PMID:8647043

Fernandez, E. (2011, October 17). High Rate of False-Positives with Annual Mammogram. UCFS news article, University of California San Francisco.

Fiumara, G., Celesti, A., Galletta, A., Carnevale, L., & Villari, M. (2018). Applying Artificial Intelligence in Healthcare Social Networks to Identity Critical Issues in Patients' Posts. In *Proceedings of the 11th International Joint Conference on Biomedical Engineering Systems and Technologies* (pp. 680–687). SCITEPRESS - Science and Technology Publications. 10.5220/0006750606800687

Focsa, M. (2010). Knowledge-based EHR Systems. In *Proceedings of the 31st Romanian National Conference on Medical Informatics "Solution-based Medical Informatics"* (pp. 64-68). Academic Press.

Foy, C., O'Sullivan, D., & O'Brien, S. (2012). Assessing the Potential of Novel Molecular Microbiological Approaches for Managing Food-borne Disease Outbreaks. The Food Standards Agency.

Fuentes, J., Bakare, M., Munir, K., Aguayo, P., Gaddour, N., Öner, Ö., & Mercadante, M. (2012). *Autism Spectrum Disorders.* Academic Press.

Fukushima, K. (1975). Cognitron: A self-organizing multi-layered neural network. *Biological Cybernetics, 20*(3-4), 121–136. doi:10.1007/BF00342633 PMID:1203338

Fuster, V., Rydén, L. E., Asinger, R. W., Cannom, D. S., Crijns, H. J., Frye, R. L., ... McNamara, R. L. (2001). ACC/AHA/ESC guidelines for the management of patients with atrial fibrillation: Executive summary a report of the American College of Cardiology/American Heart Association task force on practice guidelines and the European Society of Cardiology committee for practice guidelines and policy conferences (committee to develop guidelines for the management of patients with atrial fibrillation) developed in collaboration with the North American Society of Pacing and Electrophysiology. *Circulation*, *104*(17), 2118–2150. PMID:11673357

Gambhir, S., Malik, S. K., & Kumar, Y. (2016). Role of Soft Computing Approaches in HealthCare Domain: A Mini Review. *Journal of Medical Systems*, *40*(12), 287. doi:10.100710916-016-0651-x PMID:27796841

Gambhir, S., Malik, S. K., & Kumar, Y. (2017). PSO-ANN based diagnostic model for the early detection of dengue disease. *New Horizons in Translational Medicine*, *4*(1-4), 1–8. doi:10.1016/j.nhtm.2017.10.001

Ganji, M. F., & Abadeh, M. S. (2011). A fuzzy classification system based on ant colony optimization for diabetes disease diagnosis. *Expert Systems with Applications*, *38*(12), 14650–14659. doi:10.1016/j.eswa.2011.05.018

García, M., Ródenas, J., Alcaraz, R., & Rieta, J. J. (2016). Application of the relative wavelet energy to heart rate independent detection of atrial fibrillation. *Computer Methods and Programs in Biomedicine*, *131*, 157–168. doi:10.1016/j.cmpb.2016.04.009 PMID:27265056

Garg, P. K. (Ed.). (2013). *Chronic Pancreatitis-ECAB*. Elsevier Health Sciences.

Georgakopoulos, S. V., Iakovidis, D. K., Vasilakakis, M., Plagianakos, V. P., & Koulaouzidis, A. (2016). Weakly-supervised convolutional learning for detection of inflammatory gastrointestinal lesions. In *Imaging Systems and Techniques (IST), 2016 IEEE International Conference on* (pp. 510–514). IEEE. 10.1109/IST.2016.7738279

Ghodasra, J. H., Wang, D., Jayakar, R. G., Jensen, A. R., Yamaguchi, K. T., Hegde, V. V., & Jones, K. J. (2018). The Assessment of Quality, Accuracy, and Readability of Online Educational Resources for Platelet-Rich Plasma. *Arthroscopy*, *34*(1), 272–278. doi:10.1016/j.arthro.2017.06.023 PMID:28784239

Gialelis, J., Chondros, P., Karadimas, D., Dima, S., & Serpanos, D. (2011, October). *Identifying Chronic disease complications utilizing state of the art data fusion methodologies and signal processing algorithms*. In *International Conference on Wireless Mobile Communication and Healthcare* (pp. 256-263). Springer.

Gil, D., & Manuel, D. J. (2009). *Diagnosing Parkinson by using artificial neural networks and support vector machines* (Vol. 9). Global Journal of Computer Science and Technology.

Glasgow, R. E., Cho, M., Hutter, M. M., & Mulvihill, S. J. (2000). The spectrum and cost of complicated gallstone disease in California. *Archives of Surgery*, *135*(9), 1021–1025. doi:10.1001/archsurg.135.9.1021 PMID:10982504

Gorgel, P., Sertbas, A., & Ucan, O. N. (2009). *AWavelet-Based Mammographic Image Denoising and Enhancement with Homomorphic Filtering*. Springer Science Business Media, LLC.

Grana, M., & Jackwoski, K. (2015, November). Electronic health record: A review. In *Bioinformatics and Biomedicine (BIBM), 2015 IEEE International Conference on* (pp. 1375-1382). IEEE. 10.1109/BIBM.2015.7359879

Gravina, R., Alinia, P., Ghasemzadeh, H., & Fortino, G. (2017). Multi-sensor fusion in *body sensor networks: State-of-the-art and research challenges. Information Fusion, 35*, 68–80. doi:10.1016/j.inffus.2016.09.005

Grimson, J., Grimson, W., Berry, D., Stephens, G., Felton, E., Kalra, D., … Weier, O. W. (1998). A CORBA-based integration of distributed electronic healthcare records using the synapses approach. *IEEE Transactions on Information Technology in Biomedicine, 2*(3), 124–138. doi:10.1109/4233.735777

Groves, P., Kayyali, B., Knott, D., & Van Kuiken, S. (2013). The 'big data' revolution in healthcare. *The McKinsey Quarterly*, *2*, 3.

Gujral. (2017). Early Diabetes Detection using Machine Learning: A Review. *International Journal for Innovative Research in Science & Technology, 3*(10).

Gulshan, V., Peng, L., Coram, M., Stumpe, M. C., Wu, D., Narayanaswamy, A., ... Webster, D. R. (2016). Development and validation of a deep learning algorithm for detection of diabetic retinopathy in retinal fundus photographs. *Journal of the American Medical Association*, *316*(22), 2402–2410. doi:10.1001/jama.2016.17216 PMID:27898976

Gunčar, G., Kukar, M., Notar, M., Brvar, M., Černelč, P., Notar, M., & Notar, M. (2018). An application of machine learning to hematological diagnosis. *Scientific Reports*, *8*(1), 411. doi:10.103841598-017-18564-8 PMID:29323142

Gunn, J., Gilchrist, G., Chondros, P., Ramp, M., Hegarty, K., Blashki, G., ... Herrman, H. (2008). Who is identified when screening for depression in general practice? Findings from the Diagnosis, Management and Outcomes of Depressive Symptoms Longitudinal (diamond) Study. *The Medical Journal of Australia*, *188*(12), S119–S125. PMID:18558911

Guyon, I., & Elisseeff, A. (2003). An introduction to variable and feature selection. *Journal of Machine Learning Research*, *3*(Mar), 1157–1182.

Habashy, S. M. (2013). Identification of diabetic retinopathy stages using fuzzy C-means classifier. *International Journal of Computers and Applications*, *77*(9).

Haddadi, Healey, & McCabe. (2014). *Healthcare informatics for mental health: recent advances and the outlook for the future.* Ment. Health Found.

Hagerty, R. G., Butow, P. N., Ellis, P. M., Dimitry, S., & Tattersall, M. H. (2005). Communicating prognosis in cancer care: A systematic review of the literature. *Annals of Oncology: Official Journal of the European Society for Medical Oncology*, *16*(7), 1005–1053. doi:10.1093/annonc/mdi211 PMID:15939716

Haghi, M., Thurow, K., & Stoll, R. (2017). Wearable Devices in Medical Internet of Things: Scientific Research and Commercially Available Devices. *Healthcare Informatics Research, 23*(1), 4–15. doi:10.4258/hir.2017.23.1.4 PMID:28261526

Hajli, M. N., Sims, J., Featherman, M., & Love, P. E. D. (2015). Credibility of information in online communities. *Journal of Strategic Marketing, 23*(3), 238–253. doi:10.1080/0965254X.2014.920904

Haloi, M. (2016). *Improved microaneurysm detection using deep neural networks*. arXiv preprint arXiv: 1505.04424v2

Halonen, K. I., Leppäniemi, A. K., Lundin, J. E., Puolakkainen, P. A., Kemppainen, E. A., & Haapiainen, R. K. (2003). Predicting fatal outcome in the early phase of severe acute pancreatitis by using novel prognostic models. *Pancreatology, 3*(4), 309–315. doi:10.1159/000071769 PMID:12890993

Haroon, A., Shah, M. A., Asim, Y., Naeem, W., Kamran, M., & Javaid, Q. (2016). Constraints in the IoT: The world in 2020 and beyond. *Constraints, 7*(11).

Hedman, E., Andersson, E., Ljótsson, B., Andersson, G., Rück, C., & Lindefors, N. (2011). Cost-effectiveness of Internet-based cognitive behavior therapy vs. cognitive behavioral group therapy for social anxiety disorder: Results from a randomized controlled trial. *Behaviour Research and Therapy, 49*(11), 729–736. doi:10.1016/j.brat.2011.07.009 PMID:21851929

Heil, J., ter Waarbeek, H. L. G., Hoebe, C. J. P. A., Jacobs, P. H. A., van Dam, D. W., Trienekens, T. A. M., ... Dukers-Muijrers, N. H. T. M. (2017). Pertussis surveillance and control: Exploring variations and delays in testing, laboratory diagnostics and public health service notifications, the Netherlands, 2010 to 2013. *Eurosurveillance, 22*(28), 1–8. doi:10.2807/1560-7917.ES.2017.22.28.30571 PMID:28749331

Hidron, A., Vogenthaler, N., Santos-Preciado, J. I., Rodriguez-Morales, A. J., Franco-Paredes, C., & Rassi, A. (2010). Cardiac involvement with parasitic infections. *Clinical Microbiology Reviews, 23*(2), 324–349. doi:10.1128/CMR.00054-09 PMID:20375355

Holland, J. H. (1975). *Adaptation in Natural and Artificial Systems*. Ann Arbor, MI: University of Michigan Press.

Hongmei, Y., Yingtao, J., Jun, Z., Chenglin, P., & Li, Q. (2006). A multilayer perceptron-based medical decision support system for heart disease diagnosis. *Expert Systems with Applications, 30*(2), 272–281. doi:10.1016/j.eswa.2005.07.022

Hong, S. H., Lee, W., & AlRuthia, Y. (2016). Health care applicability of a patient-centric web portal for patients' medication experience. *Journal of Medical Internet Research, 18*(7), 1–22. doi:10.2196/jmir.5813 PMID:27450362

Hong, W. D., Chen, X. R., Jin, S. Q., Huang, Q. K., Zhu, Q. H., & Pan, J. Y. (2013). Use of an artificial neural network to predict persistent organ failure in patients with acute pancreatitis. *Clinics, 68*(1), 27–31. doi:10.6061/clinics/2013(01)RC01 PMID:23420153

Hoque, M. R., & Bao, Y. (2015). Cultural Influence on Adoption and Use of e-Health: Evidence in Bangladesh. *Telemedicine Journal and E-Health: The Official Journal of the American Telemedicine Association, 21*(10), 845–851. doi:10.1089/tmj.2014.0128 PMID:26348844

Horst, H. J., & Sinitsyn, A. (2011). An approach to structuring reasoning for interpretation of sensor data in home-based health and well-being monitoring applications. *2011 5th International Conference on Pervasive Computing Technologies for Healthcare (PervasiveHealth) and Workshops*, 47-54. 10.4108/icst.pervasivehealth.2011.246099

Horton, R. (2007). What ' s Wrong with Doctors. *The New York Review of Books, 54*(13), 66. Retrieved from http://www.nybooks.com/articles/2007/05/31/whats-wrong-with-doctors/

Hu, F., Xie, D., & Shen, S. (2013). On the application of the internet of things in the field of medical and health care. *Xplore IEEE - 2013 IEEE International Conference on Green Computing and Communications and IEEE Internet of Things and IEEE Cyber, Physical and Social Computing, GreenCom-IThings-CPSCom 2013*, 2053–2058. 10.1109/GreenCom-iThings-CPSCom.2013.384

Huang, C., Ye, S., Chen, H., Li, D., He, F., & Tu, Y. (2011). A novel method for detection of the transition between atrial fibrillation and sinus rhythm. *IEEE Transactions on Biomedical Engineering, 58*(4), 1113–1119. doi:10.1109/TBME.2010.2096506 PMID:21134807

Huang, W., Gaydos, C. A., Barnes, M. R., Jett-Goheen, M., & Blake, D. R. (2011). Cost-effectiveness analysis of Chlamydia trachomatis screening via Internet-based self-collected swabs compared to clinic-based sample collection. *Sexually Transmitted Diseases, 38*(9), 815–820. doi:10.1097/OLQ.0b013e31821b0f50 PMID:21844736

Hunter, D. J. (2005). Gene-environment interactions in human diseases. *Nature Reviews. Genetics, 6*(4), 287–298. doi:10.1038/nrg1578 PMID:15803198

Huynh, B. Q., Li, H., & Giger, M. L. (2016). Digital mammographic tumor classification using transfer learning from deep convolutional neural networks. *Journal of Medical Imaging (Bellingham, Wash.), 3*(3), 034501. doi:10.1117/1.JMI.3.3.034501 PMID:27610399

Imrie, C., Benjamin, I., Ferguson, J., McKay, A., Mackenzie, I., O'neill, J., & Blumgart, L. (1978). A single-centre double-blind trial of trasylol therapy in primary acute pancreatitis. *British Journal of Surgery, 65*(5), 337–341. doi:10.1002/bjs.1800650514 PMID:348250

Indo-Asian News Service. (2016). *In India, Deaths due to Diabetes increased by 50% in Last Decade Study*. Retrieved from https://everylifecounts.ndtv.com/india-deaths-due-diabetes-increased-50-last-decade-study-5934

Iovea, M., Neagu, M., Stefanescu, B., Mateiasi, G., Porosnicu, I., & Angheluta, E. (2015). Portable low-cost flat panel detectors for real-time digital radiography. *International Symposium on NDT in Aerospace.*

ISO/IEEE 11073-20601:2016. (2016). *Health informatics - Personal health device communication - Part 20601: Application profile - Optimized exchange protocol*, IT applications in health care technology, 2016-06, 2.

Issa, Z. F., Miller, J. M., & Zipes, D. P. (2012). *Clinical arrhythmology and electrophysiology: a companion to Braunwald's heart disease*. Elsevier Health Sciences.

Istepanian, R. S. H., Hu, S., Philip, N. Y., & Sungoor, A. (2011). The potential of Internet of m-health Things “m-IoT” for non-invasive glucose level sensing. In *2011 Annual International Conference of the IEEE Engineering in Medicine and Biology Society* (pp. 5264–5266). IEEE. 10.1109/IEMBS.2011.6091302

Itchhaporia, D., Snow, P. B., Almassy, R. J., & Oetgen, W. J. (1996). Artificial neural networks: Current status in cardiovascular medicine. *Journal of the American College of Cardiology*, *28*(2), 515–521. doi:10.1016/0735-1097(96)00174-X PMID:8800133

Iyer, P., Jasem, J., Springer, M. A., Klein, C. E., & Kabos, P. (2017). PALB2-Positive Breast Cancer in a 40-Year-Old Man. *Oncology (Williston Park, N.Y.)*, *31*(1), 50–52. PMID:28090623

Jabbour, J., Saluda, M.A., Bixler, J.N., & Maitland, K.C. (2012). Confocal Endomicroscopy: Instrumentation and Medical Applications. *Annals of Biomedical Engineering,* (40), 378-397. doi:10.100710439-011-0426-y

Jalloh, O. B., & Waitman, L. R. (2006). Improving Computerized Provider Order Entry (CPOE) usability by data mining users' queries from access logs. *AMIA ... Annual Symposium Proceedings - AMIA Symposium. AMIA Symposium*, *2006*, 379. PMID:17238367

January, C. T., Wann, L. S., Alpert, J. S., Calkins, H., Cigarroa, J. E., Conti, J. B., ... Sacco, R. L. (2014). 2014 AHA/ACC/HRS guideline for the management of patients with atrial fibrillation: A report of the American College of Cardiology/American Heart Association Task Force on Practice Guidelines and the Heart Rhythm Society. *Journal of the American College of Cardiology*, *64*(21), e1–e76. doi:10.1016/j.jacc.2014.03.022 PMID:24685669

Jiang, P., Winkley, J., Zhao, C., Munnoch, R., Min, G., & Yang, L. T. (2016). An intelligent information forwarder for healthcare big data systems with distributed wearable sensors. *IEEE Systems Journal*, *10*(3), 1147–1159. doi:10.1109/JSYST.2014.2308324

Jia, X., & Meng, M. Q.-H. (2016). A deep convolutional neural network for bleeding detection in wireless capsule endoscopy images, *38th Annual International Conference of the IEEE Engineering in Medicine and Biology Society (EMBC)*, pp. 639–642. IEEE.

Jonsson, P., & Wohlin, C. (2004), An evaluation of k-nearest neighbour imputation using likert data. *Proc. software metrics, 10th international, symposium*, 108–118.

Jonsson, B. (2002). Revealing the cost of Type II diabetes in Europe. *Diabetologia*, *45*(S1), S5–S12. doi:10.100700125-002-0858-x

Joseph, R. C., & Johnson, N. A. (2013). Big data and transformational government. *IT Professional*, *15*(6), 43–48. doi:10.1109/MITP.2013.61

Joshi, S., Shenoy, D., Vibhudendra Simha, G. G., Rashmi, P. L., ... Patnaik, L. M. (2010). Classification of Alzheimer's Disease and Parkinson's Disease by Using MachineLearning and Neural Network Methods. *2010 Second International Conference on Machine Learning and Computing*, 219-222.

Jovanovic, P., Salkic, N. N., & Zerem, E. (2014). Artificial neural network predicts the need for therapeutic ERCP in patients with suspected choledocholithiasis. *Gastrointestinal Endoscopy*, *80*(2), 260–268. doi:10.1016/j.gie.2014.01.023 PMID:24593947

Jovanović, P., Salkić, N. N., Zerem, E., & Ljuca, F. (2011). Biochemical and ultrasound parameters may help predict the need for therapeutic endoscopic retrograde cholangiopancreatography (ERCP) in patients with a firm clinical and biochemical suspicion for choledocholithiasis. *European Journal of Internal Medicine*, *22*(6), e110–e114. doi:10.1016/j.ejim.2011.02.008 PMID:22075294

Juusola, J. L., Quisel, T. R., Foschini, L., & Ladapo, J. A. (2016). The impact of an online crowdsourcing diagnostic tool on health care utilization: A case study using a novel approach to retrospective claims analysis. *Journal of Medical Internet Research*, *18*(6), 1–10. doi:10.2196/jmir.5644 PMID:27251384

Kacprzyk, M. F. (Ed.). (1992). *Fuzzy Regression Analysis. Studies in Fuzziness and Soft Computing*. Physica-Verlag HD.

Kaiser, J. F. (1990, April). On a simple algorithm to calculate the'energy'of a signal. In *Acoustics, Speech, and Signal Processing, 1990. ICASSP-90., 1990 International Conference on* (pp. 381-384). IEEE.

Kaiser, J. F. (1993, April). Some useful properties of Teager's energy operators. In *Acoustics, Speech, and Signal Processing, 1993. ICASSP-93., 1993 IEEE International Conference on* (Vol. 3, pp. 149-152). IEEE. 10.1109/ICASSP.1993.319457

Kamnitsas, K., Ledig, C., Newcombe, V. F. J., Simpson, J. P., Kane, A. D., Menon, D. K., ... Glocker, B. (2017). Efficient multiscale 3d cnn with fully connected crf for accurate brain lesion segmentation. *Medical Image Analysis*, *36*, 61–78. doi:10.1016/j.media.2016.10.004 PMID:27865153

Kapoor, V. (2006). Cholecystectomy in patients with asymptomatic gallstones to prevent gall bladder cancer-the case against. *Indian Journal of Gastroenterology*, *25*, 152–154. PMID:16877831

Karabatak, M., & Ince, M. C. (2009). An expert system for detection of breast cancer based on association rules and neural network. *Expert Systems with Applications*, *36*(2), 3465–3469. doi:10.1016/j.eswa.2008.02.064

Kariuki, J. K., Stuart-Shor, E. M., Leveille, S. G., & Hayman, L. L. (2015). Methodological Challenges in Estimating Trends and Burden of Cardiovascular Disease in Sub-Saharan Africa. *Cardiology Research and Practice*, *2015*, 1–6. doi:10.1155/2015/921021 PMID:26697260

Karthikeyan, N., & Sukanesh, R. (2012). Cloud based emergency health care information service in India. *Journal of Medical Systems*, *36*(6), 4031–4036. doi:10.100710916-012-9875-6 PMID:22865161

Kasaie, P., Sohn, H., Kendall, E., Gomez, G. B., Vassall, A., Pai, M., & Dowdy, D. W. (2017). Exploring the epidemiological impact of universal access to rapid tuberculosis diagnosis using agent-based simulation. In 2017 Winter Simulation Conference (WSC) (pp. 1097–1108). IEEE. doi:10.1109/WSC.2017.8247858

Katewa, R., Jakhar, R. S., & Barala, G. L. (2014). Mixed connective tissue disorder: A case report. *International Journal of Case Reports and Images*, *5*(9), 650–655. doi:10.5348/ijcri-2014116-CR-10427

Kaul, K., Tarr, J. M., Ahmad, S. I., Kohner, E. M., & Chibber, R. (2013). Introduction to diabetes mellitus. In *Diabetes* (pp. 1–11). Springer.

Kayyali, B., Knott, D., & Van Kuiken, S. (2013). *The big-data revolution in US health care: Accelerating value and innovation*. McKinsey & Company.

Keller, K., Unakafov, A. M., & Unakafova, V. A. (2014). Ordinal patterns, entropy, and EEG. *Entropy (Basel, Switzerland)*, *16*(12), 6212–6239. doi:10.3390/e16126212

Kershaw, C., Taylor, J. L., Horowitz, G., Brockmeyer, D., Libman, H., Kriegel, G., & Ngo, L. (2018). Use of an electronic medical record reminder improves HIV screening. *BMC Health Services Research*, *18*(1), 1–8. doi:10.118612913-017-2824-9 PMID:29316919

Kim, H. K., Cunningham, I. A., Yin, Z., & Cho, G. (n.d.). On the Development of Digital Radiography Detectors: A Review. *International Journal of Precision Engineering and Manufacturing*, *9*(4), 86-100.

Kim, J. A., Cho, I., & Kim, Y. (2008, August). CDSS (clinical decision support system) architecture in Korea. In *Convergence and Hybrid Information Technology, 2008. ICHIT'08. International Conference on* (pp. 700-703). IEEE.

Kim, J., Lee, B. J., & Yoo, S. K. (2013, July). Design of real-time encryption module for secure data protection of wearable healthcare devices. In *Engineering in Medicine and Biology Society (EMBC), 2013 35th Annual International Conference of the IEEE* (pp. 2283-2286). IEEE.

Kim, K. K., Joseph, J. G., & Ohno-Machado, L. (2015). Comparison of consumers' views on electronic data sharing for healthcare and research. *Journal of the American Medical Informatics Association*, *22*(4), 821–830. doi:10.1093/jamia/ocv014 PMID:25829461

Kinley, A., Zibrik, L., Cordeiro, J., Lauscher, H. N., & Ho, K. (2012). *TeleHealth for Mental Health and Substance Use*. Academic Press.

Kinoshita, T., Tokumasu, H., Tanaka, S., Kramer, A., & Kawakami, K. (2017). Policy implementation for methicillin-resistant *Staphylococcus aureus* in seven European countries: A comparative analysis from 1999 to 2015. *Journal of Market Access & Health Policy*, *5*(1), 1351293. doi:10.1080/20016689.2017.1351293 PMID:28804601

Kitson, A., Marshall, A., Bassett, K., & Zeitz, K. (2013). What are the core elements of patient-centred care? A narrative review and synthesis of the literature from health policy, medicine and nursing. *Journal of Advanced Nursing*, *69*(1), 4–15. doi:10.1111/j.1365-2648.2012.06064.x PMID:22709336

Knaus, W. A., Draper, E. A., Wagner, D. P., & Zimmerman, J. E. (1985). APACHE II: A severity of disease classification system. *Critical Care Medicine*, *13*(10), 818–829. doi:10.1097/00003246-198510000-00009 PMID:3928249

Kobayashi, D., Takahashi, O., Arioka, H., Koga, S., & Fukui, T. (2013). A prediction rule for the development of delirium among patients in medical wards: Chi-Square Automatic Interaction Detector (CHAID) decision tree analysis model. *The American Journal of Geriatric Psychiatry*, *21*(10), 957–962. doi:10.1016/j.jagp.2012.08.009 PMID:23567433

Kohonen, T. (1982). Self-organized formation of topologically correct featuremaps. *Biological Cybernetics*, *43*(1), 59–69. doi:10.1007/BF00337288

Kolovos, S., van Dongen, J. M., Riper, H., Buntrock, C., Cuijpers, P., Ebert, D. D., ... Bosmans, J. E. (2018). Cost effectiveness of guided Internet-based interventions for depression in comparison with control conditions: An individual-participant data meta-analysis. *Depression and Anxiety*, *35*(3), 209–219. doi:10.1002/da.22714 PMID:29329486

Komi, M., Li, J., Zhai, Y., & Zhang, X. (2017, June). Application of data mining methods in diabetes prediction. In *Image, Vision and Computing (ICIVC), 2017 2nd International Conference on* (pp. 1006-1010). IEEE. 10.1109/ICIVC.2017.7984706

Koopman Schap, M. (2003). Coping with Type II diabetes: The patient's perspective. *Diabetologia*, *45*, 302–303.

Koroukian, S. M., Basu, J., Schiltz, N. K., Navale, S., Bakaki, P. M., Warner, D. F., ... Stange, K. C. (2018). Changes in Case-Mix and Health Outcomes of Medicare Fee-for-Service Beneficiaries and Managed Care Enrollees during the Years 1992-2011. *Medical Care*, *56*(1), 39–46. doi:10.1097/MLR.0000000000000847 PMID:29176368

Kourou, K., Exarchos, T. P., Exarchos, K. P., Karamouzis, M. V., & Fotiadis, D. I. (2015). Machine learning applications in cancer prognosis and prediction. *Computational and Structural Biotechnology Journal*, *13*, 8–17. doi:10.1016/j.csbj.2014.11.005 PMID:25750696

Kraemer, K. L. (2007). The cost-effectiveness and cost-benefit of screening and brief intervention for unhealthy alcohol use in medical settings. *Substance Abuse*, *28*(3), 67–77. doi:10.1300/J465v28n03_07 PMID:18077304

Kramer, D. B., Baker, M., Ransford, B., Molina-Markham, A., Stewart, Q., Fu, K., & Reynolds, M. R. (2012a). *Security and Privacy Qualities of Medical Devices: An Analysis of FDA Postmarket Surveillance*. Public Library of Science.

Kramer, D. B., Xu, S., & Kesselheim, A. S. (2012b). Regulation of medical devices in the United States and European Union. *The New England Journal of Medicine*, *366*(9), 848–855. doi:10.1056/NEJMhle1113918 PMID:22332952

Krishnan, N. C., & Cook, D. J. (2014). Activity recognition on streaming sensor data. *Pervasive and Mobile Computing*, *10*, 138–154. doi:10.1016/j.pmcj.2012.07.003 PMID:24729780

Kruse, C. S., Kothman, K., Anerobi, K., & Abanaka, L. (2016). Adoption Factors of the Electronic Health Record: A Systematic Review. *JMIR Medical Informatics*, *4*(2), e19. doi:10.2196/medinform.5525 PMID:27251559

Kulkarni, P., Ganesan, D., Shenoy, P., & Lu, Q. (2005). SensEye : A Multi-tier Camera Sensor Network. In *MULTIMEDIA '05 Proceedings of the 13th annual ACM international conference on Multimedia, Hilton, Singapore* (pp. 229–238). Hilton, Singapore: ACM Digital Library. 10.1145/1101149.1101191

Kumar Sangwan, M., & Sangwan, V., Kumar Garg, M., Singla, D., Thami, G., & Malik, P. (2016). Gallstone disease menacing rural population in north India: A retrospective study of 576 cases in a rural hospital. *International Surgery Journal*, *2*(4), 487–491.

Kumar, A. S. (2013). Diagnosis of diabetic using Advanced Fuzzy resolution Mechanism. *International Journal of Science and Applied Information Technology*, *2*(2), 22–30.

Kumar, Y., & Sahoo, G. (2013). Prediction of different types of liver diseases using rule based classification model. *Technology and Health Care*, *21*(5), 417–432. PMID:23963359

Kushinka, S. A. (2011). *Electronic health record deployment techniques*. Retrieved from https://www.chcf.org/publication/electronic-health-record-deployment-techniques/

Kyriacos, U., Jelsma, J., & Jordan, S. (2011). Monitoring vital signs using early warning scoring systems: A review of the literature. *Journal of Nursing Management*, *19*(3), 311–330. doi:10.1111/j.1365-2834.2011.01246.x PMID:21507102

Ladavich, S., & Ghoraani, B. (2015). Rate-independent detection of atrial fibrillation by statistical modeling of atrial activity. *Biomedical Signal Processing and Control*, *18*, 274–281. doi:10.1016/j.bspc.2015.01.007

Lahiri, T., Kumar, U., Mishra, H., Sarkar, S., & Das, R. A. (2009). Analysis of ECG signals by chaos principle to help automatic diagnosis of myocardial infarction. *Journal of Scientific and Industrial Research*, *68*, 866–870.

Lake, D. E., & Moorman, J. R. (2011). Accurate estimation of entropy in very short physiological time series: The problem of atrial fibrillation detection in implanted ventricular devices. *American Journal of Physiology. Heart and Circulatory Physiology*, *300*(1), H319–H325. doi:10.1152/ajpheart.00561.2010 PMID:21037227

Lamb, S. (2017). *Improving Disease Diagnosis with Machine Learning*. Retrieved on march 15, 2018 from https://verneglobal.com/blog/improving-disease-diagnosis-with-machine-learning

Langley, P., Iba, W., & Thompson, K. (1992). An analysis of Bayesian classifiers. *Proceedings of the Tenth National Conference on Artificial Intelligence*, 223-228.

Latham, B. (2007). Sampling: What is it? *Quantitative Research Methods*, 1-13. Retrieved from http://webpages.acs.ttu.edu/rlatham/Coursework/5377(Quant))/Sampling_Methodology_Paper.pdf

Latré, B., Braem, B., Moerman, I., Blondia, C., & Demeester, P. (2011). A survey on wireless body area networks. *Wireless Networks*, *17*(1), 1–18. doi:10.100711276-010-0252-4

Laura B. (2014). *CHARLIE: a new robot prototype for improving communication and social skills in children with autism and a new single-point infrared sensor technique for detecting breathing and heart rate remotely* (PhD dissertation). University of South Carolina.

Le Fanu, J. (2011). *The rise and fall of modern medicine*. Hachette, UK.

Le Reste, J. Y., Nabbe, P., Rivet, C., Lygidakis, C., Doerr, C., Czachowski, S., ... Van Royen, P. (2015). The European general practice research network presents the translations of its comprehensive definition of multimorbidity in family medicine in ten European languages. *PLoS One*, *10*(1), 1–13. doi:10.1371/journal.pone.0115796 PMID:25607642

Leape, L. L., Brennan, T. A., Laird, N., Lawthers, A. G., Localio, A. R., Barnes, B. A., & Hiatt, H. (1991). The nature of adverse events in hospitalized patients: Results of the Harvard Medical Practice Study II. *The New England Journal of Medicine*, *324*(6), 377–384. doi:10.1056/NEJM199102073240605 PMID:1824793

Lee, C. S., & Wang, M. H. (2011). A fuzzy expert system for diabetes decision support application. *Systems, Man, and Cybernetics, Part B: Cybernetics. IEEE Transactions on*, *41*(1), 139–153.

Lee, C., Luo, Z., Ngiam, K. Y., Zhang, M., Zheng, K., Chen, G., & Yip, W. L. J. (2017). Big healthcare data analytics: Challenges and applications. In *Handbook of Large-Scale Distributed Computing in Smart Healthcare* (pp. 11–41). Cham: Springer. doi:10.1007/978-3-319-58280-1_2

Lee, K. H., Kung, S. Y., & Verma, N. (2012). Low-energy formulations of support vector machine kernel functions for biomedical sensor applications. *Journal of Signal Processing Systems for Signal, Image, and Video Technology*, *69*(3), 339–349. doi:10.100711265-012-0672-8

Lee, S., & Do, H. (2018). Comparison and Analysis of ISO/IEEE 11073, IHE PCD-01, and HL7 FHIR Messages for Personal Health Devices. *Healthcare Informatics Research*, *24*(1), 46–52. doi:10.4258/hir.2018.24.1.46 PMID:29503752

Lee, S., Huang, H., & Zelen, M. (2004). Early detection of disease and scheduling of screening examinations. *Statistical Methods in Medical Research*, *13*(6), 443–456. doi:10.1191/0962280204sm377ra PMID:15587433

LeLorier, J., Gregoire, G., Benhaddad, A., Lapierre, J., & Derderian, F. (1997). Discrepancies between meta-analyses and subsequent large randomized, controlled trials. *The New England Journal of Medicine*, *337*(8), 536–542. doi:10.1056/NEJM199708213370806 PMID:9262498

Li, J., Land, L., & Ray, P. (2008). *Humanitarian Technology Challenge (HTC)-electronic health records perspective.* A Report of Joint Project of IEEE and United Nations Foundation.

Liakat, S., Bors, K. A., Xu, L., Woods, C. M., Doyle, J., & Gmachl, C. F. (2014). Noninvasive in vivo glucose sensing on human subjects using mid-infrared light. *Biomedical Optics Express*, *5*(7), 2397. doi:10.1364/BOE.5.002397 PMID:25071973

Li, J., Talaei-Khoei, A., Seale, H., Ray, P., & MacIntyre, C. R. (2013). Health Care Provider Adoption of eHealth: Systematic Literature Review. *Interactive Journal of Medical Research*, *2*(1), e7. doi:10.2196/ijmr.2468 PMID:23608679

Lin, T., Gal, A., Mayzel, Y., Horman, K., & Bahartan, K. (2017). Non-Invasive Glucose Monitoring: A Review of Challenges and Recent Advances. *Current Trends in Biomedical Engineering and Biosciences*, *6*(5). DOI:.2017.06.555696 doi:10.19080/CTBEB

Linder, G., Sandin, F., Johansson, J., Lindblad, M., Lundell, L., & Hedberg, J. (2018). Patient education-level affects treatment allocation and prognosis in esophageal- and gastroesophageal junctional cancer in Sweden. *Cancer Epidemiology*, *52*, 91–98. doi:10.1016/j.canep.2017.12.008

Liu Y., Gadepalli K., Norouzi M., Dahl, G.E., & Stumpe, M.C. (2017). *Detecting cancer metastases on gigapixel pathology images*. CoRRabs/1703.02442

Lo'ai, A. T., Mehmood, R., Benkhlifa, E., & Song, H. (2016). Mobile cloud computing model and big data analysis for healthcare applications. *IEEE Access: Practical Innovations, Open Solutions*, *4*, 6171–6180. doi:10.1109/ACCESS.2016.2613278

Loh, W. Y., & Shih, X. (1997). Split selection methods for classification tree. *Statistica Sinica*, *7*, 815–840.

Lowres, N., Neubeck, L., Salkeld, G., Krass, I., McLachlan, A. J., Redfern, J., ... Freedman, S. B. (2014). Feasibility and cost-effectiveness of stroke prevention through community screening for atrial fibrillation using iPhone ECG in pharmacies. The SEARCH-AF study. *Thrombosis and Haemostasis*, *111*(6), 1167–1176. doi:10.1160/TH14-03-0231 PMID:24687081

Lucas, P. J., & Lucas, P. (2016). *Bayesian analysis, pattern analysis, and data mining in health care health care.* Academic Press.

Lukmanto, R. B., & Irwansyah, E. (2015). The Early Detection of Diabetes Mellitus (DM) Using Fuzzy Hierarchical Model. *Procedia Computer Science*, *59*, 312–319. doi:10.1016/j.procs.2015.07.571

Maclin, P. S., Dempsey, J., Brooks, J., & Rand, J. (1991). Using neural networks to diagnose cancer. *Journal of Medical Systems*, *15*(1), 11–19. doi:10.1007/BF00993877 PMID:1748845

Maguire, R., Ream, E., Richardson, A., Connaghan, J., Johnston, B., Kotronoulas, G., ... Kearney, N. (2015). Development of a novel remote patient monitoring system: The advanced symptom management system for radiotherapy to improve the symptom experience of patients with lung cancer receiving radiotherapy. *Cancer Nursing*, *38*(2), E37–E47. doi:10.1097/NCC.0000000000000150 PMID:24836956

Maheshwari, N., Chatterjee, G., & Rao, V. R. (2014, September). A Technology Overview and Applications of Bio-MEMS. *J. ISSS*, *3*(2), 39–59.

Mandal, I., & Sairam, N. (2012). Accurate telemonitoring of parkinson's disease diagnosis using robust inference system. *International Journal of Medical Informatics*. PMID:23182747

Manogaran, G., & Lopez, D. (2017). A survey of big data architectures and machine learning algorithms in healthcare. *International Journal of Biomedical Engineering and Technology*, *25*(2-4), 182–211. doi:10.1504/IJBET.2017.087722

Manogaran, G., & Lopez, D. (2018). Health data analytics using scalable logistic regression with stochastic gradient descent. *International Journal of Advanced Intelligence Paradigms*, *10*(1-2), 118–132. doi:10.1504/IJAIP.2018.089494

Marshall, J. C., Cook, D. J., Christou, N. V., Bernard, G. R., Sprung, C. L., & Sibbald, W. J. (1995). Multiple organ dysfunction score: A reliable descriptor of a complex clinical outcome. *Critical Care Medicine*, *23*(10), 1638–1652. doi:10.1097/00003246-199510000-00007 PMID:7587228

Marshall, R. J. (2001). The use of classification and regression trees in clinical epidemiology. *Journal of Clinical Epidemiology*, *54*(6), 603–609. doi:10.1016/S0895-4356(00)00344-9 PMID:11377121

Maxim, L. D., Niebo, R., & Utell, M. J. (2014). Screening tests: A review with examples. *Inhalation Toxicology*, *26*(13), 811–828. doi:10.3109/08958378.2014.955932 PMID:25264934

McCarthy, J. F., Marx, K. A., Hoffman, P. E., Gee, A. G., O'Neil, P., Ujwal, M. L., & Hotchkiss, J. (2004). Applications of machine learning and high-dimensional visualization in cancer detection, diagnosis, and management. *Annals of the New York Academy of Sciences*, *1020*(1), 239–262. doi:10.1196/annals.1310.020 PMID:15208196

McCulloch, W. S., & Pitts, W. (1943). A logical calculus of the ideas immanent in nervous activity. *The Bulletin of Mathematical Biophysics*, *5*(4), 115–133. doi:10.1007/BF02478259

Menon. (2016, February). *What is the Relationship between Precision Medicine & Predictive Analytics?* Editor's Note.

Merker, V. L., McDannold, S., Riklin, E., Talaei-Khoei, M., Sheridan, M. R., Jordan, J. T., ... Vranceanu, A. M. (2018). Health literacy assessment in adults with neurofibromatosis: Electronic and short-form measurement using FCCHL and Health LiTT. *Journal of Neuro-Oncology*, *136*(2), 335–342. doi:10.100711060-017-2657-8 PMID:29119424

Minue, S., Bermudez-Tamayo, C., Fernandez, A., Martin-Martin, J. J., Benitez, V., Melguizo, M., ... Montoro, R. (2014). Identification of factors associated with diagnostic error in primary care. *BMC Family Practice*, *15*(1), 92. doi:10.1186/1471-2296-15-92 PMID:24884984

Miotto, R., Wang, F., Wang, S., Jiang, X., & Dudley, J. T. (2017). Deep learning for healthcare: Review, opportunities and challenges. *Briefings in Bioinformatics*. doi:10.1093/bib/bbx044 PMID:28481991

Mishra & Silakari. (2012). Predictive Analytics: A Survey, Trends, Applications, Oppurtunities & Challenges. *International Journal of Computer Science and Information Technologies, 3*(3), 4434-4438.

Mitchell, T. (1997). *Machine Learning*. New York: McGraw Hill.

Montague, E., & Perchonok, J. (2012). Health and wellness technology use by historically underserved health consumers: Systematic review. *Journal of Medical Internet Research, 14*(3), e78. doi:10.2196/jmir.2095 PMID:22652979

Moorhead, S., Johnson, M., Maas, M., & Swanson, E. (2018). *Nursing Outcomes Classification (NOC)-E-Book: Measurement of Health Outcomes*. Elsevier. Retrieved from https://books.google.de/books?hl=de&lr=&id=LYlIDwAAQBAJ&oi=fnd&pg=PP1&dq=define+health+outcomes&ots=bOTv_XytcU&sig=hqWEjophQarxuLKuIOw7ea6XdNY#v=onepage&q=definehealthoutcomes&f=false

Moser, R. H. (1956). Diseases of medical progress. *The New England Journal of Medicine, 255*(13), 606–614. doi:10.1056/NEJM195609272551306 PMID:13369682

Mulyani, Y., Rahman, E. F., & Riza, L. S. (2016). A new approach on prediction of fever disease by using a combination of Dempster Shafer and Naïve bayes. In Science in Information Technology (ICSITech) (pp. 367-371). IEEE.

Muniaraj, M. (2014). Fading chikungunya fever from India: Beginning of the end of another episode? *The Indian Journal of Medical Research, 139*(3), 468. PMID:24820844

Murad, R., Oliver, M., & Kelly, M. (2017). *Differences between screening and diagnostic tests and case finding*. Retrieved March 18, 2018, from https://www.healthknowledge.org.uk/public-health-textbook/disease-causation-diagnostic/2c-diagnosis-screening/screening-diagnostic-case-finding

Murcia-Robayo, R. Y., Jouanisson, E., Beauchamp, G., & Diaw, M. (2018). Effects of staining method and clinician experience on the evaluation of stallion sperm morphology. *Animal Reproduction Science, 188*, 165–169. doi:10.1016/j.anireprosci.2017.11.021

Murphy, R. R. (1996). Biological and cognitive foundations of intelligent sensor fusion. *IEEE Transactions on Systems, Man, and Cybernetics. Part A, Systems and Humans, 26*(1), 42–51. doi:10.1109/3468.477859

Muthukaruppan, S., & Er, M. J. (2012). A hybrid particle swarm optimization based fuzzy expert system for the diagnosis of coronary artery disease. *Expert Systems with Applications, 39*(14), 11657–11665. doi:10.1016/j.eswa.2012.04.036

Nabar, A., & Pathan, I. (2016). Pathophysiology of Atrial Fibrillation-current Concepts. *The Journal of the Association of Physicians of India, 64*(8), 11–15. PMID:28812335

Nachega, J. B., Skinner, D., Jennings, L., Magidson, J. F., Altice, F. L., Burke, J. G., ... Theron, G. B. (2016). Acceptability and feasibility of mHealth and community-based directly observed antiretroviral therapy to prevent mother-to-child HIV transmission in South African pregnant women under Option B+: An exploratory study. *Patient Preference and Adherence*, *10*, 683–690. doi:10.2147/PPA.S100002 PMID:27175068

Namdeo, A., & Bhadoriya, S. S. (2016). A Review on Image Enhancement Techniques with its Advantages and Disadvantages. *International Journal for Science and Advance Research & Development*, *2*(5).

Nath, C., Huh, J., Adupa, A. K., & Jonnalagadda, S. R. (2016). Website Sharing in Online Health Communities: A Descriptive Analysis. *Journal of Medical Internet Research*, *18*(1), e11. doi:10.2196/jmir.5237 PMID:26764193

Negra, R., Jemili, I., & Belghith, A. (2016). Wireless body area networks: Applications and technologies. *Procedia Computer Science*, *83*, 1274–1281. doi:10.1016/j.procs.2016.04.266

Nelson, H. D., O'Meara, E. S., Kerlikowske, K., Balch, S., & Miglioretti, D. (2016). Factors associated with rates of false-positive and false-negative results from digital mammography screening: An analysis of registry data. *Annals of Internal Medicine*, *164*(4), 226–235. doi:10.7326/M15-0971 PMID:26756902

Nguyen, T., Khosravi, A., Creighton, D., & Nahavandi, S. (2015). Classification of healthcare data using genetic Fuzzy Logic system and wavelets. *Expert Systems with Applications*, *42*(4), 2184–2197. doi:10.1016/j.eswa.2014.10.027

Nieman, A.-E., de Mast, Q., Roestenberg, M., Wiersma, J., Pop, G., Stalenhoef, A., ... van der Ven, A. (2015, November). … van der Ven, A. (2009). Cardiac complication after experimental human malaria infection: A case report. *Malaria Journal*, *8*(1), 277. doi:10.1186/1475-2875-8-277 PMID:19958549

O'Connor, J. M., Das, M., Didier, C., Mah'd, M., & Glick, S. J. (2010). Development of an Ensemble of Digital Breast ObjectModels. *IWDM*, *2010*, 54–61.

OECD. (2017). *Health at a Glance 2017*. OECD Publishing. doi:10.1787/health_glance-2017-

Ohno-Machado, L. (1996). *Medical applications of artificial neural networks: connectionist models of survival* (Doctoral dissertation). Stanford University.

Ohno-Machado, L. (2013). Sharing data for the public good and protecting individual privacy: Informatics solutions to combine different goals. *Journal of the American Medical Informatics Association: JAMIA*, *20*(1), 1. doi:10.1136/amiajnl-2012-001513 PMID:23243087

Oldach, B. R., & Katz, M. L. (2014). Health literacy and cancer screening: A systematic review. *Patient Education and Counseling*, *94*(2), 149–157. doi:10.1016/j.pec.2013.10.001 PMID:24207115

Oneview. (2018). *The Eight Principles of Patient-Centered Care*. Retrieved from https://www.oneviewhealthcare.com/the-eight-principles-of-patient-centered-care/

Ong, M. K. (2016). Effectiveness of Remote Patient Monitoring After Discharge of AMA Intern Med Hospitalized Patients With Heart Failure: The Better Effectiveness After Transition–Heart Failure (BEAT-HF) Randomized Clinical Trial. *Jama Interm Med., 314*(19), 2034–2044. doi:10.1001/jama.2015.7712

On, R., & In, E. (2010). Editorial Note on the Processing. *Storage, 14*(4), 895–896. PMID:20687242

Opeyemi, O., & Justice, E. O. (2012). Development of Neuro-fuzzy System for Early Prediction of Heart Attack. *International Journal of Information Technology and Computer Science, 4*(9), 22–28. doi:10.5815/ijitcs.2012.09.03

Ordóñez, F. J., & Roggen, D. (2016). Deep convolutional and lstm recurrent neural networks for multimodal wearable activity recognition. *Sensors (Basel), 16*(1), 115. doi:10.339016010115 PMID:26797612

Orhan, E., Yumusak, N., & Temurtas, F. (2012). Diagnosis of chest diseases using artificial immune system. *Expert Systems with Applications, 39*(2), 1862–1868. doi:10.1016/j.eswa.2011.08.064

Ozcift, A. (2011). Random forests ensemble classifier trained with data resampling strategy to improve cardiac arrhythmia diagnosis. *Computers in Biology and Medicine, 41*(5), 265–271. doi:10.1016/j.compbiomed.2011.03.001 PMID:21419401

Palaniappan, S., & Awang, R. (2008), Intelligent heart disease prediction system using data mining techniques. *Proc. 2008 IEEE/ACS International Conference on Computer Systems and Applications,* 108–11.

Paliwal, G., & Bunglowala, A. (2017). Software Product Lines for Mobile Patient Monitoring Systems Using FoDA a Grammar. *Biochem Ind J., 11*(2), 112.

Paliwal, G., & Kiwelekar, A. W. (2013, March). A comparison of mobile patient monitoring systems. In *International Conference on Health Information Science* (pp. 198-209). Springer. 10.1007/978-3-642-37899-7_17

Paliwal, G., & Kiwelekar, A. W. (2015). A Product Line Architecture for Mobile Patient Monitoring System. In *Mobile Health* (pp. 489–511). Cham: Springer. doi:10.1007/978-3-319-12817-7_22

Paolotti, D., Carnahan, A., Colizza, V., Eames, K., Edmunds, J., Gomes, G., ... Vespignani, A. (2014). Web-based participatory surveillance of infectious diseases: The Influenzanet participatory surveillance experience. *Clinical Microbiology and Infection, 20*(1), 17–21. doi:10.1111/1469-0691.12477 PMID:24350723

Papacosta, E., & Nassis, G. P. (2011). Saliva as a tool for monitoring steroid, peptide and immune markers in sport and exercise science. *Journal of Science and Medicine in Sport, 14*(5), 424–434. doi:10.1016/j.jsams.2011.03.004 PMID:21474377

Papoutsi, C., Reed, J. E., Marston, C., Lewis, R., Majeed, A., & Bell, D. (2015). Patient and public views about the security and privacy of Electronic Health Records (EHRs) in the UK: Results from a mixed methods study. *BMC Medical Informatics and Decision Making, 15*(1), 86. doi:10.118612911-015-0202-2 PMID:26466787

Parker, P. D., Heiney, S. P., Friedman, D. B., Felder, T. M., Estrada, R. D., Harris, E. H., & Adams, S. A. (2018). How are health literacy principles incorporated into breast cancer chemotherapy education? A review of the literature. *Journal of Nursing Education and Practice*, *8*(6), 77. doi:10.5430/jnep.v8n6p77

Park, J., Lee, S., & Jeon, M. (2009). Atrial fibrillation detection by heart rate variability in Poincare plot. *Biomedical Engineering Online*, *8*(1), 38. doi:10.1186/1475-925X-8-38 PMID:20003345

Patidar, S., Pachori, R. B., & Acharya, U. R. (2015). Automated diagnosis of coronary artery disease using tunable-Q wavelet transform applied on heart rate signals. *Knowledge-Based Systems*, *82*, 1–10. doi:10.1016/j.knosys.2015.02.011

Patrick, E. A., & Fischer, F. P. III. (1970). A generalized k-nearest neighbor rule. *Information and Control*, *16*(2), 128–152. doi:10.1016/S0019-9958(70)90081-1

Pawar, P., Jones, V., Van Beijnum, B. J. F., & Hermens, H. (2012). A framework for the comparison of mobile patient monitoring systems. *Journal of Biomedical Informatics*, *45*(3), 544–556. doi:10.1016/j.jbi.2012.02.007 PMID:22406009

Pei, M., Wu, X., Guo, Y., & Fujita, H. (2017). Small bowel motility assessment based on fully convolutional networks and long short-term memory. *Knowledge-Based Systems*, *121*, 163–172. doi:10.1016/j.knosys.2017.01.023

Peng, H., Long, F., & Ding, C. (2005). Feature selection based on mutual information criteria of max-dependency, max-relevance, and min-redundancy. *IEEE Transactions on Pattern Analysis and Machine Intelligence*, *27*(8), 1226–1238. doi:10.1109/TPAMI.2005.159 PMID:16119262

Pereira, J., Porto-Figueira, P., Cavaco, C., Taunk, K., & Camara, J.S. (2015). Breath Analysis as a Potential and Non-Invasive Frontier in Disease Diagnosis: An Overview. *Metabolites, 5*(1), 3–55. doi:10.3390/metabo5010003

Petrenas, A., Marozas, V., Sornmo, L., & Lukosevicius, A. (2012). An echo state neural network for QRST cancellation during atrial fibrillation. *IEEE Transactions on Biomedical Engineering*, *59*(10), 2950–2957. doi:10.1109/TBME.2012.2212895 PMID:22929362

Phillips, M., Cataneo, R. N., Ditkoff, B. A., Fisher, P., Greenberg, J., Gunawardena, Rahbari-Oskoui, F., & Wong, C. (2003). *Volatile Markers of Breast Cancer in the Breath.* Blackwell Publishing. doi:1075-122X/03/$15.00/0

Piccart, M., Lohrisch, C., Di Leo, A., & Larsimont, D. (2001). The predictive value of HER2 in breast cancer. *Oncology*, *61*(Suppl 2), 73–82. doi:10.1159/000055405 PMID:11694791

Poleshchuk, E. (2012). *A fuzzy linear regression model for interval type-2 fuzzy sets. NAFIPS 2012.* Fuzzy Information Processing Society.

Polikar, R. (2006). Ensemble based systems in decision making. *IEEE Circuits and Systems Magazine*, *6*(3), 21–45. doi:10.1109/MCAS.2006.1688199

Potter, B. J., & Le Lorier, J. (2015). Taking the pulse of atrial fibrillation. *Lancet*, *386*(9989), 113–115. doi:10.1016/S0140-6736(14)61991-7 PMID:25960109

Pratt, H., Coenen, F., Broadbent, D., Harding, S. P., & Zheng, Y. (2016). Convolutional neural networks for diabetic retinopathy. *Procedia Computer Science*, *90*, 200–205. doi:10.1016/j.procs.2016.07.014

Pronovost, P., & Vohr, E. (2010). *Safe patients, smart hospitals: how one doctor's checklist can help us change health care from the inside out*. Penguin.

PubMed Health. (2016). *Benefits and risks of Screening Tests*. Retrieved from https://www.ncbi.nlm.nih.gov/pubmedhealth/PMH0072602/

Pusiol, T., Lavezzi, A. M., Radice, F., Alfonsi, G., & Matturri, L. (2014). Unsuspected imported malaria in a case of sudden infant death. *World Journal of Clinical Infectious Diseases*, *4*(2), 5–8. doi:10.5495/wjcid.v4.i2.5

Qian, R., & Long, Y. (2017). Wearable Chemosensors: A Review of Recent Progress. *ChemistryOpen*, *7*(2), 118–130. doi:10.1002/open.201700159 PMID:29435397

Quaglini, S. (2008, September). Process mining in healthcare: a contribution to change the culture of blame. In *International Conference on Business Process Management* (pp. 308-311). Springer.

Quinlan, J. R. (1986). Induction of decision tree. *Machine Learning*, *1*(1), 81–106. doi:10.1007/BF00116251

Quinlan, J. R. (1993). *C4.5: Programs for machine learning*. Morgan Kaufman Publishers Inc.

Quinn, J. A., Nakasi, R., Mugagga, P., Byanyima, P., . . . Andama, A. (2016). *Deep convolutional neural networks for microscopy-based point of care diagnostics*. arXiv preprint arXiv:1608.02989

Raghupathi, W., & Raghupathi, V. (2014). Big data analytics in healthcare: Promise and potential. *Health Information Science and Systems*, *2*(1), 3. doi:10.1186/2047-2501-2-3 PMID:25825667

Rahmawati, D., & Huang, Y. P. (2016). Using C-support vector classification to forecast dengue fever epidemics in Taiwan. In System Science and Engineering (ICSSE) (pp. 1-4). IEEE.

Rakotomamonjy, A. (2003). Variable selection using SVM-based criteria. *Journal of Machine Learning Research*, *3*(Mar), 1357–1370.

Rana, A. K. M. M., Wahlin, A., Lundborg, C. S., & Kabir, Z. N. (2008). Impact of health education on health-related quality of life among elderly persons: Results from a community-based intervention study in rural Bangladesh. *Health Promotion International*, *24*(1), 36–45. doi:10.1093/heapro/dan042 PMID:19136677

Ranson, J. H. C. (1974). Prognostic signs and the role of operative management in acute pancreatitis. *Surgery, Gynecology & Obstetrics*, *139*, 69–81. PMID:4834279

Ravì, D., Wong, C., Deligianni, F., Berthelot, M., Andreu-Perez, J., Lo, B., & Yang, G. Z. (2017). Deep learning for health informatics. *IEEE Journal of Biomedical and Health Informatics*, *21*(1), 4–21. doi:10.1109/JBHI.2016.2636665 PMID:28055930

Read, J. R., Sharpe, L., Modini, M., & Dear, B. F. (2017). Multimorbidity and depression: A systematic review and meta-analysis. *Journal of Affective Disorders*, *221*, 36–46. doi:10.1016/j.jad.2017.06.009 PMID:28628766

Remais, J. V., Zeng, G., Li, G., Tian, L., & Engelgau, M. M. (2013). Convergence of non-communicable and infectious diseases in low- and middle-income countries. *International Journal of Epidemiology*, *42*(1), 221–227. doi:10.1093/ije/dys135 PMID:23064501

Renner, P. (2009). *Why most EMR implementations fail: How to protect your practice and enjoy successfully implementation.* Retrieved from http://www.emrindustry.com/wpcontent/uploads/2014/04/StreamlineMD_WhitePaper_1B.pdf

Renshaw, A. A., & Gould, E. W. (2013). Reducing false-negative and false-positive diagnoses in anatomic pathology consultation material. *Archives of Pathology & Laboratory Medicine*, *137*(12), 1770–1773. doi:10.5858/arpa.2013-0012-OA PMID:24283857

Reyes-Ortiz, J. L., Oneto, L., Samà, A., Parra, X., & Anguita, D. (2016). Transition-aware human activity recognition using smartphones. *Neurocomputing*, *171*, 754–767. doi:10.1016/j.neucom.2015.07.085

Rezaeibagha, F., Win, K. T., & Susilo, W. (2015). A systematic literature review on security and privacy of electronic health record systems: Technical perspectives. *Health Information Management: Journal of the Health Information Management Association of Australia*, *44*(3), 23–38. doi:10.1177/183335831504400304 PMID:26464299

Riahi-Madvar, H., Ayyoubzadeh, S. A., Khadangi, E., & Ebadzadeh, M. M. (2009). An expert system for predicting longitudinal dispersion coefficient in natural streams by using ANFIS. *Expert Systems with Applications*, *36*(4), 8589–8596. doi:10.1016/j.eswa.2008.10.043

Riazul Islam, S. M., Daehan Kwak, Humaun Kabir, M., Hossain, M., & Kyung-Sup Kwak. (2015). The Internet of Things for Health Care: A Comprehensive Survey. *IEEE Access: Practical Innovations, Open Solutions*, *3*, 678–708. doi:10.1109/ACCESS.2015.2437951

Richardson, J. E., & Ancker, J. S. (2015). Public Perspectives of Mobile Phones' Effects on Healthcare Quality and Medical Data Security and Privacy: A 2-Year Nationwide Survey. *AMIA ... Annual Symposium Proceedings - AMIA Symposium. AMIA Symposium*, *2015*, 1076–1082. PMID:26958246

Richman, J. S., & Moorman, J. R. (2000). Physiological time-series analysis using approximate entropy and sample entropy. *American Journal of Physiology. Heart and Circulatory Physiology*, *278*(6), H2039–H2049. doi:10.1152/ajpheart.2000.278.6.H2039 PMID:10843903

Riesbeck, C. K., & Schank, R. C. (2013). *Inside case-based reasoning*. Psychology Press.

Rieta, J. J., Ravelli, F., & Sornmo, L. E. I. F. (2013). Advances in modeling and characterization of atrial arrhythmias. *Biomedical Signal Processing and Control*, *8*(6), 956–957. doi:10.1016/j.bspc.2013.10.008

Rigla, M., García-Sáez, G., Pons, B., & Hernando, M. E. (2018). Artificial Intelligence Methodologies and Their Application to Diabetes. *Journal of Diabetes Science and Technology*, *12*(2), 303–310. doi:10.1177/1932296817710475 PMID:28539087

Roberts, G. (2015). Improving Health Literacy to Reduce Health Inequalities. *UCL Institute for Health Equity*. Retrieved from file:///Users/janereeve/Documents/Janes Documents/EGA Module 4/M4 Documents/Improving Health Literacy to Reduce Health Inequalities.webarchive

Ródenas, J., García, M., Alcaraz, R., & Rieta, J. J. (2015). Wavelet entropy automatically detects episodes of atrial fibrillation from single-lead electrocardiograms. *Entropy (Basel, Switzerland)*, *17*(9), 6179–6199. doi:10.3390/e17096179

Rodvold, D. M., McLeod, D. G., Brandt, J. M., Snow, P. B., & Murphy, G. P. (2001). Introduction to artificial neural networks for physicians: Taking the lid off the blackbox. *The Prostate*, *46*(1), 39–44. doi:10.1002/1097-0045(200101)46:1<39::AID-PROS1006>3.0.CO;2-M PMID:11170130

Ronao, C. A., & Cho, S. B. (2016). Human activity recognition with smartphone sensors using deep learning neural networks. *Expert Systems with Applications*, *59*, 235–244. doi:10.1016/j.eswa.2016.04.032

Saeed, H., Saleem, Z., Naeem, R., Shahzadi, I., & Islam, M. (2018). Impact of health literacy on diabetes outcomes: A cross-sectional study from Lahore, Pakistan. *Public Health*, *156*, 8–14. doi:10.1016/j.puhe.2017.12.005 PMID:29353668

Safavian, S. R., & Landgrebe, D. (1991). A survey of decision tree classifier methodology. *IEEE Transactions on Systems, Man, and Cybernetics*, *21*(3), 660–674. doi:10.1109/21.97458

Sahoo, G., Anoop, J., & Kumar, Y. (2014). Seminal quality prediction using data mining methods. *Technology and Health Care*, *22*(4), 531–545. PMID:24898862

Saidi, T., & Douglas, T. S. (2018). Medical device regulation in South Africa: The Medicines and Related Substances Amendment Act 14 of 2015. *South African Medical Journal*, *108*(3), 168–170. doi:10.7196/SAMJ.2018.v108i3.12820

San Roman, J. A., Vilacosta, I., Castillo, J. A., Rollan, M. J., Hernández, M., Peral, V., ... Fernández-Avilés, F. (1998). Selection of the optimal stress test for the diagnosis of coronary artery disease. *Heart (British Cardiac Society)*, *80*(4), 370–376. doi:10.1136/hrt.80.4.370 PMID:9875115

Santosh Kumar, P. S. (2017). *Malaria, dengue and chikungunya in India – An update*. Indian J Med Spec. doi:10.1016/j.injms.2017.12.001

Sanz, J. A., Galar, M., Jurio, A., Brugos, A., Pagola, M., & Bustince, H. (2014). Medical diagnosis of cardiovascular diseases using an intervalvalued fuzzy rule-based classification system. *Applied Soft Computing*, *20*, 103–111. doi:10.1016/j.asoc.2013.11.009

Saquib, N., Saquib, J., & Ioannidis, J. P. A. (2015). Does screening for disease save lives in asymptomatic adults? Systematic review of meta-analyses and randomized trials. *International Journal of Epidemiology*, *44*(1), 264–277. doi:10.1093/ije/dyu140 PMID:25596211

Sarkar, S., Ritscher, D., & Mehra, R. (2008). A detector for a chronic implantable atrial tachyarrhythmia monitor. *IEEE Transactions on Biomedical Engineering*, *55*(3), 1219–1224. doi:10.1109/TBME.2007.903707 PMID:18334416

Savelieva, I., & Camm, A. J. (2000). Clinical relevance of silent atrial fibrillation: Prevalence, prognosis, quality of life, and management. *Journal of Interventional Cardiac Electrophysiology*, *4*(2), 369–382. doi:10.1023/A:1009823001707 PMID:10936003

Schazmann, B., Morris, D., Slater, C., Beirne, S., Fay, C., Reuveny, R., & Diamond, D. (2010). A wearable electrochemical sensor for the real-time measurement of sweat sodium concentration. *Analytical Methods*, *2*(4), 342–348. doi:10.1039/b9ay00184k

Scher, D. L. (2012). *How Patient-Centric Care Differs from Patient-Centered Care*. Retrieved from https://davidleescher.wordpress.com/2012/03/03/how-patient-centric-care-differs-from-patient-centered-care-2/

Schmalfuss, F., & Kolominsky-Rabas, P. L. (2013). Personalized medicine in screening for malignant disease: A review of methods and applications. *Biomarker Insights*, *8*, 9–14. doi:10.4137/BMI.S11153 PMID:23471146

Schroeder, J. (1994). Signal Processing via Fourier-Bessel Series Expansion. *Digital Signal Processing*, *3*(2), 112–124. doi:10.1006/dspr.1993.1016

Schwartz, A. G., Bailey-Wilson, J. E., & Amos, C. I. (2018). 6 – Genetic Susceptibility to Lung Cancer. *IASLC Thoracic Oncology*, 46–51. doi:10.1016/B978-0-323-52357-8.00006-8

Sentell, T. L., Tsoh, J. Y., Davis, T., Davis, J., & Braun, K. L. (2015). Low health literacy and cancer screening among Chinese Americans in California: A cross-sectional analysis. *BMJ Open*, *5*(1), e006104. doi:10.1136/bmjopen-2014-006104 PMID:25564140

Shaji, S., Ramesh, M. V., & Menon, V. N. (2016). Real-time processing and analysis for activity classification to enhance wearable wireless ecg. In *Proceedings of the Second International Conference on Computer and Communication Technologies* (pp. 21-35). Springer. 10.1007/978-81-322-2523-2_3

Shannon, C. (1948). A mathematical theory of communication. *The Bell System Technical Journal, 27*, 379-423.

Shapiro, A.F. (2006). *Fuzzy regression models*. Retrieved on 10.4.2013 from file:///C:/Users/mcaesar/Downloads/arch06v40n1-ii%20(1).pdf

Sharma, M., & Aggarwal, H. (2016). EHR adoption in India: Potential and the challenges. *Indian Journal of Science and Technology*, *9*(34). doi:10.17485/ijst/2016/v9i34/100211

Sharma, N. (2015). Patient centric approach for clinical trials: Current trend and new opportunities. *Perspectives in Clinical Research*, *6*(3), 134. doi:10.4103/2229-3485.159936 PMID:26229748

Shaukat, K., Masood, N., Mehreen, S., & Azmeen, U. (2015). Dengue Fever Prediction: A Data Mining Problem. *Journal of Data Mining in Genomics & Proteomics*.

Sheer, D. L. (2012). *How Patient-Centric Care Differs from Patient-Centered Care*. Retrieved from https://davidleescher.wordpress.com/2012/03/03/how-patient-centric-care-differs-from-patient-centered-care-2/

Shirazi, S. H., Umar, A. I., Haq, N., Naz, S., & Razzak, M. I. (2015). Accurate microscopic red blood cell image enhancement and segmentation. In *International Conference on Bioinformatics and Biomedical Engineering* (pp. 183–192). Springer International Publishing. 10.1007/978-3-319-16483-0_18

Shirazi, S. H., Umar, A. I., Naz, S., & Razzak, M. I. (2016). Efficient leukocyte segmentation and recognition in peripheral blood image. *Technology and Health Care*, *24*(3), 335–347. doi:10.3233/THC-161133 PMID:26835726

Shmueli, G., & Koppius, O. R. (2011). Predictive analytics in information systems research. *Management Information Systems Quarterly*, *35*(3), 553–572. doi:10.2307/23042796

Sikchi, S. S., Sikchi, S., & Ali, M. S. (2013). Fuzzy Expert Systems (FES) for Medical Diagnosis. *International Journal of Computer Applications, 63*(11), 7-17.

Sikchi, S. S., Sikchi, S., & Ali, M. S. (2012). Design of fuzzy expert system for diagnosis of cardiac diseases. *International Journal of Medical Science and Public Health*, *2*(1), 56–61. doi:10.5455/ijmsph.2013.2.56-61

Silber, E. N., & Katz, L. N. (1982). *Heart Disease*. New York: MacMillan Publishing Co.

Simes, R. J. (1985). Treatment selection for cancer patients: Application of statistical decision theory to the treatment of advanced ovarian cancer. *Journal of Chronic Diseases*, *38*(2), 171–186. doi:10.1016/0021-9681(85)90090-6 PMID:3882734

Simon, P. (2013). *Too big to ignore: the business case for big data* (Vol. 72). John Wiley & Sons.

Simpson, R. J. S., & Pearson, K. (1904). Report on certain enteric fever inoculation statistics. *British Medical Journal*, 1243–1246. PMID:20761760

Sindhwani, V., Rakshit, S., Deodhare, D., Erdogmus, D., Principe, J. C., & Niyogi, P. (2004). Feature selection in MLPs and SVMs based on maximum output information. *IEEE Transactions on Neural Networks*, *15*(4), 937–948. doi:10.1109/TNN.2004.828772 PMID:15461085

Sirinukunwattana, K., Raza, S. E. A., Tsang, Y. W., Snead, D. R., Cree, I. A., & Rajpoot, N. M. (2016). Locality sensitive deep learning for detection and classification of nuclei in routine colon cancer histology images. *IEEE Transactions on Medical Imaging*, *35*(5), 1196–1206. doi:10.1109/TMI.2016.2525803 PMID:26863654

Siriyasatien, P., Phumee, A., Ongruk, P., Jampachaisri, K., & Kesorn, K. (2016). Analysis of significant factors for dengue fever incidence prediction. *BMC Bioinformatics*, *17*(1), 166. doi:10.118612859-016-1034-5 PMID:27083696

Sivarajah, U., Kamal, M. M., Irani, Z., & Weerakkody, V. (2017). Critical analysis of Big Data challenges and analytical methods. *Journal of Business Research*, *70*, 263–286. doi:10.1016/j.jbusres.2016.08.001

Slavin, R. E. (1986). Best-evidence synthesis: An alternative to meta-analytic and traditional reviews. *Educational Researcher*, *15*(9), 5–11. doi:10.3102/0013189X015009005

Smith, M., Szongott, C., Henne, B., & Von Voigt, G. (2012, June). *Big data privacy issues in public social media.* In *Digital Ecosystems Technologies (DEST),* 2012 6th IEEE International Conference on (pp. 1-6). IEEE. 10.1109/DEST.2012.6227909

Somorjai, R. L., Dolenko, B., & Baumgartner, R. (2003). Class prediction and discovery using gene microarray and proteomics mass spectroscopy data: Curses, caveats, cautions. *Bioinformatics (Oxford, England)*, *19*(12), 1484–1491. doi:10.1093/bioinformatics/btg182 PMID:12912828

Song, J. G., Zeng, W. H., Xu, Y., & Xu, W. X. (2011, May). The Improvement of Neural Network Cascade-correlation Algorithm and its Application in Picking Seismic First Break. *73rd EAGE Conference and Exhibition incorporating SPE EUROPEC 2011*. 10.3997/2214-4609.20149418

Sørensen, K., Van den Broucke, S., Fullam, J., Doyle, G., Pelikan, J., Slonska, Z., & Brand, H. (2012). Health literacy and public health: A systematic review and integration of definitions and models. *BMC Public Health*, *12*(1), 80. doi:10.1186/1471-2458-12-80 PMID:22276600

Sriram, T. V. S., Rao, M. V., Narayana, G. V. S., & Kaladhar, D. S. V. G. K. (2014). Diagnosis of Parkinson Disease Using Machine Learning and Data Mining Systems from Voice Dataset. In *Proceedings of the 3rd International Conference on Frontiers of Intelligent Computing: Theory and Applications (FICTA)*. Springer.

Starfield, B. (2011). Is patient-centered care the same as person-focused care? *The Permanente Journal*, *15*(2), 63–69. doi:10.7812/TPP/10-148 PMID:21841928

Stegemann, S., Ternik, R. L., Onder, G., Khan, M. A., & van Riet-Nales, D. A. (2016). Defining Patient Centric Pharmaceutical Drug Product Design. *The AAPS Journal*, *18*(5), 1047–1055. doi:10.120812248-016-9938-6 PMID:27317470

Steinmetz, L. M., & Jones, A. (2016). *Sensing a revolution*. Academic Press.

Stephenson, A., McDonough, S. M., Murphy, M. H., Nugent, C. D., & Mair, J. L. (2017). Using computer, mobile and wearable technology enhanced interventions to reduce sedentary behaviour: A systematic review and meta-analysis. *The International Journal of Behavioral Nutrition and Physical Activity*, *14*(1), 105. doi:10.118612966-017-0561-4 PMID:28800736

Strong, K., Wald, N., Miller, A., & Alwan, A. (2005a). Current concepts in screening for noncommunicable disease: World Health Organization Consultation Group Report on methodology of noncommunicable disease screening. *Journal of Medical Screening, 12*(1), 12–19. doi:10.1258/0969141053279086 PMID:15825234

Strong, K., Wald, N., Miller, A., & Alwan, A. (2005b). Current concepts in screening for noncommunicable disease : World Health Organ .... *The Library, 12*(1), 12–19.

Summers, M. J., Madl, T., Vercelli, A. E., Aumayr, G., Bleier, D. M., & Ciferri, L. (2017). Deep Machine Learning Application to the Detection of Preclinical Neurodegenerative Diseases of Aging. *DigitCult-Scientific Journal on Digital Cultures, 2*(2), 9–24.

Su, X., Tong, H., & Ji, P. (2014). Activity recognition with smartphone sensors. *Tsinghua Science and Technology, 19*(3), 235–249. doi:10.1109/TST.2014.6838194

Talaei-Khoei, A., Ray, P., Parameshwaran, N., & Lewis, L. (2012). A framework for awareness maintenance. *Journal of Network and Computer Applications, 35*(1), 199–210. doi:10.1016/j.jnca.2011.06.011

Tanaka & Asai. (1982). Linear regression analysis with fuzzy model. IEEE Transactions and Systems, Man and Cybernetics, 12(6), 159-171.

Tateno, K., & Glass, L. (2001). Automatic detection of atrial fibrillation using the coefficient of variation and density histograms of RR and ΔRR intervals. *Medical & Biological Engineering & Computing, 39*(6), 664–671. doi:10.1007/BF02345439 PMID:11804173

Tavares, J., & Oliveira, T. (2017). Electronic Health Record Portal Adoption: A cross country analysis. *BMC Medical Informatics and Decision Making, 17*(1), 97. doi:10.118612911-017-0482-9 PMID:28679423

Terry, N. (2016). Will the Internet of Health Things Disrupt Healthcare? *Vanderbilt Journal of Entertainment & Technology Law, 19*(2), 28–31. doi:10.2139srn.2760447

Thirugnanam, M., Kumar, P., Srivatsan, S. V., & Nerlesh, C. (2012). Improving the prediction rate of diabetes diagnosis using fuzzy, neural network, case based (fnc) approach. *Procedia Engineering, 38*, 1709–1718. doi:10.1016/j.proeng.2012.06.208

Thomas, E. J., Studdert, D. M., Burstin, H. R., Orav, E. J., Zeena, T., Williams, E. J., & Brennan, T. A. (2000). Incidence and types of adverse events and negligent care in Utah and Colorado. *Medical Care, 38*(3), 261–271. doi:10.1097/00005650-200003000-00003 PMID:10718351

Thombs, B. D., de Jonge, P., Coyne, J. C., & Whooley, M. A., Frasure-Smith, N., Mitchell, A. J., … Ziegelstein, R. C. (2008). Clinician's Corner Depression Screening and Patient Outcomes in Cardiovascular Care A. *Systematic Reviews, 300*(18).

Thomopoulos, S. C. (1990). Sensor integration and data fusion. *Journal of Field Robotics, 7*(3), 337–372.

Thrall, J. H., Li, X., Li, Q., Cruz, C., Do, S., Dreyer, K., & Brink, J. (2018). Artificial Intelligence and Machine Learning in Radiology: Opportunities, Challenges, Pitfalls, and Criteria for Success. *Journal of the American College of Radiology*, *15*(3), 504–508. doi:10.1016/j.jacr.2017.12.026 PMID:29402533

Traczynski, J., & Udalova, V. (2018). Nurse practitioner independence, health care utilization, and health outcomes. *Journal of Health Economics*, *58*, 90–109. doi:10.1016/j.jhealeco.2018.01.001 PMID:29475093

Traverso, G., Ciccarelli, G., Schwartz, S., Hughes, T., Boettcher, T., Barman, R., & Swiston, A. (2015). Physiologic status monitoring via the gastrointestinal tract. *PLoS One*, *10*(11), e0141666. doi:10.1371/journal.pone.0141666 PMID:26580216

Travis, G. (2016, May). Medical Device Regulation: A comparison of the United States and the European Union. *The Journal of the American Academy of Orthopaedic Surgeons*, *24*(8), 537–543. doi:10.5435/JAAOS-D-15-00403 PMID:27195383

Tricoli, A., Nasiri, N., & De, S. (2017). Wearable and miniaturized sensor technologies for personalized and preventive medicine. *Advanced Functional Materials*, *27*(15), 1605271. doi:10.1002/adfm.201605271

Trung, T. Q., & Lee, N.-E. (2016). Flexible and Stretchable Physical Sensor Integrated Platforms for Wearable Human-Activity Monitoringand Personal Healthcare. *Advanced Materials (Deerfield Beach, Fla.)*, *28*(22), 4338–4372. doi:10.1002/adma.201504244 PMID:26840387

Tsanas, A., Little, M. A., McSharry, P. E., & Ramig, L. O. (2010). Accurate telemonitoring of parkinsons diseaseprogression by noninvasive speech tests. *IEEE Transactions on Biomedical Engineering*, *57*(4), 884–893. doi:10.1109/TBME.2009.2036000 PMID:19932995

Tsaur, R. C., Wang, H. F., & Yang, J.-C. O. (2002). Fuzzy regression for seasonal time series analysis. *International Journal of Information Technology & Decision Making*, *1*, 165–175. doi:10.1142/S0219622002000117

Tseng, F. M., & Tzeng, G. H. (2002). A fuzzy seasonal ARIMA model for forecasting. *Fuzzy Sets and Systems*, *126*(3), 367–376. doi:10.1016/S0165-0114(01)00047-1

Tsuyuki, R. T., & Krass, I. (2013). What is patient-centred care? [que sont les soins axes sur le patient?]. *Canadian Pharmacists Journal*, *146*(4), 177–180. doi:10.1177/1715163513494591

Tu, M. C. (2009). A comparative study of medical data classification methods based on decision tree and bagging algorithms. *Proc. IEEE 8th international conference on dependable, autonomic and secure, computing*, 183–187. 10.1109/DASC.2009.40

Turney, D. (1995). Cost-sensitive classification: Empirical evaluation of a hybrid genetic decision tree induction algorithm. *Journal of Artificial Intelligence Research*, 369–409.

Unertl, K. M., Johnson, K. B., & Lorenzi, N. M. (2011). Health information exchange technology on the front lines of healthcare: Workflow factors and patterns of use. *Journal of the American Medical Informatics Association*, *19*(3), 392–400. doi:10.1136/amiajnl-2011-000432 PMID:22003156

Upstill-Goddard, R., Eccles, D., Fliege, J., & Collins, A. (2012). Machine learning approaches for the discovery of gene-gene interactions in disease data. *Briefings in Bioinformatics*, *14*(2), 251–260. doi:10.1093/bib/bbs024 PMID:22611119

US Centers for Medicare and Medicaid Services. (2017). *National health expenditure data*. Author.

Utgoff, P. E. (1988). ID5: An incremental ID3. *Proc. of the fifth National Conference on Machine Learning*, 107–120.

Utgoff, P. E. (1989). Incremental induction of decision trees. *Machine Learning*, *4*(2), 161–186. doi:10.1023/A:1022699900025

Uy, C., Lopez, J., Trinh-Shevrin, C., Kwon, S. C., Sherman, S. E., & Liang, P. S. (2017). Text Messaging Interventions on Cancer Screening Rates: A Systematic Review. *Journal of Medical Internet Research*, *19*(8), e296. doi:10.2196/jmir.7893 PMID:28838885

Van Nguyen, T., Woo, Y. C., & Choi, D. (2009, April). Ccbr: Chaining case based reasoning in context-aware smart home. In *Intelligent Information and Database Systems, 2009. ACIIDS 2009. First Asian Conference on* (pp. 453-458). IEEE. 10.1109/ACIIDS.2009.20

Vapnik, V. (1982). *Estimation of Dependences Based on Empirical Data*. New York: Springer Verlag.

Varma, K. V., Rao, A. A., Lakshmi, T. S. M., & Rao, P. N. (2014). A computational intelligence approach for a better diagnosis of diabetic patients. *Computers & Electrical Engineering*, *40*(5), 1758–1765. doi:10.1016/j.compeleceng.2013.07.003

Vendrell, E., Morales, C., Risques, R. A., Capella, G., & Peinado, M. A. (2005). Genomic determinants of prognosis in colorectal cancer. *Cancer Letters*, *221*(1), 1–9. doi:10.1016/j.canlet.2004.08.023 PMID:15797621

Vendy, R. (2017, November). *EU MDR and Clinical Evidence: What You Need to Know*. Retrieved from https://www.meddeviceonline.com/doc/eu-mdr-and-clinical-evidence-what-you-need-to-know-0001

Vincent, J. L., Moreno, R., Takala, J., Willatts, S., De Mendonça, A., Bruining, H., … Thijs, L. G. (1996). *The SOFA (Sepsis-related Organ Failure Assessment) score to describe organ dysfunction/failure*. Academic Press.

Viswanathan, H., Baozhi, C., & Pompili, D. (2012). Research challenges in computation, communication, and context awareness for ubiquitous healthcare. *Communications Magazine, IEEE*, *50*(5), 92–99. doi:10.1109/MCOM.2012.6194388

Vos De, C. B., Pisters, R., Nieuwlaat, R., Prins, M. H., Tieleman, R. G., Coelen, R. J. S., ... Crijns, H. J. (2010). Progression from paroxysmal to persistent atrial fibrillation: Clinical correlates and prognosis. *Journal of the American College of Cardiology*, *55*(8), 725–731. doi:10.1016/j.jacc.2009.11.040 PMID:20170808

Wald, N. J., & Morris, J. K. (1996). Editorials What is case-finding? *Journal of Medical Screening*, *3*(1), 1996. doi:10.1177/096914139600300101 PMID:8861041

Waller, M. A., & Fawcett, S. E. (2013). Data science, predictive analytics, and big data: A revolution that will transform supply chain design and management. *Journal of Business Logistics*, *34*(2), 77–84. doi:10.1111/jbl.12010

Wang, Z., Kang, Y., Zhao, Y., & Qu, Q. (2014). Breast tumor detection in digital mammography based on extreme learning machine. Neurocomputing, 128, 175-184.

Wang, A., Lin, F., Jin, Z., & Xu, W. (2016). Ultra-low power dynamic knob in adaptive compressed sensing towards biosignal dynamics. *IEEE Transactions on Biomedical Circuits and Systems*, *10*(3), 579–592. doi:10.1109/TBCAS.2015.2497304 PMID:26800548

Wang, L. X. (1999). Article. *Fuzziness and Knowledge-Based Systems*, *7*, 83–98. doi:10.1142/S0218488599000076

Wang, Y., Kung, L., & Byrd, T. A. (2018). Big data analytics: Understanding its capabilities and potential benefits for healthcare organizations. *Technological Forecasting and Social Change*, *126*, 3–13. doi:10.1016/j.techfore.2015.12.019

Wan, J., Zou, C., Ullah, S., Lai, C.-F., Zhou, M., & Wang, X. (2013). Cloud-enabled wireless body area networks for pervasive healthcare. *IEEE Network*, *27*(5), 56–61. doi:10.1109/MNET.2013.6616116

Weblogs-WordPress. (2016). *Is screening different to case finding in high risk groups*. Retrieved March 18, 2018, from https://gregfellpublichealth.wordpress.com/2016/02/20/is-screening-different-to-case-finding-in-high-risk-groups/

Weed, L. (2017). *History of EHR*. Retrieved from http://v2020eresource.org/home/newsletter/SM116

Wellbery, C. (2011). Flaws in Clinical Reasoning: A Common Cause of Diagnostic Error. *American Family Physician*, *84*(9), 1042–1044. PMID:22046946

Wen, K.-Y., Kreps, G., Zhu, F., & Miller, S. (2010). Consumers' perceptions about and use of the internet for personal health records and health information exchange: Analysis of the 2007 Health Information National Trends Survey. *Journal of Medical Internet Research*, *12*(4), e73. doi:10.2196/jmir.1668 PMID:21169163

Wessler, M. (2013). *Big data analytics for dummies*. John Wiley & Sons.

Westerlund, M., Leminen, S., & Rajahonka, M. (2014). Designing business models for the internet of things. *Technology Innovation Management Review*, *4*(7).

Weston, A. D., & Hood, L. (2004). Systems biology, proteomics, and the future of health care: Toward predictive, preventative, and personalized medicine. *Journal of Proteome Research*, *3*(2), 179–196. doi:10.1021/pr0499693 PMID:15113093

Whalen, M., Maliszewski, B., Sheinfeld, R., Gardner, H., & Baptiste, D. (2018). Outcomes of an Innovative Evidence-Based Practice Project: Building a Difficult-Access Team in the Emergency Department. *Journal of Emergency Nursing: JEN, 1–5*. doi:10.1016/j.jen.2018.03.011 PMID:29704977

WHO. (2016). Multimorbidity. In *Technical Series on Safer Primary Care* (pp. 1–28). World Health Organization. Retrieved from http://apps.who.int/iris/bitstream/handle/10665/252275/9789241511650-eng.pdf;jsessionid=563FC8FC1EB37789B5F44978759EF4C4?sequence=1

Widrow, B., & Hoff, M. E. (1960). *Adaptive switching circuits (No. TR-1553-1)*. Stanford Univ.

Widrow, B., Rumelhart, D. E., & Lehr, M. A. (1994). Neural networks: Applications in industry, business and science. *Communications of the ACM, 37*(3), 93–106. doi:10.1145/175247.175257

Williams, P. A. H., & McCauley, V. (2016). Always connected: The security challenges of the healthcare Internet of Things. In *2016 IEEE 3rd World Forum on Internet of Things (WF-IoT)* (pp. 30–35). IEEE. 10.1109/WF-IoT.2016.7845455

Williams, R., Van Gaal, L., & Lucioni, C. (2002). Assessing the impact of complications on the costs of Type II diabetes. *Diabetologia, 45*(S1), S13–S17. doi:10.100700125-002-0859-9

Williams, S. J. (2017). *Improving Healthcare Operations*. Cham: Springer International Publishing; doi:10.1007/978-3-319-46913-3

Wilson, A. D. (2015). Advances in Electronic-Nose Technologies for the Detection of Volatile Biomarker Metabolites in the Human Breath. *Metabolites,* (5), 140-163. doi:10.3390/metabo5010140

Wilson, J. M. G., Jungner, G., & Organization, W. H. (1968). *Principles and practice of screening for disease*. Academic Press.

Wilson, H. J. (2013). Wearables in the Workplace. *Harvard Business Review*, 1–6.

Wilson, J. M., & Jungner, Y. G. (1968). Principles and practice of screening for disease. *Boletin de La Oficina Sanitaria Panamericana. Pan American Sanitary Bureau, 65*(4), 281–393. doi:10.1001/archinte.1969.00300130131020

Wilson, R. M., Harrison, B. T., Gibberd, R. W., & Hamilton, J. D. (1999). An analysis of the causes of adverse events from the Quality in Australian Health Care Study. *The Medical Journal of Australia, 170*(9), 411–415. PMID:10341771

Wimmer, G., Hegenbart, S., Vecsei, A., & Uhl, A. (2016). Convolutional neural network architectures for the automated diagnosis of celiac disease. In *International Workshop on Computer-Assisted and Robotic Endoscopy* (pp. 104–113). Springer.

Wolterink, J. M., Leiner, T., de Vos, B. D., van Hamersvelt, R. W., Viergever, M. A., & Isgum, I. (2016). Automatic coronary artery calcium scoring in cardiac ct angiography using paired convolutional neural networks. *Medical Image Analysis*, *34*, 123–136. doi:10.1016/j.media.2016.04.004 PMID:27138584

Wolterink, J. M., Leiner, T., Viergever, M. A., & Isgum, I. (2015). Automatic coronary calcium scoring in cardiac ct angiography using convolutional neural networks. In *International Conference on Medical Image Computing and Computer-Assisted Intervention* (pp. 589–596). Springer. 10.1007/978-3-319-24553-9_72

World Health Organization (WHO). (2016). *Ten facts on malaria*. Retrieved from http://www.who.int/features/factfiles/malaria/en/

World Health Organization (WHO). (2018). About Diabetes. Retrieved from http://www.who.int/diabetes/action_online/basics/en/index3.html

World Health Organization. (2007). *Anopheline Species Complexes in South and South-East Asia*. SEARO Technical Publication No. 57.

World Health Organization. (2016). *Diagnostic Errors. Technical Series on Safer Primary Care*. Retrieved from http://apps.who.int/iris

Wu, J.-H., Wang, S.-C., & Lin, L.-M. (2007). Mobile computing acceptance factors in the healthcare industry: A structural equation model. *International Journal of Medical Informatics*, *76*(1), 66–77. doi:10.1016/j.ijmedinf.2006.06.006 PMID:16901749

Xie, D. X., Wang, R. Y., & Chinnadurai, S. (2018). Readability of online patient education materials for velopharyngeal insufficiency. *International Journal of Pediatric Otorhinolaryngology*, *104*, 113–119. doi:10.1016/j.ijporl.2017.09.016 PMID:29287850

Yadav, G., Kumar, Y., & Sahoo, G. (2012). Predication of Parkinson's disease using data mining methods: A comparative analysis of tree, statistical and support vector machine classifiers. *Proceedings of National Conference on Computing and Communication Systems (NCCCS)*, 1–8. 10.1109/NCCCS.2012.6413034

Yang, C., Zhang, S., Yao, L., & Fan, L. (2018). *Evaluation of risk factors for false-negative results with an antigen-specific peripheral blood-based quantitative cell assay (T-SPOT. TB) in the diagnosis of active tuberculosi : A large-scale retrospective study in China*. Academic Press. doi:10.1177/0300060518757381

Yang, G., Hipwell, J. H., Hawkes, D. J., & Arridge, S. R. (2012). Numerical Methods for Coupled Reconstruction and Registration inDigital Breast Tomosynthesis. *Annals of the BMVA*, 1-29.

Yang, J. B., Shen, K. Q., Ong, C. J., & Li, X. P. (2008, October). Feature selection via sensitivity analysis of MLP probabilistic outputs. In *Systems, Man and Cybernetics, 2008. SMC 2008. IEEE International Conference on* (pp. 774-779). IEEE. 10.1109/ICSMC.2008.4811372

Yang, G. Z., Andreu-Perez, J., Hu, X., & Thiemjarus, S. (2014). Multi-sensor fusion. In *Body sensor networks* (pp. 301–354). Springer London. doi:10.1007/978-1-4471-6374-9_8

Yang, G., Xie, L., Mäntysalo, M., Zhou, X., Pang, Z., Xu, L., & Da. (2014). A Health-IoT platform based on the integration of intelligent packaging, unobtrusive bio-sensor, and intelligent medicine box. *IEEE Transactions on Industrial Informatics*, *10*(4), 2180–2191. doi:10.1109/TII.2014.2307795

Yao, S., Swetha, P., & Zhu, Y. (2018). Nanomaterial-Enabled Wearable Sensors for Healthcare. *Advanced Healthcare Materials*, *7*(1), 1700889. doi:10.1002/adhm.201700889 PMID:29193793

Yeh, J. Y., Wu, T. H., & Tsao, C. W. (2011). Using data mining techniques to predict hospitalization of hemodialysis patients. *Decision Support Systems*, *50*(2), 439–448. doi:10.1016/j.dss.2010.11.001

Yin, H., & Jha, N. K. (2017). A Health Decision Support System for Disease Diagnosis Based on Wearable Medical Sensors and Machine Learning Ensembles. *IEEE Transactions on Multi-Scale Computing Systems*, *3*(4), 228–241. doi:10.1109/TMSCS.2017.2710194

Yong, M., Xin, H., & Yu, K. (2008). Metabonomic analysis of hepatitis B virus-induced liver failure: Identification of potential diagnostic biomarkers by fuzzy support vector machine. *Journal of Zhejiang University. Science. B.*, *9*(6), 474–481. doi:10.1631/jzus.B0820044 PMID:18543401

Yoo, I., Alafaireet, P., Marinov, M., Pena-Hernandez, K., Gopidi, R., Chang, J. F., & Hua, L. (2012). Data mining in healthcare and biomedicine: A survey of the literature. *Journal of Medical Systems*, *36*(4), 2431–2448. doi:10.100710916-011-9710-5 PMID:21537851

Yuan, B. (2014). *Context-aware real-time assistant architecture for pervasive healthcare.* Academic Press.

Yuan, B., & Herbert, J. (2014). Context-aware hybrid reasoning framework for pervasive healthcare. *Personal and Ubiquitous Computing*, *18*(4), 865–881. doi:10.100700779-013-0696-5

Yu, C., Yang, J., Pang, C., Dai, M., Wang, Z.-S., & Wang, Y.-W., … Lu, Y. (2017). Behavior analysis of epidemiological patients for medical site treatment from a spatial perspective. In *2017 International Conference on Machine Learning and Cybernetics (ICMLC)* (pp. 311–316). IEEE. 10.1109/ICMLC.2017.8107782

Z¨ohrer, F., Harz, M. T., B¨odicker, A., Seyffarth, H., Schilling, K. J., Tab´ar, L., & Hahn, H. K. (2010). *Interactive Multi-scale Contrast Enhancement of Previously Processed Digital Mammograms.* Springer-Verlag Berlin Heidelberg.

Zadeh, L. A. (2004). *Fuzzy Logic Systems: Origin, Concepts, and Trends*. Retrieved November 29, 2015, from http://wi-consortium.org/wicweb/pdf/Zadeh.pdf

Zadeh, L. A. (1965). Fuzzy sets. *Information and Control*, *8*(3), 338–353. doi:10.1016/S0019-9958(65)90241-X

Zadeh, L. A. (2009). Toward extended Fuzzy Logic—A first step. *Fuzzy Sets and Systems*, *160*(21), 3175–3181. doi:10.1016/j.fss.2009.04.009

Zafar, M. Z. (2016). A Case Study: Pneumonia. *Occupational Medicine & Health Affairs*, *4*, 242. doi:10.4172/2329-6879.1000242

Zhang, T. (2004, July). Solving large scale linear prediction problems using stochastic gradient descent algorithms. In *Proceedings of the twenty-first international conference on Machine learning* (p. 116). ACM. 10.1145/1015330.1015332

Zhang, Y., Qiu, M., Tsai, C. W., Hassan, M. M., & Alamri, A. (2017). Health-CPS: Healthcare cyber-physical system assisted by cloud and big data. *IEEE Systems Journal*, *11*(1), 88–95. doi:10.1109/JSYST.2015.2460747

Zhao, W., Wang, C., & Nakahira, Y. (2012). Medical application on internet of things. *IET Conference Publications IET International Conference on Communication Technology and Application, ICCTA 2011 Elsevier, 2011*(586 CP), 660–665. Retrieved from http://www.scopus.com/inward/record.url?eid=2-s2.0-84864915621&partnerID=tZOtx3y1

Zhou, X., Ding, H., Ung, B., Pickwell-MacPherson, E., & Zhang, Y. (2014). Automatic online detection of atrial fibrillation based on symbolic dynamics and Shannon entropy. *Biomedical Engineering Online*, *13*(1), 18. doi:10.1186/1475-925X-13-18 PMID:24533474

Zhu, R., Zhang, R., & Xue, D. (2015). Lesion detection of endoscopy images based on convolutional neural network features. In *Image and Signal Processing (CISP), 2015 8th International Congress on* (pp. 372–376). IEEE. 10.1109/CISP.2015.7407907

Zhu, X., Liu, W., Shuang, S., Nair, M., & Li, C. Z. (2017). Intelligent tattoos, patches, and other wearable biosensors. In Medical Biosensors for Point of Care (POC) Applications (pp. 133-150). Academic Press. doi:10.1016/B978-0-08-100072-4.00006-X

Zhu, J., Xie, Q., & Zheng, K. (2015). An improved early detection method of type-2 diabetes mellitus using multiple classifier system. *Information Sciences*, *292*, 1–14. doi:10.1016/j.ins.2014.08.056

Zhu, Y. (2011). Automatic detection of anomalies in blood glucose using a machine learning approach. *Journal of Communications and Networks (Seoul)*, *13*(2), 125–131. doi:10.1109/JCN.2011.6157411

Zimmerman, H. J. (1991). *Fuzzy Set Theory and its Applications*. Boston: Kluwer Academic. doi:10.1007/978-94-015-7949-0

Zink, M. D., Marx, N., Crijns, H. J. G. M., & Schotten, U. (2018, December). Opportunities and challenges of large-scale screening for atrial fibrillation. *Herzschrittmachertherapie + Elektrophysiologie*, 57–61. doi:10.100700399-017-0550-y

Zolezzi, M., Eltorki, Y. H., Almaamoon, M., Fathy, M., & Omar, N. E. (2018). Outcomes of patient education practices to optimize the safe use of lithium: A literature review. *Mental Health Clinician*, *8*(1), 41–48. doi:10.9740/mhc.2018.01.041 PMID:29955544

About the Contributors

Thierry Edoh is an associate researcher at the University of Bonn (Germany)/ department of pharmacy, visiting associate lecturer at the Institute of Mathematics and Physics (IMSP)/University Abomey-Calavi, (Benin-Africa), visiting lecturer at IUT Lokossa (Benin-Africa), and an associate researcher at Technical University of Munich/department of Applied Software Engineering (Germany). He has 20+ years of work experiences in software architecture, design, and implementation. He has worked with Siemens, BMW, for several years. He received his Diploma in computer sciences from the Technical University of Munich in Germany and hold a Ph.D. at the German Federal Army University, where he worked for several years on the improvement of rural health care provision and access to healthcare in developing countries using ITC systems. He completed a Post Doctoral research works at the University of Bonn, dept. of Drug Regulatory Affairs (institute of pharmacy). His research interests are mobile computing, pervasive health and health informatics, telehealth and IoT in medical applications. He is an expert in telemedicine/telehealth-care, health informatics, and bio-Informatics. He is also working on an Information system in Drug Regulatory Affairs, and he is the initiator and general chair of the international conference of rural and elderly health informatics (IREHI-2017 and IREHI-2018).

Pravin Pawar is a Senior Scientist at Philips Research and he has 15+ years of comprehensive international research and software development experience in the cutting-edge informatics projects worldwide. He received education from premier institutions - IIT Bombay (M.Tech. CSE), University of Twente (Ph.D. CSE) and credited with 5 filed patents, 50 peer reviewed publications and one book. His research interests are health informatics, data analytics, machine learning, deep learning, clinical data management, mobile computing, big data applications, service-oriented computing. He has leadership and management experience in academia, research institutes and software industry. He likes to travel and experience different cultures.

Sagar P. Mohammad is a Senior Systems Architect at Philips Research. He received his B.Tech. in Biomedical Engineering from Cochin University of Science and Technology and M.Tech. in Electronic Systems from the department of Electrical Engineering, Indian Institute of Technology Bombay. He has filed patent to his credit. He started his career with Defence Research and Development Organisation and led the Sensors and Instrumentation group of the Defence Bio-engineering and Electromedical laboratory. He then moved to Wipro Technologies and was Architect for Integrated Medical Device programs. Over the 20+ years of his professional career, he was instrumental in development of various medical devices & healthcare solutions. His interests include design for safety, design for reliability, wireless sensor networks, and IoT. He is a member of the The Institute of Electrical and Electronics Engineers (IEEE), The Photonics Society of India(PSI), and The Biomedical Engineering Society of India (BMESI).

* * *

Annappa B. is currently working as an Associate Professor in the Department of Computer Science and Engineering, National Institute of Technology Karnataka, Surathkal, Mangalore, India. He has more than 25 years of experience in teaching and research. He holds Ph.D. and M.Tech. in Computer Science and Engineering from National Institute of Technology Karnataka Surathkal and B.E. in Computer Science and Engineering from Govt. B.D.T. College of Engineering, Davangere, Karnataka affiliated Mysore University, Karnataka. He is a Fellow of Institution of Engineers (India), Senior member of IEEE, Senior member of ACM and Life member of Computer Society of India, Cloud Computing Innovation Council of India (CCICI) and Indian Society of Technical Education. He is the current Chair of IEEE Computer Society Chapter, India Council and Chair of IEEE Mangalore subsection. He was the former secretary of IEI Mangaluru Local center. His research interests include Cloud computing, Big Data Analytics, Distributed Computing, Software Engineering and Process Mining. He has published more than 100 papers in International conferences and Journals. He was the Organizing Chair of International conference ADCONS-2013 and he is in the Program Committees of many International conferences and reviewer of Journals. He visited various Institutes of Higher learning abroad for Academic and Research interactions including University of British Columbia, Canada, University of Manitoba, Canada, Kumamoto University Japan, Penn State University, USA, Carnegie Mellon University, USA, Ohio State University, USA, University of Cincinnati, USA, University of Dayton, USA, Wright State University, USA.

Abhishek Banerjee received the B.Tech. and M.Tech degree in Information Technology from the West Bengal University of Technology, Kolkata, India, in 2006 and 2009 respectively. Since 2011, he has been with the Department of Computer Science & Engineering, Pailan College of Management & Technology, as Assistant professor. His current research interests include Data mining, Image processing. He has 4 publication in national and international journals.

Aaquil Bunglowala is currently working as Associate Dean at School of Technology Management & Engineering, NMIMS-Indore Campus. A meritorious scholar during his academics and topper during his M. Tech, he has over 24 years of experience in industry and academics on various profiles. His expertise lies in Advanced Logic and VLSI design. He is actively involved in research and has contributed more than 49 research papers in national / international journals and conferences. He has been reviewer of McGraw Hill publications and on editorial board and Program Chair of various National/international conferences and journals.

Parag Chatterjee received the B.Tech. degree in Computer Science & Engineering from the Karnatak University, Dharwad, India, in 1998 and received M.Tech. degree from IIEST Shibpur, Kolkata, India, in 2007. Since 2007, he has been with the Department of Computer Science & Engineering, Pailan College of Management & Technology, as Associate professor. His current research interests include Data Warehousing, Data mining and Wireless sensor. He has 2 publications in national and international journals.

Shalini Gambhir graduated from the department of Information Technology, Kurukshetra University in 2007. She qualified GATE exam and took her M.Tech degree from Computer Science and Engineering department GGSIPU University in 2009. She is currently a Full Time Ph.D Scholar at SRM university and had worked as an assistant professor Computer Science at GGSIPU University. Her interest areas include artificial intelligence, pattern recognition, machine learning, intelligent diagnosis systems and data mining.

Sujitkumar Hiwale holds a professional degree in medicine (MBBS) and has a master‘s degree in Medical Science and Technology (MMST) from the Indian Institute of Technology (IIT), Kharagpur, India. Currently he is working as a senior research scientist at the Philips Research India.

Yugal Kumar is presently working as Assistant Professor (Senior Grade) in Department of Computer Science & Engineering at Jaypee University of Information Technology (JUIT), Waknaghat, Himachal Pradesh, India. He has more than 10 years of teaching and research experience at reputed colleges and universities of India. He has completed his Ph.D. in Computer Science & Engineering from Birla institute of Technology, Mesra, Ranchi. His primary area of research includes meta-heuristic algorithms, data clustering, swarm intelligence, pattern recognition, medical data international journals and conferences of repute. He is serving as editorial review board member of various journals including Soft Computing, Neurocomputing, Computer Methods and Programs in Biomedicine, PLOSE ONE, Journal of Advanced Computational Intelligence and Intelligent Informatics and Journal of Information Processing System.

Upendra Kumar has done schoolings (10th and 10+2) from Govt. Inter College, Allahabad, India with First Honors. He graduated in B. Tech. (Information Technology) from UPTU Lucknow, India with First Honors (75.60% marks) and received M. Tech. (Information Technology) from Indian Institute of Information Technology, Allahabad, India with 9.19/10 CGPI. Currently, he has completed his Ph. D. in the faculty of Computer Science & Engineering under supervision of Dr. Tapobrata Lahiri, IIIT Allahabad, India. During M.Tech program, he got the placement opportunity in Tata Consultancy Services Limited and joined as an Assistant Engineer in 2008. He worked in various corporate projects for 4 years in TCS as a Java/ J2EE developer: i) Automation System for Ministry of Corporate Affairs from Dec, 2008 to Sep, 2009, ii) Passport Seva Project for India from Sep, 2009 to June, 2011 iii) SMB Education Project from July, 2011 to Aug, 2012. Owing to his research interest and also coding skill, during his post graduation, he worked on Biomedical Signal Processing, especially ECG to develop automatic diagnosis of heart diseases. In continuation with this he got the opportunity to be registered in Ph. D. program from UPTU Lucknow and research working place at IIIT Allahabad. He also got opportunity to work as a Research Engineer, in Knowledge Flow Limited, Indian Institute of Technology, Delhi on Real Time Image Processing projects offered from Dr. Anirban Das, Head & Founder Member, from Aug, 2012 to till now. He developed various industrial projects like Home Automation and Security Surveillance System, Perimeter Protection and Security System and Sensor based Interactive Robot. He also developed some android programming based applications for robotics. As for his teaching experience, he worked as a Lecturer in Department of Computer Science and Information Technology, SIET, Allahabad from August 2004 to June 2006. He attended and completed various training programs and workshops during his Ph. D work: i) Training Course on "Robotics and Embedded in C" by Robosapians India Pvt. Ltd., Noida (01-15, Dec, 2012), ii) Training on "Initial

Learning Program" by TCS, Tiruvanatpuram, Kerala (Aug-Sept, 2008), iii) "5th IEEE Conference on Wireless Communication and Sensor Networks" (Held at IIIT-Allahabad 2008), iv) Workshop on "Network and Information Security: Emerging Challenges and Practices", held at Ansal Technical Campus, Lucknow (05-08 Dec, 2013). Currently he is working as assistant professor in CSE department in Institute of Engineering and Technology Lucknow 226021 UP, India

Manoj Kumar M. V. completed his Ph.D. from the department of computer science and engineering at National Institute of Technology Karnataka, Surathkal, Mangalore, India. He did his masters from Bapuji Institute of Engineering and Technology, Davanagere, India and is graduated from Vishweshwaraiah Technology University, Belgaum, India. His research interest is in data and process mining, mobile application, and statistical data analysis. R-programming is one of his key interest and building mobile apps is his hobby. He has been a resource person in various workshops on mobile application development and data analysis. He is currently working on a problem related to concept drift, in the context of process mining. He has a good number of publications in international journals and conferences. He has worked as a research scholar under Dr. Annappa, associate professor, NITK and he is currently working as an associate professor, in the department of information science and engineering, NITTE Meenakshi, Bangalore, Karnataka, India.

Gaurav Paliwal is currently working as Assistant Professor in Department of Computer Engineering at R. C. Patel Institute of Technology, Shirpur. His area of interest are Health Informatics, Product Line Architecture, Mobile Patient Monitoring, Domain Modeling, Wearable Healthcare Devices and Bioinformatics in Computer Science.

Shivnarayan Patidar was born in Badnawar, Dhar, Madhya Pradesh India, in 1983. He received the B.E. degree in Biomedical engineering (BME) from the Shri G.S.I.T.S., Indore, India, in 2006, and the M.Tech (BME) and Ph.D (Electrical engineering) from the Indian Institute of Technology (IIT) BHU and IIT Indore in 2008 and 2015, respectively. Prior to PhD, he worked as an assistant professor in the Department of Biomedical engineering at Chameli Devi Group of Institutions, Indore, for four years. After PhD, he worked in Uniken Systems at Pune, India, as a senior research engineer. In 2015, he joined the Department of Electronics and communication engineering, National Institute of Technology Goa, as an Assistant Professor. His current research interests include biomedical signal/ image analysis and processing, time-frequency analysis, multi-resolution analysis, machine learning and other soft computing techniques.

Gopal Purkait received the B.Tech. and M.Tech degree in Computer Science & Engineering from the University of Calcutta, Kolkata, India, in 2012 and 2014 respectively. Since 2014, he has been with the Department of Computer Science & Engineering, Pailan College of Management & Technology, as Assistant professor. His current research interests include Data mining, Image processing and Wireless sensor. He has 3 publications in national and international journals.

Ashish Sharma was born in Indore, Madhya Pradesh India. He received the B.E. degree in Biomedical engineering and M.E. degree in Electrical engineering from the Shri G.S. Institute Technology and Science, Indore, India, in 2007, and 2010 respectively. Currently he is working towards PhD degree in biomedical signal processing from the department of Electronics and communication engineering, National Institute of Technology Goa, India. His current research interests include biomedical signal and image analysis and processing, time-frequency analysis, artificial intelligence and machine learning.

Dharmpal Singh received his Bachelor of Computer Science and Engineering and Master of Computer Science and Engineering from West Bengal University of Technology. He has about seven years of experience in teaching and research. At present, he is with JIS College of Engineering, Kalyani, and West Bengal, India as an Assistant Professor. Currently, he is pursuing PhD in University of Kalyani. He has about sixteen publications in national and international journals and conference proceedings.

Likewin Thomas did his Ph.D. and masters from the field of computer science and engineering at National Institute of Technology Karnataka, Surathkal, Mangalore. He is graduated from Vishweshwaraiah Technology University, Belgaum in the year 2004. His research interest is in the field of machine learning and its application in the clinical area, and process mining. He holds more than 11 years of teaching and research experience and has worked as a research scholar under Dr. Annappa, associate professor, NITK. He has been a resource person and a keynote speaker at many workshops and conferences. He along with Dr. Annappa has organized a workshop on machine learning and its application at an IEEE international conference, EmergiTech 2016, held at Mauritius. He is keen on understanding the image processing techniques in the clinical field. He is interested in contributing his researching excellence to the betterment and management of healthcare sectors. He is currently working as an associate professor, in the department of computer science and engineering, PESITM, Shivamogga, Karnataka, India.

Index

E

F

H

I

J

K

M

N

P

R

S

T

W

www.ingramcontent.com/pod-product-compliance
Lightning Source LLC
LaVergne TN
LVHW080608300926
849162LV00005B/1081